Retroviruses and Human Pathology

Experimental Biology and Medicine

Retroviruses and Human Pathology, edited by ***Robert C. Gallo, Dominique Stehelin, and Oliviero E. Varnier***, *1985*

Directed Drug Delivery, edited by ***Ronald T. Borchardt, Arnold Repta, and Valentino Stella***, *1985*

Immune Regulation, edited by ***Marc Feldmann and N. A. Mitchison***, *1985*

Human T Cell Clones: *A New Approach to Immune Regulation,* edited by ***Marc Feldmann, Jonathan R. Lamb, and James N. Woody,*** *1985*

Inositol and Phosphoinositides: *Metabolism and Regulation,* edited by ***John E. Bleasdale, Joseph Eichberg, and George Hauser,*** *1985*

Growth, Cancer, and the Cell Cycle, edited by ***Philip Skehan and Susan J. Friedman,*** *1984*

Ir Genes: *Past, Present, and Future,* edited by ***Carl W. Pierce, Susan E. Cullen, Judith A. Kapp, Benjamin D. Schwartz, and Donald C. Shreffler,*** *1983*

Methods in Protein Sequence Analysis, edited by ***Marshall Elzinga,*** *1982*

Inflammatory Diseases and Copper, edited by ***John R. J. Sorenson,*** *1982*

Membrane Fluidity: *Biophysical Techniques and Cellular Regulation,* edited by ***Morris Kates and Arnis Kuksis,*** *1980*

International Symposium:

RETROVIRUSES AND HUMAN PATHOLOGY

Edited by

Robert C. Gallo,
Dominique Stehelin,
and Oliviero E. Varnier

Humana Press · Clifton, New Jersey

Crescent Manor
PO Box
Clifton, NJ 07015 USA

Printed in the United States of America.

Library of Congress Cataloging in Publication Data
Main entry under title:

Retroviruses and Human Pathology.

(Experimental biology and medicine)
Proceedings of the International Symposium on Retroviruses and Human Pathology, held in San Terenzo di Lerici (La Spezia), Italy at the Villa Marigola, Centro studi della cassa di risparmio della Spezia on Sept. 24-26, 1984; organized by the Istituto di microbiologia dell'Universita and Istituto nazionale per la ricerca sul cancro, Genoa, Italy.
Includes indexes.
1. Retroviruses—Congresses. 2. Oncogenes—Congresses. 3. Carcinogenesis—Congresses. I. Gallo, Robert C. II. Stehelin, Dominique. III. Varnier, Oliviero E. IV. International Symposium on Retroviruses and Human Pathology (1984: Lerici, Italy) V. Universita di Genova. Istituto di microbiologia. VI. Istituto nazionale per la ricerca sul cancro (Italy) VII. Series: Experimental biology and medicine (Clifton, NJ) [DNLM: 1. Oncogenes—congresses. 2. Retroviridae—congresses. 3. Tumor Virus Infections—pathology—congresses.

QW 166 R4375 1984]
QR414.5.R47 1985 616.07'1 85-31692
ISBN 0-89603-098-9

Acknowledgments

This volume contains the proceedings of the International Symposium on Retroviruses and Human Pathology held in San Terenzo di Lerici (La Spezia), Italy at the Villa Marigola, Centro Studi della Cassa di Risparmio della Spezia on September 24–26, l984. The symposium was organized by:

Istituto di Microbiologia dell'Universita
and
Istituto Nazionale per la Ricerca sul Cancro
Genova, Italia

under the auspices of:

Universita' degli Studi di Genova
Assessorato della Sanita, Regione Liguria
Comune di Lerici
Cassa di Risparmio della Spezia
Cassa di Risparmio di Genova e Imperia
Consiglio Nazionale delle Ricerche
Ministero della Pubblica Istruzione
Ministero degli Affari Esteri

Front cover and title page logo designed by: ***Marco Matricardi***

Preface

For decades retroviruses have been riding the crest of a wave of experimental research directed toward the identification of an infectious agent of human neoplastic diseases. In the early l970s, several scientists successfully demonstrated the presence of retroviruses in numerous animal species and proved their etiological role in some related diseases. Corresponding findings in humans were somewhat discouraging. Although financial support for this line of research declined, a few dedicated retrovirologists survived and continued to collect more biological information and technological expertise that opened a new approach to the search for a human retrovirus.

The rewards came with the discovery that the genes responsible for neoplastic transformation (oncogenes) are of cellular origin and can be shuttled about by retroviruses, and with the identification of a new family of Human T-cell Lymphotrophic retroViruses (HTLV) from patients with diseases ranging from leukemia to the acquired immunodeficiency syndrome (AIDS).

An understanding of the role and significance of retroviruses in human pathology requires basic knowledge of the major animal systems studied. With this perspective in mind, we present here a survey that includes general overviews, minireviews on each animal system studied with selected experimental reports and, finally, a stimulating review of the field of human retrovirology by many of the pioneer scientists who created it.

We are especially grateful to Profs. C. A. Romanzi and G. C. Schito for promoting the organization of the Symposium. On behalf of the Symposium Committee, we thank E. Boeri, L. Casarino, G. P. Gesu, M. Malnati, R. Mangione, G. Melioli, A. Merli, O. Muratore, C. M. Repetto, M. Ricchetti, F. Sessarego, C. Tarantola, and G. Tudor, who participated in the organization of the meeting. We also expend our appreciation to D. Bernini for her expert secretarial assistance, P. Magni for her photography, A. Dagnino for her typing, and K. Anderson for her valuable editorial assistance in the preparation of this volume. We are indebted to S. P. Raffanti for his constant and enthusiastic help.

Robert C. Gallo
Dominique Stehelin
Oliviero E. Varnier

Contents

Section 4. Retroviruses and Oncogenes

Conference Participants

Kari Alitalo, Institute of Virology, University of Helsinki, Helsinki, Finland
Bruno Azzarone, Laboratory of Cellular Pathology, ICIG, Villejuif, France
Uldis Banders, August Kirchenstein Institute of Microbiology, Latvian SSR Academy of Sciences, Riga, USSR
Mariano Barbacid, NCI, Frederick Cancer Research Facility, Frederick, Maryland, USA
Ottavia Barbieri, Istituto Nazionale per la Ricerca sul Cancro, Genova, Italia
Francoise Barre-Sinoussi, Viral Oncology Unit, Institut Pasteur, Paris, France
Ann Bayley, University Teaching Hospital, Losaka, Zambia
Mauro Bendinelli, Istituto di Igiene, Pisa, Italia
Arrigo Benedetto, Laboratorio di Virologia, Ospedale S. Camillo, Roma, Italia
Elke Beth, Divisione di Virologia Oncologica, Napoli, Italia
Generoso Bevilaqua, Istituto di Anatomia Patologica, University of Pisa, Pisa, Italia
Lidia Boffa, Istituto Nazionale pe la Ricerca sul Cancro, Genova, Italia
Francoise Brun-Vezinet, Laboratoire Central, Virologie, Hopital Claude Bernard, Paris, France
Arsene Burny, Department di Biologie Moleculaire, University of Brussels, Rhode St. Genese, Belgium
Claire-M. Calberg-Bacq, Institute of Microbiology, Liege, Belgium
Letizia Calegari, Istituto di Microbiologia, Genova, Italia
Robert Callahan, Laboratory of Tumor Immunology and Biology, NCI, Bethesda, Maryland, USA
Angelo Castro, Istituto di Microbiologia, Catania, Italia
Franco Celada, Cattedra di Immunologia, Genova, Italia
Rachanee Cheingsong-Popov, Institute of Cancer Research, London, England
Jean Claude Chermann, Unite d'Oncologie Virale, Institut Pasteur, Paris, France
Luigi Chieco-Bianchi, Cattedra di Oncologia, Padova, Italia
Roel Coutinho, Municipal Health Service, Amsterdam, The Netherlands
Aren Dalen, Department of Virology, University of Trondheim, Trondheim, Norway

Mukkattu Ramachandra Das, Centre for Cellular and Molecular Biology, Hyderabad, India
Carlo de Giuli-Morghen, Centro di Citofarmacologia del CNR, Milano, Italia
Brigitte Debuire, INSERM, IRCL, Lille, France
Giuseppe Della Porta, Istituto Nazionale Tumori, Milano, Italia
Ferdinando Dianzani, Istituto di Virologia, Roma, Italia
Amedea Donelli, Laboratorio di Ematologia Sperimentale, University of Modena, Modena, Italia
Robert Downing, PHCS CAMR, Salisbury, England
Renato Dulbecco, The Salk Institute, San Diego, California, USA
Giovanni Emilia, Laboratorio di Ematologia Sperimentale, Modena, Italia
Giovanni Fadda, Istituto di Microbiologia, Sassari, Italia
Sergio Ferrari, Laboratorio di Ematologia Sperimentale, Modena Italia
Roland Friedrich, Institute of Immunobiology, Freiburg, Federal Republic of Germany
Ursula Friedrich, Institute of Immunobiology, Freiburg, Federal Republic of Germany
Robert C. Gallo, National Institutes of Health, Bethesda, Maryland, USA
Louis Gazzolo, Unite de Virologie, INSERM, Lyon, France
C. J. Gibbs, Jr., National Institutes of Health, Bethesda, Maryland, USA
Gaetano Giraldo, Divisione di Virologia Oncologica, Napoli, Italia
Jaap Goudsmit, Virology Department, University of Amsterdam, Amsterdam, The Netherlands
Nicole Hanania, Institut Gustave Roussy, IRSC, Villejuif, France
J. Hilgers, Division of Genetics, The Netherlands Cancer Institute, Amsterdam, The Netherlands
Monica Hollstein, International Agency for Cancer Research, Lyon, France
Yoji Ikawa, Riken Institute, Saitama, Japan
Harry Ioachim, College of Physicians and Surgeons, Columbia University, New York, USA
Giorgio Ivaldi, Istituto di Fisiologia Generale, Sassari, Italia
Ole Jan Iversen, Department of Microbiology, University of Trondheim, Trondheim, Norway
Daniel Jamaer, Institute of Blood Transfusion, Leuven, Belgium
Michel Janowski, Centre d'Etude de l'Energie Nucleaire, Mol, Belgium
Osvald Jarrett, Department of Veterinary Pathology, University of Glasgow, Glasgow, Scotland
Slavenka Kam-Hansen, Department of Neurobiology, Huddinge, Sweden
Newton Khoobyarian, University of Illinois, Chicago, Illinois, USA
Erik Larsson, Patologiska Institutionen, University of Uppsala, Uppsala, Sweden

Jay A. Levy, Cancer Research Institute, University of California, San Francisco, California, USA
Marie-Henriette Loucheux-Lefebre, INSERM Unite I24, Lille, France
Giovanni Melioli, Istituto di Microbiologia, Genova, Italia
Annamaria Molina, Istituto di Microbiologia, Siena, Italia
Pier Carlo Montecucchi, Farmitalia Carlo Erba, Milano, Italia
Carlo Moscovici, Tumor Virology Laboratory, University of Florida, Gainesville, Florida, USA
O. Muratore, Institute of Microbiology, University of Genova, Genova, Italia
Bjorn A. Nexo, Novo Research Institute, Bagsvaerd, Denmark
Giuseppe Nicoletti, Istituto di Microbiologia, Catania, Italia
Nils Oker-Blom, University of Helsinki, Helsinki, Finland
Sandra Panem, US Environmental Protection Agency, Washington, DC, USA
Maya Parfanovich, Institute of Virology, Moscow, USSR
Silvio Parodi, Istituto Nazionale per la Ricerca sul Cancro, Genova, Italia
Nadine Pavloff, Institut G. Roussy, Villejuif, France
Giorgio Prodi, Istituto di Cancerologia, Bologna, Italia
Ulf Rapp, National Cancer Institute, Frederick, Maryland, USA
Suraiya Rasheed, Department of Pathology, University of Southern California School of Medicine, Los Angeles, California, USA
M. Robert-Guroff, National Cancer Institute, Bethesda, Maryland, USA
Jacquelines Robert-Lezenes, INSERM U 248, Paris, France
Carmine Alfredo Romanzi, Istituto di Microbiologia, Genova, Italia
Lorenzo Rossi, Istituto Nazionale per la Ricerca sul Cancro, Genova, Italia
Tommaso Rosso, Istituto di Scienze Biochimiche, Napoli, Italia
Antonio Sanna, Istituto di Microbiologia, Roma, Italia
Leonardo Santi, Istituto Nazionale per la Ricerca sul Cancro, Genova, Italia
Gian Carlo Schito, Istituto di Microbiologia, Genova, Italia
Licia Selleri, Laboratorio di Ematologia Sperimentale, University of Modena, Modena, Italia
Marianne Semmel, Institut G. Roussy, Villejuif, France
Roulette William Smith, Institute for Postgraduate Interdisciplinary Studies, Palo Alto, California, USA
Dominique Stehelin, Institut Pasteur, Lille, France
Horacio Guillermo Suarez, Laboratoire de Genetique Cellulaire, IRSC, Villejuif, France
William A. Suk, Northrup Services Inc., Research Triangle Park, North Carolina, USA
John M. Taylor, Fox Chase Cancer Center, Philadelphia, Pennsylvania
Gianna Tempera, Istituto di Microbiologia, Catania, Italia

Lise Thiry, Institute Pasteur du Brabant, Brussels, Belgium
T. G. Todorov, Institute of General and Comparative Pathology, Sofia, Bulgaria
Gian Paolo Tonini, Istituto Giannina Gaslini, Genova, Italia
Giuseppe Torelli, Laboratorio di Ematologia Sperimentale, University of Modena, Modena, Italia
Adolfo Turano, Istituto di Microbiologia, Brescia, Italy
Antti Vaheri, Department of Virology, University of Helsinki, Helsinki, Finland
Oliviero E. Varnier, Istituto di Microbiologia, University of Genova, Genova, Italia
W. L. E. Vasmel, Central Laboratory of the Netherlands, Amsterdam, The Netherlands
Xin Li Wen, Institut Curie, Orsay, France
F. Wong-Staal, National Cancer Institute, Bethesda, Maryland, USA
Volker Wunderlich, Central Institute for Cancer Research, Berlin, East Germany
Tsubura Yoshihiko, Nara Medical College, Kashihara City, Japan

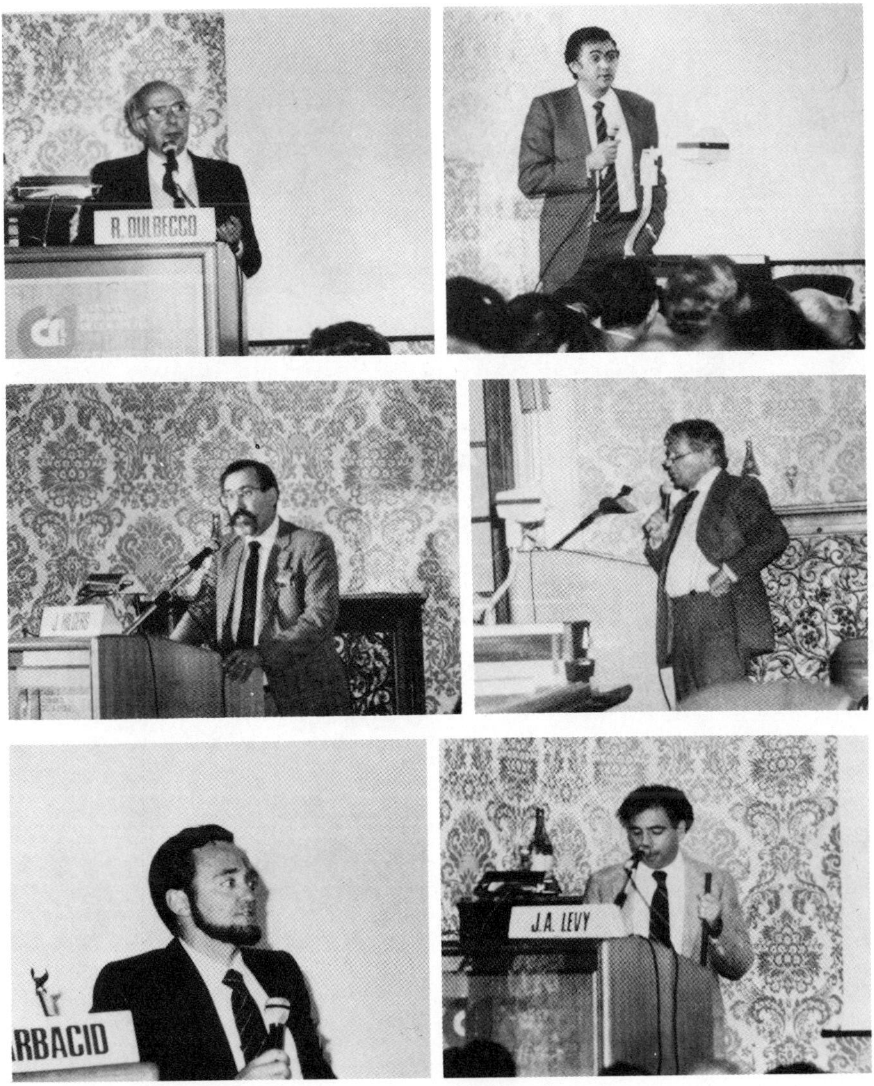

Top row: R. Dulbecco, J. C. Chermann
Second row: J. Hilgers, C. Moscovici
Bottom row: M. Barbacid, J. A. Levy

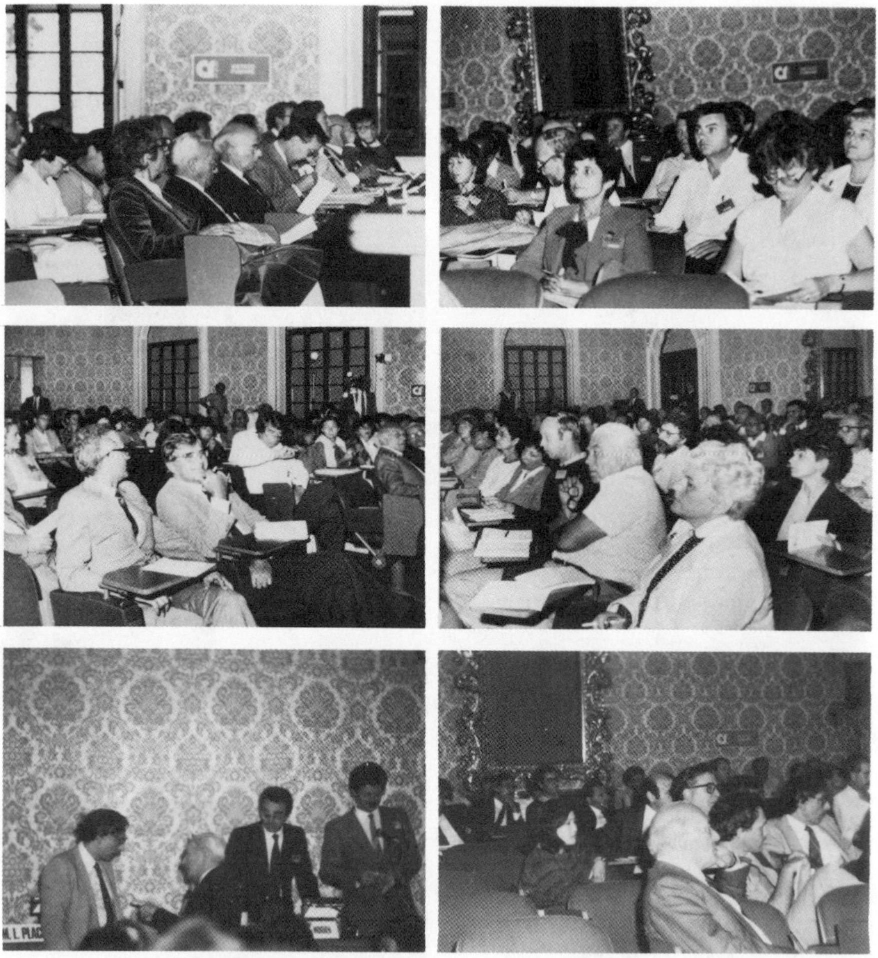

Top row: A. M. Molina, A. Sanna, R. Dulbecco, J. Hilgers, R. Cheingsong-Popov, F. Celada, S. Rasheed, R. Callahan, J. C. Chermann, F. Barre-Sinoussi

Second row: G. Della Porta, G. Prodi, A. Burny, U. T. Banders, T. G. Todorov, M. Parfanovic, L. Selleri

Bottom row: R. C. Gallo, A. Sanna, C. De Giuli-Morghen, O. E. Varnier, F. Wong-Stahl, C. A. Romanzi, A. Turano, D. Stehelin, R. C. Gallo

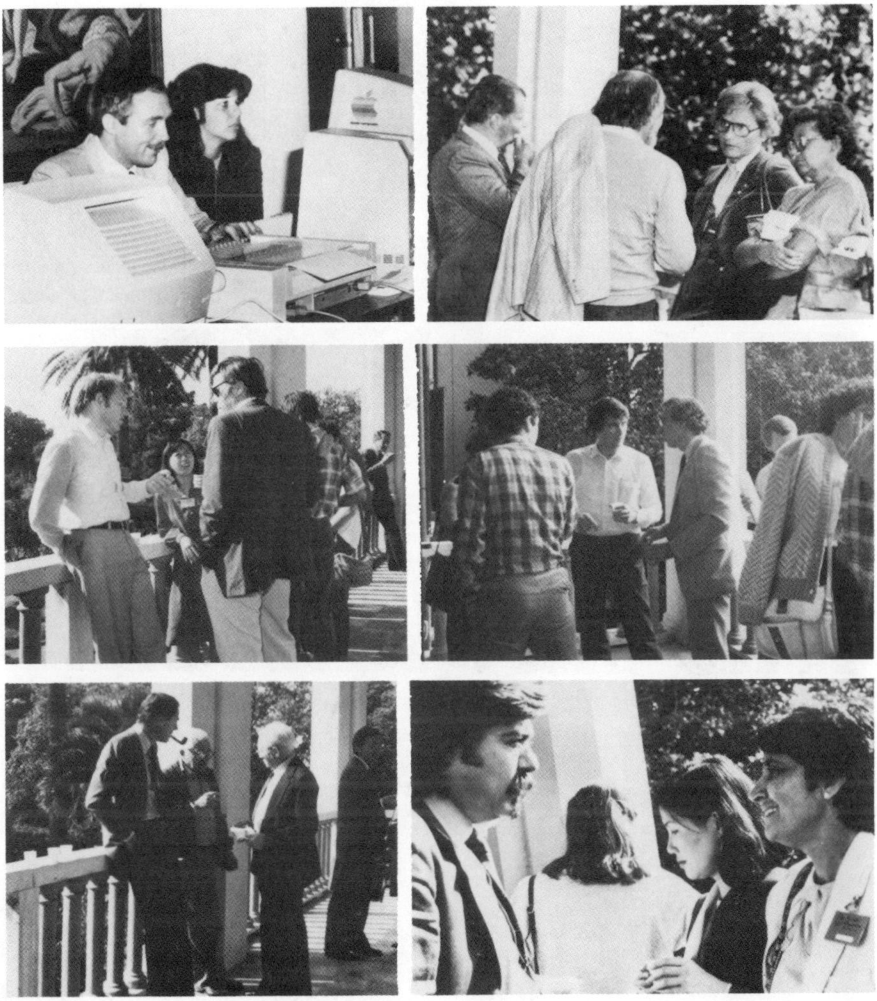

Top row: C. Tarantola, D. Bernini, G. C. Schito, F. Celada, A. M. Molina, L. Calegari

Second row: B. A. Nexo, R. Cheingsong-Popov, A. Vaheri, A. Burny, R. C. Gallo

Bottom row: F. Dianzini, A. Benedetto, A. Sanna, G. W. Canonica, F. Wong-Stahl, S. Rasheed

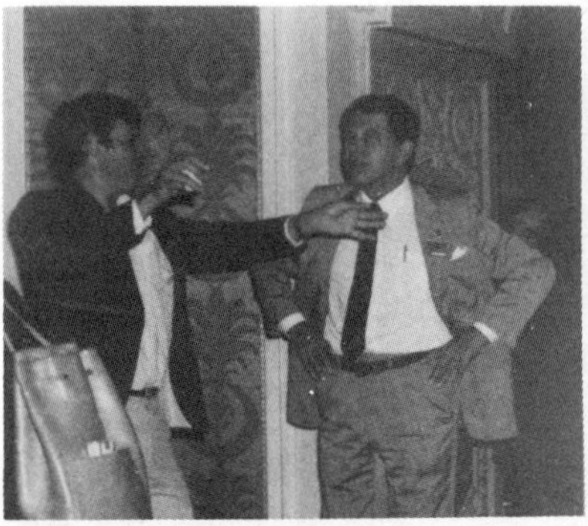
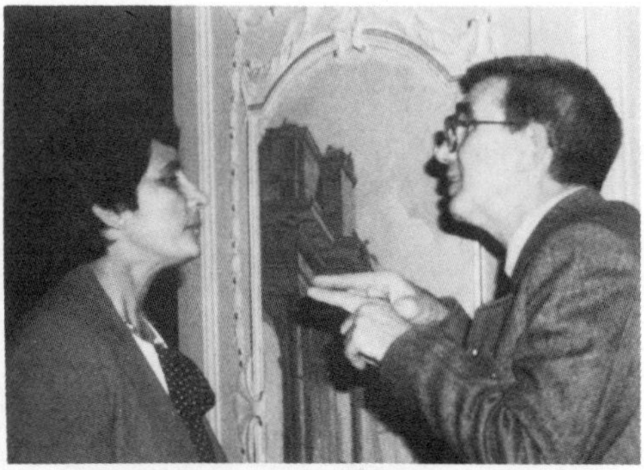
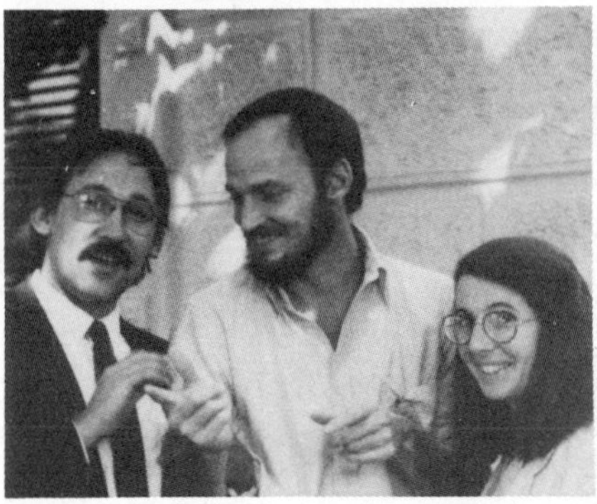
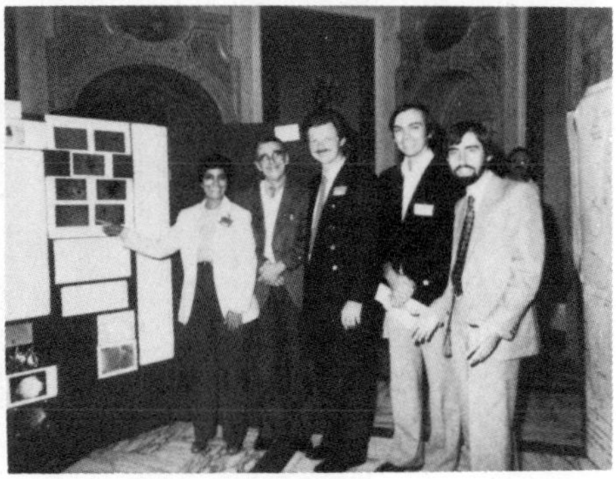
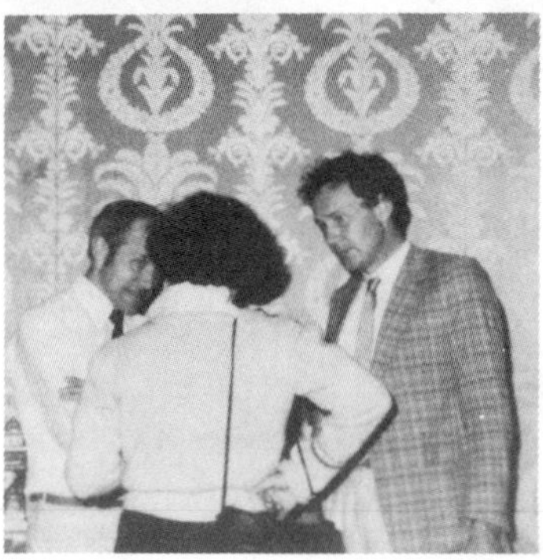
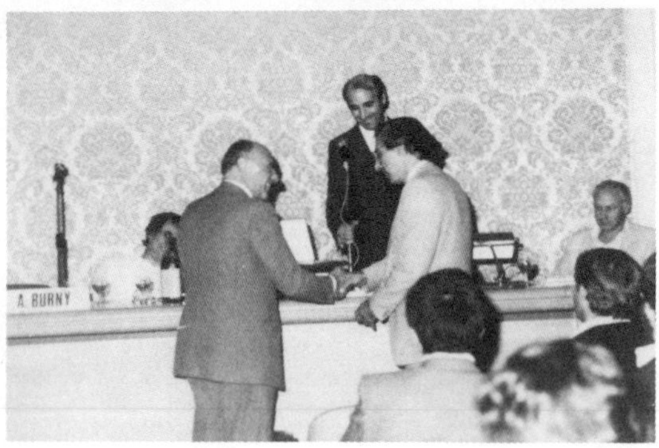

Top row: A. Vaheri, N. Oker-Blom, S. Rasheed, G. Ivaldi

Second row: G. Melioli, T. Weinert, K. Anderson, S. Rasheed, G. Ivaldi, O. E. Varnier, S. P. Raffanti, O. Muratore

Bottom row: J. M. Taylor, S. Panem, D. Stehelin, L. Santi, R. C. Gallo, L. Chieco-Bianchi, O. Jarrett

INTRODUCTION

The Role of Retroviruses

OPENING REMARKS

As Rector of the University of Genoa, I am very pleased to welcome you all and thank you for your participation at this meeting.

We decided to organize this symposium because we believe that recent findings in the field herald an upsurge of interest in the role retroviruses play in human pathology.

For years retrovirologists have worked with several animal models, identifying endogenous and exogenous viral agents which cause malignant and non-malignant diseases. This research on the biology and molecular biology of these genetic elements provided the fundamental information which led to the discovery and identification of the oncogenes and human retroviruses.

It is no coincidence that this symposium has been organized in Genoa, where retroviruses have been studied at the Institute of Microbiology for more than ten years. The study of retroviruses has been the major research interest of our virology laboratory. My personal interest in this project was originally stimulated by the similarities between xenotropic retroviruses and bacteriophages, on which I was working at the time, and I supported this program even when fndings were limited to the realm of classical virology.

I am very glad to find among you not only the most outstanding scientists in this field but also many young researchers. This means that interest, love and curiosity for the unknown is still alive. This large and qualified audience provides the best possible guarantee for the success of this symposium.

Now let me wish you a successful meeting and a pleasant stay in Lerici. I hope you find here the same inspiration that prompted Shelley and D. H. Lawrence to stop and work in these beautiful surroundings.

Carmine A. Romanzi
Rector, University of Genova

RETROVIRUSES IN NEOPLASIA YESTERDAY, TODAY AND TOMORROW

N. Oker-Blom[1], S. Pfeifer-Ohlsson[2] and K. Alitalo[3].

1. University of Helsinki, Finland, 2. Department of Microbiology, University of Umea, Sweden[1], and 3. Department of Virology, University of Helsinki, Finland.

".....
Qué es la vida? Un frenesi.
Qué es la vida? Una illusion
una sombra, una ficcion,
y el mayor bien es pequeno;
que toda la vida es sueno,
y los suenos, suenos son."
Calderon de la Barca

Some advances in retrovirus research are summarized, with emphasis, on the correlation between oncogenes and cellular genes governing proliferation and differentiation. The significance of these recent findings for the understanding of neoplastic and normal developmental processes is briefly discussed.

The history of modern cancer research can be said to have seen its first light through the discovery of the Rous sarcoma virus in 1911 by Peyton Rous (32). Although a long time elapsed before this important finding was recognized, it led during the following decades to the search for other viruses as possible causes of cancer, and many RNA and DNA viruses causing both benign and malignant neoplastic lesions in animals were isolated. The discovery of the mammary tumor agent and the vertically transmitted leukemia in inbred mice stressed the importance of the genetic background of cancer, which also had been suggested already in the beginning of the century (9).

The ideas of the pioneers of yesterday could be summarized as expressed by Francisco Duran-Reynals in a review from 1950 (14) in which he concludes that "... a theoretical cause of cancer should be endowed with the following fundamental properties: (1) It should exhibit an affinity for cells and induce them to grow while multiplying along with them. 2) It should be specific for cells so that many different lesions are produced. 3) It should be able to remain in a latent state in tissues and be conditioned by genetic and surrounding conditions such as those of age. 4) It should be capable of existing either in a free or occult state ".

Since then a vast number of new retroviruses, among them the acute leukemia viruses and recently also finally a retrovirus from man (31), have been isolated and characterized.

As far as the understanding of the mechanism of retrovirus action is concerned, a new era began, however, with the painstaking creation of temperature sensitive mutants, the discovery of the reverse transcriptase (5,38) the hypothesis that retroviral genes exist in the germline of all species (18,39) and finally by the preparation of radioctive DNA probes representative for different regions of the retroviral genome (35,36) followed by the demonstration that the retroviral genes responsible for transformation, the viral or v-oncogenes, have a cellular counterpart, the cellular oncogenes, c-oncogenes or proto-oncogenes, in normal.vertebrate DNA (for reviews, see 7,8). Today we now know about two dozen different oncogenes (Table 1). Most of these have been identified by studies of acutely transforming retroviruses, which have captured cellular oncogenes into their genome.

Table 1. CURRENTLY KNOWN ONCOGENES

RETROVIRUS (example)	ONCOGENE	CELLULAR LOCATION	FUNCTION OF PROTEIN	CLASS
RSV	src	Plasma membrane		Class 1a
Y73V	yes	Plasma membrane		(Cytoplasmatic
GR-FeSV	fgr	Plasma membrane		tyrosine protein
Ab-MuLV	abl	Plasma membrane	Tyrosine-specific	kinases)
FuSV	fps/fes	Cytoplasm	protein kinases	
		(plasma membrane?)	(fgr contains	
ST- and	fes/fps	Cytoplasm	sequences homologous	
GA-FeSV		(cytoskeleton?)	to actin)	
UR2V	ros			
AEV	erb-B	Plasma and cyto-	EGF receptor's cyto-	Class 1b
		plasmic membranes	plasmic domain	(Class 1a-related
SM-FeSV	fms	Plasma and cyto-	Cytoplasmic domain of	proteins)
		plasmic membranes	a growth factor receptor?	
MH-2V	mil/raf	Cytoplasm	?	
3911-MSV	raf/mil	Cytoplasm	?	
Mo-MSV	mos	Cytoplasm	?	
SSV	sis	Secreted	PDGF-like growth factor	Class 2 (Growth factors)

Table 1. CURRENTLY KNOWN ONCOGENES (continued-2)

RETROVIRUSES (example)	ONCOGENE	CELLULAR LOCATION	FUNCTION OF PROTEIN	CLASS
Ra-MSV	Ha-ras	Plasma membrane	GTP-binding proteins	Class 3 (Cytoplasmatic
Ki-MSV	Ki-ras	Plasma membrane		GTP-binding ? kinases)
FBJ-MuSV	fos	Nucleus	?	Class 4
OK-10V	myc	Nucleus	Nuclear matrix protein	(Nuclear
AMV	myb	Nucleus	?	phosphoproteins)
SKSV	ski	Nucleus?	?	
REV	rel	?	?	Unclassified
AEV	erb-A	?	?	
E26V	ets	?	?	

Table 1. CURRENTLY KNOWN ONCOGENES (continued-3)
ONCOGENES NOT FOUND IN RETROVIRUSES

TUMOR CELLS WHERE FOUND	ONCOGENE	CELLULAR LOCATION	FUNCTION OF PROTEIN	CLASS
Neuroblastoma	N-ras	Plasma membrane	GTP-binding	Class 3
Neuroblastoma	N-myc	?	?	Class 4
B-cell lymphoma	B-lym	Nucleus	?	Unclassified
N-methyl-N'-nitro-N-nitrosoguanidine-transformed osteosarcoma cell line	met	?	?	Unclassified

Nontransforming retroviruses (the leukosis viruses) have contributed to the understanding of how cellular oncogenes are activated in maligant disease, via their capacity to integrate near and promote the transcription of specific proto-oncogenes (16). Transfection studies with human tumor DNA have demonstrated conclusively that the same cellular oncogenes, which are integrated into retroviruses, can also induce transformation without a viral intermediate, possibly through changes in oncogene (mutations or chromosomal rearrangements) or through regulatory changes leading to altered expression (8,20,22,33,34).

From studies on different retroviral isolates, it has been demonstrated that the same cellular oncogenes have been rescued from different species in several cases. Oncogenes display strong evolutionary conservation and have been found in widely divergent organisms from yeast to man (7). At a more distant level it has been shown that oncogenes fall into a few families of different functional groups (see Classes in Table 1) having possible common ancestral origins (e.g. src, abl, are homologous to only one gene in *Drosophila*). Distant functional reatedness has even been found between viral oncogenes of some DNA tumour viruses and the oncogenes of some RNA tumor viruses, for example adenovirus 1a and polyoma large T antigen complement ras oncogene functions in conferring serum independence and immortalization, while myc and polyoma middle t complement each other in inducing anchorage independence and morphological transformation (23). The identification of oncogenes into different functional groups, as well as the co-operation between oncogenes in malignant transformation, has reinforced the long-held view that carcinogenesis is a multistage process (10,26).

The key steps in the maturation of cells in a cell lineage involve proliferation and differentiation processes. In light of the capacity of acutely transforming retroviruses to interfere with these steps in the transformed target cells, the potential oncogene progenitors may code for proteins at different levels of the interdigitated chain of events leading to growth and/or differentiation(6,17). Such a chain could be regulated at several possible sites including the level of polypeptide growth factors and their cellular receptors, as well as a linked intracellular messenger system leading to controlled expression of specific genes (17,20,41).

Recently it was learned that the platelet-derived growth factor (PDGF) is encoded by the c-sis oncogene, by comparing amino acid sequence homology between PDGF and the sequence deduced from the simian sarcoma v-onvogene (v-sis) (12,40).

Furthermore, by employing a similar strategy, the erbB oncogene of the avian eryhroblastosis retrovirus has now been demonstrated to be a truncated version of the epidermal growth factor (EGF) receptor (13). This protein displays a tyrosine kinase activity, a feature it shares with most, if not all, growth factor receptors (17,41). It is, in this context, therefore interesting to note that a

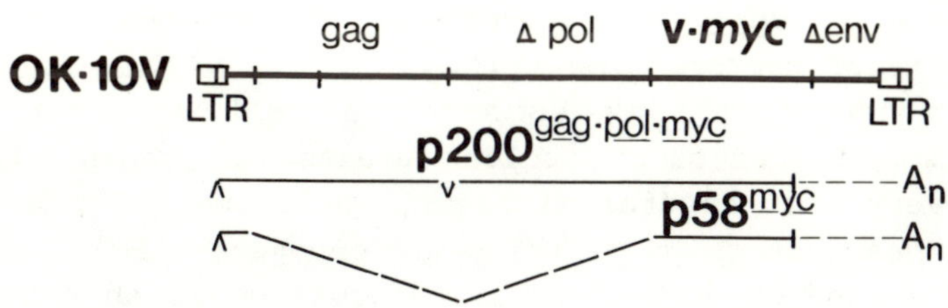

Figure 1. The structure and genomic strategy of the OK-10V provirus. The viral oncogene v-myc is expressed through two different mRNAs, a genomic-length RNA and a spliced subgenomic RNA from which proteins of 200.000 and 58.000 m.w. are produced, respectively (2, 29, 30); LTR: long terminal repeat; An: polyadenylation signal.

large number of retroviral oncogene protein products display tyrosine kinase activity (8,17) The function associated with such an activity is at present unknown, but it could possibly be involved in mediating a growth signal (c.f. 17,41). Thus we can conclude that the sequence of events following a growth stimulus involves proto-oncogene products at both the growth factor, the growth factor receptor and subsequent levels. A tumorigenic process could therefore be based upon an overproduction of the growth factor or an alteration in the receptor so that the cell behaves as it if were constantly exposed to the growth signal. The v-sis ocnogene of simian sarcoma virus is an example of the first situation and the v-erb B oncogene of the avian erythroblastosis virus of the second situation.

It will be exiting to learn whether association with hormone receptors will be a general property of the ras proteins. With regard to the function of the ras proteins in tumorigenesis, several laboratories have demonstrated that the transforming function most often resides close to the N-terminus with a single point mutation resulting in an amino acid change in both the retrovirus and human tumor ras oncogenes (see 23 for a review). The exact molecular function exerted by this change in amino acid sequence is unknown. However, it inactivates the GTPase activity of ras proteins (24).

An important link between the cell membrane growth signal and subsequent nuclear events was shown with the discovery that several mitogens, including PDGF, are able to induce expression of the c-myc oncogenes (20).

The case of OK10 virus transformation is an example of the activity of the myc oncogene (25,26,28). (Fig. 1) The viral oncogene v-myc is expressed through two different mRNA:s, a genomic length RNA and a spliced subgenomic RNA from which proteins of 200,000 and 58,000 m.w. are produced, respectively (2,29,30). Immunoprecipitation of the transforming proteins of three myelocytomatosis viruses shows that the v-myv proteins have molecular weights of 110,000, 200,000 and 58,000 in the different

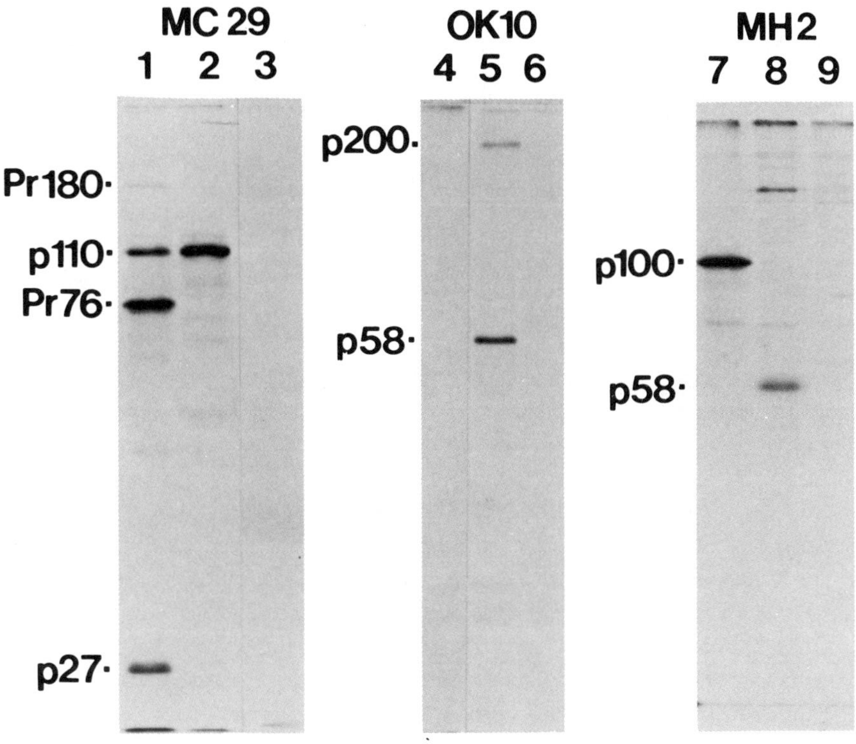

Figure 2. Immunoprecipitation of the transforming proteins of 3 myelocytomatosis viruses. The MC-29 labelled gel presents an electrophoretic analysis of immunoprecipitates from ^{35}S-methionine labelled extracts of Q8 quail cells transformed with MC-29 virus (1). The OK-10 gel shows proteins precipitated from the 9C cell line transformed by OK-10 virus (27) and MH-2 proteins precipitated from MH-2 virus transformed cells. Lanes 1, 4 and 7: the proteins precipitated with antiserum against retroviral structural proteins. Lanes 2, 5 and 8: proteins precipitated with anti-myc protein antiserum. Lanes 3, 6 and 9 show a control precipitation with anti-myc antiserum that was blocked prior to its use with the immunogen. Pr180, p76 and p27 denote structural proteins originating from the

Figure 2 (continued)
genome of a helper virus. p100 is a fusion protein containing sequences from tha gag gene and a recently identified oncogene v-mil (v-raf) (37). The v-myc proteins have m.w. of 110.000, 200.000 and 58.000 in the different virus-transformed cells (cf. Fig. 1 for OK-10 virus).

---

virus transformed cells (Fig. 2). In contrast to most of the other transforming proteins mentioned, the myc protein is located in the nucleus mainly, the OK10 $p58^{v\text{-}myc}$ and avian c-myc proteins serving as examples (Fig. 3 and 4). This seems to be the case in all species tested. The protein is supposed to have DNA binding properties (11) but is also a component of the nuclear matrix (15) and changes its distribution in mitotic cells (42). Therefore it presumably acts in a regulatory or pleiotropic fashion (4, H. Persson and P. Leder, personal communication).

One might therefore conceive that the myc oncogene could represent a key point in the cell cycle common to mitogenic pathways of many cell types. This may explain the ability of the viral myc oncogene to transform a variety of target cells of different histogenic origin. It may also account for the variety of neoplasias with abnormal expression of the c-myc oncogene. The latter is exemplified by a number of malignant diseases with chromosomal translocations and or amplifications involving the myc gene (3,21,22) suggesting that the oncogene is instrumental in tumor formation. To date, the molecular function of the myc protein is not known -- it could for example serve as a transcriptional regulator of specific genes, or indirectly influence gene expression by modulating chromatin organization. Since the myc protein appears to be expressed early in the G1 phase of the cell cycle, it is conceivable that other, as yet unknown functions, complementing the functions of the myc protein, are necessary in order to forward the cell through the cell cycle (4,17,20,41). In summary, the v-onc genes are

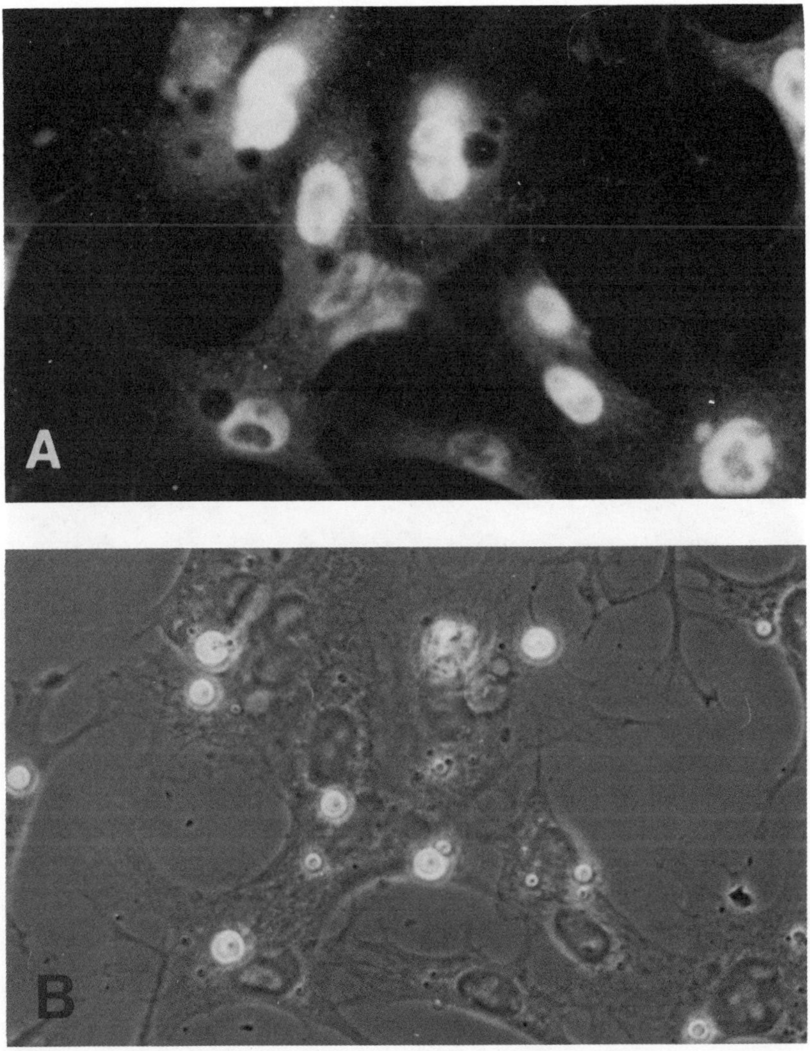

Figure 3. Immunofluorescence (A) and phase contrast (B) microscopy of v-myc proteins in OK-10 virus-transformed quail cells (9C ref. 27). There is mostly nuclear and some cytoplasmatic staining. The nuclear fluorescence excludes nucleolae (2).

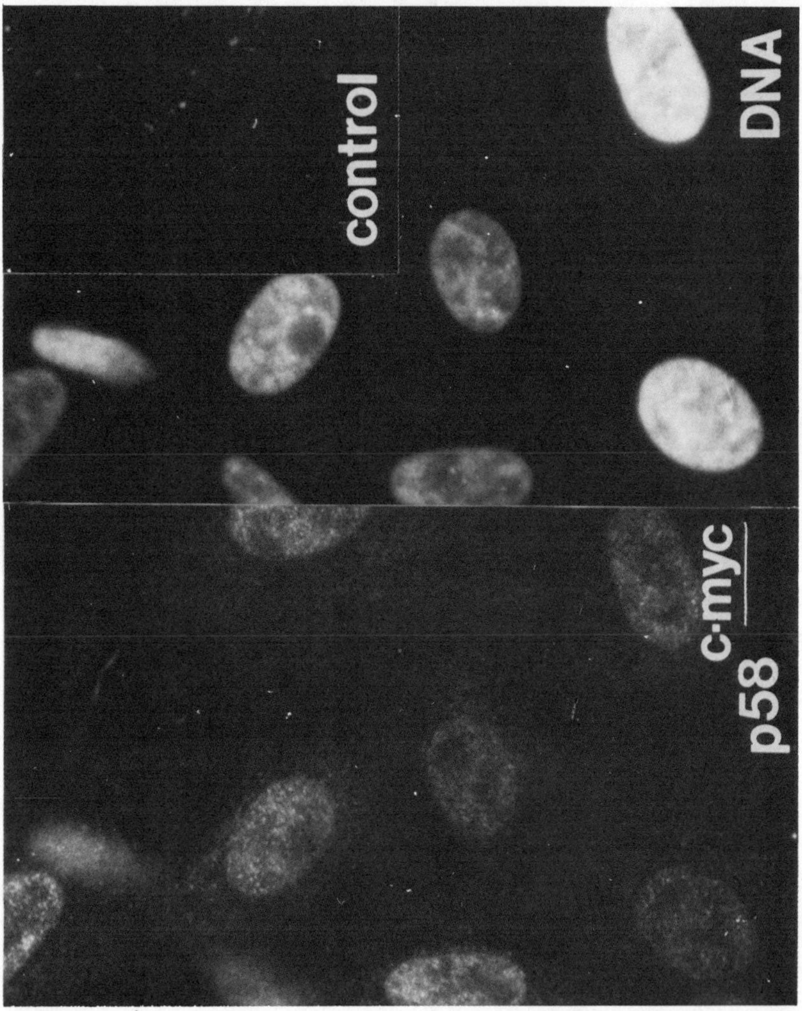

Figure 4. Fluorescent staining for the v-myc protein ($p58^{c-myc}$) and DNA in normal quail cells. Note a granular pattern of indirect immunofluorescence for c-myc protein. Control staining was performed with preimmune rabbit serum (42).

derivatives of important cellular genes governing proliferation and differentiation at the levels of :1) the growth factor 2) the growth factor receptor 3) proteins associated with growth factor receptors 4) cytoplasmic protein kinases 5) growth factor-induced nuclear proteins.

And what about the future-tomorrow? Decades of intensive research on retroviruses have layed not only the foundations for modern cancer research, but have also paved the way for understanding the complex mechanism involved in normal developmental processes. Many questions remain, such as for instance: How do the tumor producing DNA viruses fit into the picture? Could "ordinary" viruses contain oncogene-like sequences? By which mechanism do retroviruses which do not contain oncogenes induce "conversion" and prolonged life span of fibroblasts in vitro without causing transformation? And, finally, are acutely transforming retroviruses just artifacts, and should we instead of speaking about viruses as a cause of cancer speak about cancer as a cause of viruses?

It is an interesting puzzle. Many, probably most, of the pieces may already be available, but are difficult to put in place . Let us hope, however, that the dream of solving the problem of normal versus malignant growth will not remain just a dream.

REFERENCES

1. Alitalo, K., Bishop, J.M., Smith, D.H., Chen, E.Y., Colby, W.W. & Levinson, A.D. (1983) Proc. Natl. Acad. Sci. USA 80, 100-104.
2. Alitalo, K., Ramsay, G., Bishop, J.M., Pfeifer-Ohlsson, S., Colby, W.W. & Levinson A.D., (1983) Nature 306, 274-277.
3. Alitalo, K., Schawab, M., Lin, C.C., Varmus, H.E. & Bishop, M. (1983) Proc. Natl. Acad. Sci. USA 80, 1707-1711.
4. Armelin, H.A., Armelin, M.C.S, Kelly, K., Stewart, T., Leder, P., Cochran, B.H. & Stiles, C.D. (1984) Nature

310, 655-660.

5. Baltimore, D. (1970) Nature 226, 1209-1211.
6. Beug, H., Hayman, M.J. & Graf, T. (1982) Cancer Surveys 1, 205-277.
7. Bishop, J.M. (1983) Ann. Rev. Biochem. 52, 301-354.
8. Bishop; J.M. (1983) Cell 32, 1018-1020.
9. Boveri, T. (1914) Zur Frage der Erstehung Maligner Tumoren. Fische Verlag, Jena.
10. Cairns, J. (1981) Nature 289, 353-357.
11. Donner, P., Greiser-Wilke, I. & Moelling, J. (1982) Nature 296, 262-266.
12. Doolittle, R.F., Hunkapiller, M.W., Hood, L.E., Devare, S.G., Robbins, K.C., Aronson, S.A. & Antoniades, H.N. (1983) Science 221, 275-277.
13. Downward, J., Yarden, Y., Mayes, E., Scrace, G., Totty, N., Stockwell, P., Ullrich, A., Schelssinger, J. & Waterfield, M.D. (1984) Nature 307, 521-527.
14. Duran-Reynals, F. (1950) Am. J. Med. 8, 490-511.
15. Eisenman, R.N., Tachibana, C.Y., Abrams, H.D. & Hann, S.R. (1984) submitted.
16. Hayward, W.S., Neel, B.G. & Astrin, S.M. (1981) Nature 290, 475-480.
17. Heldin, C.H. & Westermark, B. (1984) Cell 37, 9-20.
18. Huebner, R.J., & Todaro, G.J. (1969) Proc. Natl. Acad. Sci. USA 54, 1087-1094.
19. Kamata, T. & Feramisco, J. (1984) Nature 310, 147-149.
20. Kelly K., Cochran, G.H., Stiles, C.D. & Leder, P. (1983) Cell 35, 603-610.
21. Klein, G. (1981) Nature 294, 313-318.
22. Klein, G. (1983) Cell 32, 311-315.
23. Land, H., Parada, L.F. & Weinberg, R.A. (1983) Science 222, 771-778.
24. McGrath, J.P., Capon, D.J., Goeddel, D.B. & Levinson, A.D. (1984) Nature 310, 644-649.
25. Oker-Blom, N., Hortling, L., Kallio, A., Nurmiaiho, E.L. & Westermarck, H. (1978) J. Gen. Virol. 40, 623-633.
26. Oker-Blom, N., Hortling, L., Kallio, A., Nurmiaiho, E.L. & Westermarck, H. (1978) J. Gen. Virol. 40,

623-633.

27. Pfeifer, S. (1984) Intervirology 21, 121-133.
28. Pfeifer, S., Kallio, A., Vaheri, A., Petterson, R. & Oker-Blom, N. (1980) Int. J. Cancer. 25, 235-242.
29. Pfeifer, S., Petterson, R.K., Kallio, A., Oker-Blom, N. & Vaheri, A. (1981) J. Virol. 40, 533-540.
30. Pfeifer, S., Zabielski; J., Ohlsson, R., Frykberg, L., Knowles, J., Petterson, R. , Oker-Blom, N., Philipson, L., Vaheri, A. & Vennstrom, B. (1983) J. Virol. 46, 347-354.
31. Poiesz, B.J., Ruscetti, F.W., Gazdar, A.F., Bunn, P.A., Minna, J.D. & Gallo, R.C. (1980) Proc. Natl. Acad. Sci. USA 77, 7415-7419.
32. Rous, P. (1911) J. Exp. Med. 13, 379-384.
33. Siebenlist, U., Hennighausen, L., Battey, J. & Leder, P. (1984) Cell 37, 381-391.
34. Spandidos, D.A. & Wilkie, NM. (1984) Nature 310, 469-475.
35. Spector, D., Varmus, H.E. & Bishop, J.M. (1978) Proc. Natl. Acad. Sci. USA 75, 4102-4106.
36. Stehelin, D., Varmus, H.E., Bishop, J.M. & Vogt, P.K. (1976) Nature 260, 170-173.
37. Sutrate, P., Bonner, T.I., Rapp, U.R., Jansen, H.W., Patschinsky, T. & Bister, K. (1984) Nature 309, 85-88.
38. Temin, H.M. & Mizutami, S. (1970) Nature 226, 1211-1213.
39. Todaro, G.J., & Huebner, R.J. (1972) Proc. Natl. Acad. Sci. USA 69, 1009-1015.
40. Waterfield, M.D., Scrace, T., Whittle, N., Strobant, P., Johnsson, A., Wasteson, A., Westermark, B., Heldin, G.H., Huang J.D. & Deuel T.F. (1983) Nature 304, 35-39.
41. Westermark, B., Heldin, G.H., Ek, B., Johnsson, A., Mellstrom, K., Nister, M. & Wasteson, A. (1983) In Growth and Maturation Factors, 1, G. Guroff, ed. (New York. John Wiley and Sons.) pp. 73-115.
42. Winqvist, R., Saksela, K. & Alitalo, K. (1984) EMBO J., in press.

THE ROLE OF RETROVIRUSES IN NATURE

R. DULBECCO
The Salk Institute, La Jolla California

This article reviews the evolution of thinking about the role of retroviruses in Nature. The observations initially suggested that integrated retroviral genomes (retrogenomes) are bona fide cellular genes which can generate the genomes of viral particles. Today, on the basis of several kinds of observation, we recognize that retrogenomes derive from infection of early embryos. Retrogenomes do not perform any crucial role for the organism, except for staving off infection by some retroviruses. The biological significance of retroviruses is that of transposons. They are of a special kind, in which transposition is based on reverse transcription. This characteristic explains their biological effect, from inactivation of genes, to activation and transduction of genes. The cancer-inducing activity is in part related to their activation and transduction of oncogenes, and in part to other biological properties which are briefly discussed. Retrogenomes are in the cellular genome for their own persistence and reproduction. The biological significance of retrogenomes, as well as of other transposons using reverse transcription, is mostly evolutionary.

Questions about the role of retroviruses in Nature were raised as soon as the characteristic behavior of these viruses was discovered. The viruses were first recognized as agents of leukemias or solid tumors in chicken and mice. What seemed most puzzling was their ability to enter the genomes of animal species and to persist there indefinitely through successive generations, during which they were transmitted like Mendelian genes. The genes of retroviral genomes integrated in the cellular genome were found sometimes to be expressed. This was shown by the appearance of proteins specificed by viral genes at the surface of the cells. With suitable treatment -- such as exposure of the cells to BudR (1,2) -- the integrated genomes could be mobilized with the result that retroviral particles were released. An example of such integrated normally silent but activable genome is the avian RAV 0 (3).

These findings raised questions about the nature and role of retroviruses. It seemed possible that in the experiment of induction of virus release by BudR, cellular genes were induced to become retroviral genomes. It seemed also that these genomes should perform functions essential for the cells that harbored them. And because retroviruses cause tumors, it was proposed that normal cellular genes capable of evolving into retroviral genomes, are the cause of cancer.

Today, some twenty years later, our perspective is different. We recognize that retroviruses go through a cycle that involves both the extracellular retrovirus particles, and the viral genome integrated in the cellular DNA. The integrated genome, which persists through many generations and is inherited like a Mendelian gene, is often called a provirus. I will refer to it as "retrogenome". We know now that retrogenomes are not essential for the species that harbor them. The most direct evidence is the existence of a strain of healthy chickens that is entirely free of them (4). A similar conclusion could be reached by recognizing that, if the persistence of retrogenomes were dependent on some important role for the animals carrying them, all three genes of a retrogenome, the gag, the pol and the env genes, should be essential for the host species. In fact the induction of retrovirus production by BudR shows that each of these genes is conserved. We have no reason, however, to believe that they perform functions essential for the host. The alternative interpretation is that all three genes are essential for the propagation of the virus generated from the retrogenomes present in the cells. The conservation of the genes would then be attributed to the functions they perform for the virus rather than for the host cell. In this alternative view the emphasis shifts from the cellular to the viral role of these genes. In other words, the conservation of the three retroviral genes suggests that retrogenomes are not permanent residents of the host DNA but that they are adventitious, and come in from time to time from the outside, through the regular cycle of infection and multiplication of viral particles.

There is ample evidence showing that retrogenomes were derived at one time or another from infectious viral particles. The most convincing evidence comes from experiments in which retroviruses are injected into mouse embryo. Some of these embryos then give rise to lineages which carry the injected retrovirus genome in a permanently integrated and heritable form. Thirteen strains carrying retroviral genomes integrated at different sites and inherited as Mendelian genes were obtained in this way (5). This experiment dramatically confirms the inference drawn from the study of congenital infection in animals. Congenital infection of the progeny occurs if in the mother the retrogenome is activated to release viral particles during the early stages of development of the embryo. If there is viremia and retroviral particles reach the embryo, it becomes infected. Viral genomes become then established in the genomes of cells of the infected embryos as retrogenomes, which persist in the adult animal deriving from the embryo. Retrogenomes that fail to spontaneously produce viral particles -- like the chicken RAV 0 (3) -- do not give rise to congenital infection (6,7).

Additional strong evidence for the origin of retrogenomes by infection derived from studies with AKR mice. All the mice of this strain are known to contain two retrogenomes, Ak -1 and Ak -2, at fixed locations in the genome (8). In crosses, these proviruses are inherited in a Mendelian fashion. In large animal colonies new additional localizations have however been recognized in some mice (9,10). Almost certainly these derive from infection of embryos with virus formed by the spontaneous activation of the two resident retrogenomes.

How frequently the genome of an animal is colonized by a new retrogenome can be deduced from these observations as well as from the comparative study of retroviruses present in different species. The picture that emerges is that the propensity for spreading varies greatly from one retrogenome to another. The differences probably depend on the opportunities a retrogenome has to generate infectious virus and to invade an embryo. Clearly the two AKR retrogenomes mentioned above have existed in that strain since it was established, but new ones have crept in since then at the rate of one per about thirty generations (10). A retrovirus common to cats and baboons, the RD-114, probably originated in primates, seems to have invaded the cat germ line several million years ago (11). Once inserted in the cell's genome, it persisted in a rather stable way. Clearly, retrogenomes are not readily lost, and the divergence of their sequences is not especially rapid. Divergence however occurs, because, the animal gene contains sequences closely related to retrogenomes, which derived from them by deletion and mutation.

Especially interesting among the retrogenomes that persist in mice are those of the xenotropic class. These retrogenomes, when activated, generate viral particles that do not multiply in mouse cells, but in cells of other species, such as mink. It might seem that the existence of these retrogenome contradicts the thesis that retrogenomes are always the result of integrations that occurred in relatively recent times as a result of infection. This is because the virus generated by xenotropic retrogenomes cannot infect animals of the same species in which they reside. It is, however, possible that these proviruses became xenotropic as a result of a mutation of a mouse gene that made infection impossible. Since the occurrence of that mutation these retrogenomes have been prisoners of the cellular genomes. They can escape and infect new cells only through the intervention of the experimenter who offers them cells of a suitable species. In recent years xenotropic retrogenomes have however gained a new meaning because, as we will see below, they can donate part of their sequences to ecotropic retrovirus genomes (which are capable of infecting the cells of the mice that harbor them). This recombination has important consequences.

Another interesting special class of retrogenomes are those that generate the so-called intracysternal A-particles. There are about 1000 copies of these retrogenomes in the mouse genome (12). These genomes represent a special class: they are not homologous to other retrogenomes (13) and are simpler. They have, however, the same general organization. The stability of these genomes suggests that, although they do not generate infectious particles able to infect other cells, they are also maintained by the cycle of transcription, enclosure in a particle, reverse transcription and integration.

The molecular analysis of the retrogenomes shows that they are related to other mobile DNA sequences, which are present in the genome of all organisms. As Temin first pointed out, retrogenomes are organized very much like transposing elements (14). The closest similarity is to bacteria transposons. In them a small group of genes is bounded by two equal sequences: the insertion sequences (IS). In retrogenomes the genes are bound by the long terminal repeats, or LTRs. Like an IS, an LTR is in turn bounded by two short inverted repeats. Moreover, two short repeats, which derive from duplication of the sequence preexisting in the host DNA before integration, flank the retrogenome as they flank a transposon.

The LTRs flanking the retrogenomes, like the repeat sequences of transposons, contain sequences for initiation and control of transcription, such as promoters, terminators, enhancers, and polyadenylation sites (15) Some retrogenomes, like those of the mammary tumor virus, have developed the ability to respond to steroid hormones (16,17). In general the LTRs respond to regulatory signals appropriate for the cells in which the retrogenome is expressed.

The analogy between retrogenomes and transposons is striking and strongly implies a relatedness of the two types of genome. In transposons some of the genes enclosed between the various repeats are needed for replication, whereas others are of host origin. The ability to incorporate copies of cellular DNA, more or less at random, is the outstanding function of transposons. Host genes found in bacterial transposons are those with a favorable effect on the host. For instance, if a bacterium is in an environment containing antibiotics, transposons contain genes that confer resistance to the antibiotics. Transposons carrying such genes are useful to the host bacteria and are selected for selection acts on the bacteria and indirectly selects the transposons. Any kind of gene, however, could end up in a transposon. In retrogenomes all three regular genes are involved in transposition. Two of them (gag and env) allow the formation of infectious viral particles enclosing RNA trascripts of the retrogenomes. The third gene (pol) is needed for the reverse transcription that generates a DNA copy of the genome capable of integration. As we will see below, sometimes a retrogenome also contains host genes. They are selected for because they make the cells neoplastic.

The ability to acquire viral characteristics makes possible the propagation of retrogenomes. It allows RNA copies of the transposon to leave as viral particles the cells in which they originated to spread to many other cells, and to colonize their DNAs. So the function of a retrogenome, like that of a transposon, is to increase in number and to spread. This view of retrogenomes is opposite to the old one, according to which retrogenomes had to supply needed functions to the host cells. The old view retains, however some validity because at least one integrated, incomplete retrogenome (known as the Fv-4 resistance gene) defends the cells against infection by infecting retroviruses (18). It acts by causing the synthesis of its own envelope glycoprotein, which invades the plasma membrane of the cells, preventing infection with retroviruses coming from the outside (19). Many other retrogenomes may similarly contribute to resistance to retrovirus infection because chicken free of functional retrogenomes are extremely susceptible to infections by retroviruses (20). This role of retrogenomes, however, only limits the spreading of other retroviruses; without retroviruses it would have no beneficial role at all.

The mechanism by which retroviruses spread from one cellular genome to another distinguishes them from other transposons. Retrogenomes spread through RNA intermediates, whereas all other transponsons spread by DNA translocation. Retrogenomes seem unable to transpose directly in DNA form. They underwent a special evolution based on reverse transcription. All transponsons are transcribed into RNA as a means of expressing the functions of their genes, but these RNAs are an end product. Only in retroviruses the possibility of reverse transcription makes the RNA an intermediate in the transposition cycle.

Some light on how retroviruses evolved is thrown by the recent demonstration of certain families of repeated sequences present in the mouse genome. One family contains sequences related to the mammary tumor virus retrogenome, even in animals that do not carry any complete retrogenome of this kind (21). This family cannot therefore have been produced by dissemination of copies of the retrogenome. Another family is made up of sequences with considerable homology to retroviral LTRs (22). It is possible that these are the sequences from which the evolution of retrogenomes began. The genomes of intracysternal A-particles may have an intermediate position. They are bounded by repeated sequences (23) and specify a reverse transcriptase, although much less efficiently than that of retroviruses (24).

Transposition by reverse transcription is not used exclusively by retroviruses. The copia transposing elements of Drosophilia (which are structurally similar to retrogenmes (25)) may use a simlar method of transposition (26). Reverse transcription is not therefore exclusive of retroviruses. It is also used in the replication of at least another virus, that of hepatitis B. There may be an even more general use of reverse transcription as suggested by a special class of pseudogenes. Their characteristics clearly show that they originated by reverse transcripion of cellular messengers, followed by integration of the DNA product in the cell genome (27). Whether the enzyme carrying out this transposition is viral or cellular is undetermined.

An important facet of retrovirus biology is that integration of a retrogenome in the cellular DNA is important not only for the perpetuation of the retrovirus but also for the function of neighboring cellular genes. They can be damaged through either inactivation or activation. The inactivation of genes is clearly demonstrated by the d mutation in DBA mice (28): mutant animals have a retrogenome inserted within the gene, whereas wild type animals do not. Rare animals that revert to wild type have lost the retrogenome (28). These revertants are interesting for the biology of retroviruses because the loss of the retrogenome occurs by recombination between the two LTRs that bound it at either end, leaving a single LTR as only vestige (29). The excised part of the retrogenome is not reintegrated anywhere else. This is because the excised DNA has only one LTR, and two are needed for integration. In fact in the normal retroviral cycle the only product of reverse transcription that can integrate is a DNA circle with two LTRs (30). This reflects the general property of transposons, which always have two repeat sequences at their ends; they seem to be essential for trasposition. In fact, no transposon uses as intermediate in transposition, a circle generated by recombination between the repeated ends. They transpose by a more complex mechanism, which causes the integration of a new copy at a new site in the host genome, leaving the older copy at its previous place.

Retroviral genomes can activate genes by inserting near them. This is a relatively recent acquisition in our understanding of how the cellular genome can be perturbed by insertions. Essential for activation are the LTRs (31) and especially the promoters and enhancers they contain. An LTR sitting at the 5' end of a non-transcribed gene may cause it to be transcribed, and one sitting at either end of a weakly transcribed gene may enhance transcription by the action of its enhancer, provided, of course, that the enhancer is active in the type of cell in which these events take place.

Activation of adjacent cellular genes by LTR insertion near them is one of the mechanisms by which retroviruses perform their oncogenic role (32). The cellular genes thus activated belong to a special class devoted to control of cell growth and differentiation. Once activated they become oncogenes, i.e., cancer agents. These normal genes are known as proto-oncogenes. How much this mechanism contributes to the cancer inducing ability of retroviruses is hard to say. Insertion of LTRs near the c-myc proto-oncogene is also found in avian (32) as well as murine (33) B lymphomas, and also in some murine T lymphomas (34). The activation of the proto-oncogene may not however be the sole factor in tumor production because bursal lymphomas of chicken also contain other activated oncogenes (35).

Cellular proto-oncogenes become activated also when they become incorporated into retrogenomes. This is the mechanism by which acutely transforming retroviruses are generated. The mechanism of incorporation has not been elucidated. Because incorporation of DNA sequences is a general property of transposons, it is surprising that retrogenomes also possess it. Under the control of the viral LTR, the incorporated gene is expressed at a high rate in all cells in which the LTRs are active as enhancers. Among these cells some are of a type in which the proto-oncogene would not be normally expressed. The gene is then expressed in an inappropriate cell.

High inappropriate expression of the oncogene is not, however, the main mechanism by which proto-oncogenes are activated. Artificially constructed viruses in which a proto-oncogene replaces the altered form present in the transforming viral particles may not transform (36). In these (and perhaps in all) cases an alteration of the sequence of the proto-oncogene is essential for generating a cancer-inducing ability. Such an alteration, usually as a deletion, may occur during the transposition of the gene to the retrogenome. It can also occur in the form of mutations, subsequent to the transposition. Mutations are formed frequently during reverse transcription (36), because the reverse transcriptase, being a primitive enzyme, lacks the sophisticated error-correcting property of the DNA replicase. In either case the structural changes of the proto-oncogene, which is not a cancer-causing agent, convert it into an active cancer-inducing oncogene. Structural alterations often occur also when an LTR becomes localized near a proto-oncogene. Thus the consequences of LTR insertion may be more complex than just increasing transcription (37).

Although the unaltered retrogenome itself may have no cancer-inducing activity, some recombinant retrogenomes, not carrying oncogenes, do. Among mouse retroviruses such recombinants are known as mink-cell focus-forming viruses -- or MCFs. They are so named because, in contrast to the usual mouse retroviruses, they can infect cells derived from minks and other species. Well-known examples are the MCFs of the AKR virus which induce thymomas in the mice (38). These retroviruses have the property of growing in cells of a foreign species because they contain a segment from the envelope gene of an xenotropic retrogenome in their own envelope gene. They have a mixed envelope, which makes them dual-tropic, that is, able to grow in cells from both mice and other species.

How the recombinants are formed is not clear, but the

mechanism is likely to be similar to that causing incorporation of proto-oncogene sequences into retrogenomes. AKR MCFs have oncogenic activity only if they retain a piece of the ecotropic genome at their 3'-end (39). Why only these recombinants are oncogenic is not clearly known. The altered precursor of the envelope protein produced by these viruses may not be processed; the abnormal glycoprotein would then perturb the function of some normal membrane protein. Perhaps the recombinant glycoprotein itself, even if normally processed, may be able to perturb the function.

A yet different mechanism of cell transformation without incorporation of proto-oncogene is characteristic of a class of retroviruses that were isolated from human T cell neoplasias:the human T-cell leukemia viruses (HTLV) (40). These viruses, which are implicated in the origin of the T-cell neoplasias, can immortalize human T cells in vitro (41). Their genome contains a region --called the X region -- that is absent in other retroviruses (42). This region has a long open reading frame, which appears to specify a protein. The function of this molecule is to activate the LTR of the HTLV, and probably also the enhancer sequences of other genes (43). The X-region is probably another gene of the transposing element that promotes transposition by increasing its transcription. Its action on other genes would be accidental. Whether and how this function is involved in the immortalization of the cells and possibly in T cell neoplasia remains to be determined.

This survey of the mechanisms by which retroviruses induce cancer shows that they are all secondary events. No unaltered retrovirus has the primary function of inducing cancer. The reason is probably evolutionary. A hereditarily transmitted retrogenome has no advantage in eliciting cancer at an early stage of development of the host animal because the retrogenome needs the animal in order to be perpetuated by it. The formation of a cancer-inducing genome takes place only months after the birth of the animal, after the animal has reproduced, transmitting the viral genome to its progeny. The cancer-inducing genomes thus persist only for the life of the individuals they affect. In fact, retrogenomes carrying an oncogene arise rarely and are eliminated by the death of their animal host, unless they are perpetuated by the experimenter. The formation of MCF recombinants also occurs fairly late in the life of the host animal, after much multiplication of the unaltered virus has taken place. A similar time lag exists for the insertion of LTRs near a proto-oncogene. In all cases the animal has ample chance to reproduce before being killed by the cancer. Evolutionary considerations may also explain why structural alterations of pre-oncogenes are important and possibly essential for making them active oncogenes. The point is that the species could not exist with an oncogene active at all times.

We can conclude that retrogenomes are a highly specialized example of DNA sequences with a tendency to spread throughout the animal genome, without any relationship to the sequences or function of the DNA in which they integrate. They do not serve the needs of the host genome but only of their own perpetuation. Retrogenomes can spread among somatic cells at great speed, using the method of viral transmission. The greatest significance of retroviruses, retrogenomes, and the families of sequences related to them is probably evolutionary. Like all transposing elements they contribute in an important way to shuffling around DNA sequences, duplicating them and creating new assortments. They may have the additional role of transferring genes from one species to another. What we observe through the process of carcinogenesis is merely a window on this much broader scenario.

REFERENCES

1. Aaronson, S.A., Todaro, G.J. and Scolnick, E.M. (1971) Science 174:157-159.

2. Lowy, D.R., Rowe, W.P., Teich, N., and Hartley, J.W. (1971) Science 174:155-156.
3. Robinson, H.L., and Eisenman, R.N. (1984) Science 225;417-419
4. Astrin, S.W., Buss, E.G. and Hayward, W.S. (1980) Nature 282:339-340.
5. Jaenisch, R., Jahner, D., Nobis, P., Simon, I., Lohler, J., Harbers, K., and Grotkopp, D. (1981) Cell 24:519-529.
6. Dougherty, R.M. and DiStefano, H.S. (1967) Cancer Res. 27:322-332.
7. Rubin, H., Fanshier, L., Cornelius, A. and Hughes, W.F. (1962) Virology 17:143-156.
8. Rowe, W.P. (1972) J. Exp. Med. 136:1272-1285.
9. Herr, W. and Gilbert, W. (1982) Nature 296:865-868.
10. Quint, W., van der Putten, H., Janssen, F. and Berns, A. (1982) J. of Virol. 41:901-908.
11. Benveniste, R.E., and Todaro, G.J. (1974) Nature 252:456-459.
12. Lueders, K.K. and Kuff, E.L. (1980) Proc. Natl. Acad. Sci. USA 77:3571-3575.
13. Lueders, K.K. and Kuff, E.L. (1979) J. Virol. 30:225-231.
14. Temin, H. (1980) Cell 21:599-600.
15. Ju, G. and Skalka, A.M. (1980) Cell 22:379-386.
16. Majors, J. and Varmus, H.E. (1983) Pro. Natl. Acad. Sci. USA. 80:5866-5870.
17. Huang, A.L., Ostrowski, M.C., Berard, D. and Hager, G.L. (1981) Cell 27:245-255.
18. Kozak, C.A., Gromet, N.J., Ikeda, H. and Buckler, C.E. (1984) Proc. Natl. Acad. Sci. USA 81:834-837.
19. Ikeda, H. and Odaka, T. (1983) Virology 128:127-139.
20. Robinson, H.L., Astrin, S.W., Senior, A.M., Salazar, F.H. (1981) J. Virol. 40:745-751.
21. Callahan R., Drohan, W., Gallahan, D., D'Hoostelaere, L. and Potter, M. (1982) Proc. Natl. Acad. Sci. USA 79:4113-4117.
22. Wirth, T., Gloggler, K., Baumruker, T., Schmidt, M. and Horak, I. (1983) Proc. Natl. Acad. Sci. USA

80:3327-3330.

23. Cole, M.D., Ono, M. and Huang, R.C.C. (1981) J. Virol. 38:680-687.
24. Wong-Staal, F., Reitz, M.S., Trainor, C.D. and Gallo, R.C. (1975) J. Virol. 16:887-896.
25. Kugimiya, W., Ikenaga, H. and Saigo, K. (1983) Proc. Natl. Acad. Sci. USA 80:3193-3197.
26. Flavell, A.J. (1984) Nature 310:514-516.
27. Hollis, G.F., Hieter, P.A., McBride, O.W., Swan, D. and Leder, P. (1982) Nature 296:321-325.
28. Jenkins, N.A., Copeland, N.G., Taylor, B.A. and Lee, B.K. (1981) Nature 293:370-374.
29. Copeland, N.G., Hutchison, K.W. and Jenkins, N.A. (1983) Cell 33:379-387.
30. Panganiban, A.T. and Temin, H.M. (1984). Cell 36:673-679.
31. Varmus, H.E. (1982) Science 216:812-820.
32. Hayward, W.S., Neel, B.G., and Astrin, S.M. (1980) Nature 290:475-480.
33. Steffen, D. (1984) Proc. Natl. Acad. Sci. USA 81:2097-2101.
34. Corcoran, L.M., Adams, J.M., Dunn, A.R. and Cory, S. Cell 37:113-122.
35. Cooper, G.M. and Neiman, P.E. Nature 287:656-659.
36. Iba, H., Takeya, T., Cross, F.R., Hanafusa, T. and Hanafusa, H. (1984) Proc. Natl. Acad. Sci. USA 81:4424-4428.
37. Westaway, D., Payne, G. and Varmus, H.E. (1984) Proc. Natl. Acad. Sci. USA 81:843-847.
38. Fischinger, P.J., Nomura, S. and Bolognesi, D.P. (1975) Proc. Natl. Acad. Sci. USA 72:5150-5155.
39. Chattopadhyay, S.K., Cloyd, M.W., Linemeyer, D.L., Lander, M.R., Rands, E. and Lowy, D.R. (1982) Nature 295:25-31.
40. Poiesz, B.J., Ruscetti, F.W., Gazdar, A.F., Bunn, P.A., Minna, J.D., and Gallo, R.C. (1980) Proc. Natl. Acad. Sci. USA 77:7415-7419.
41. Miyoshi, I., Kubonishi, I., Yoshimoto, S., Akagi, T., Ohtsuki, Y., Shiraishi, Y., Nagata, K. and Hinuma, Y.

(1981). Nature 294:770-771.
42. Seiki, M., Hattori, S., Hirayama, Y. and Yoshida, M. (1983) Proc. Natl. Acad. Sci. USA 80:3618-3622.
43. Sodroski, J.G., Rosen, C.A. and Haseltine, W.A. (1984) Science 225:381-385.

W. P. ROWE MEMORIAL LECTURE

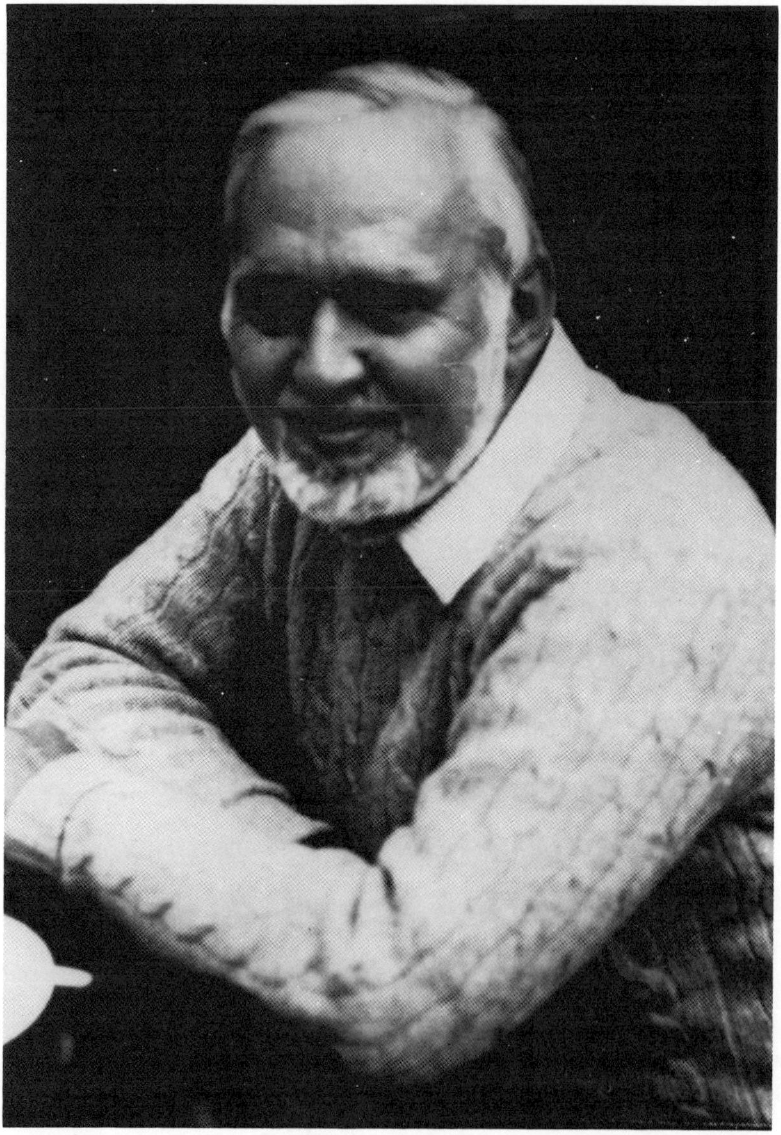

Wallace P. Rowe, M.D. (2.20.1926–7.4.1983)

CHANGING DOGMAS IN RETROVIROLOGY

J. A. Levy,

Department of Medicine, Cancer Research Institute, University of California, School of Medicine, San Francisco, CA

In the past 80 years since the first recognition of viruses, now known as retroviruses, basic tenets or dogmas about these infectious agents have been stated. Many of them have been challenged and reversed by the constant acquirement of new information on their biologic properties and diversified functions. Ten dogmas in retrovirology have been selected for discussion. By reviewing the new developments in retrovirology, one can appreciate changes that occur in basic scientific truths and the need to constantly challenge dogmas to test their validity and applicability.

It is a pleasure to present the Wallace P. Rowe Memorial Lectureship. Many of you know of the outstanding contributions that Wally made to the field of viruses, in general, and, in particular, tumor viruses. His interest in retroviruses led to major advances in the field which progressed at a much more rapid rate than would have been possible without his efforts (Table 1). He was, to me, a brilliant scientist, a dedicated teacher and a good friend.

TABLE 1 CONTRIBUTIONS BY WALLACE P. ROWE TO RETROVIROLOGY

---

1. Successful cultivation of mouse leukemia viruses in tissue culture and the development of the complement fixation (COMUL) test.

2. Isolation of mouse sarcoma viruses (MSV) in tissue culture, and definition of 2-hit kinetics of cell transformation. Recognition of the role of non-transforming mouse type C viruses in focus formation and rescue of MSV.

3. Definition of N and B tropism and its relationship to the Fv-1 genetic locus.

4. Development of the XC plaque assay for detection of mouse type C retroviruses.

5. Identification of non-producing mouse leukemia virus-infected cells. Activation of infectious virus by chemical and physical agents.

6. Identification of endogenous AKv genes.

7. Characterization of amphotropic mouse retroviruses.

8. Identification of dual-tropic (MCF) retroviruses.

9. Definition of the genetic control of endogenous retrovirus expression.

Many of these studies were done in collaboration with Dr. Robert Huebner and Dr. Janet Hartley.

As a tribute to Wally, who was constantly challenging dogmas in virology, I dedicate this lecture to "the changing dogmas of retrovirology". I initially made a list of about twenty dogmas - a term, by the way, which Webster defines as " point of view or tenet put forth as authoritative without adequate grounds, or something held as an established opinion". From these I have selected ten to discuss in a somewhat chronologic order and comment on how they have changed (Table 2). Many of them deal with the system that Wally worked with and which I know best, the mouse retroviruses. They cover the "rules of thumb" that I encountered in 1967 when I came to work at the National Institute of Health (NIH) with Robert Huebner, Wallace Rowe, and Janet Hartley on mouse leukemia and sarcoma viruses. They obviously will reflect a bias, but I hope will serve to illustrate how rapidly a field of study can change and how the rules of today can become so quickly outdated. Most importantly, they will indicate the range of biologic activities of these agents and hopefully provide insights into new approaches for their study.

Retroviruses, although not known by that name at that time, were first discovered, as you know, because of their oncogenic properties. the credit for the identification of the first retrovirus generally goes to Ellermann and Bang who, in 1908, showed that chicken leukemia could be transmitted by filtrates (1). However, the major impetus for virus research in tumors came in 1911, when Peyton Rous of the Rockerfeller Institute, induced solid tumors in susceptible strains of chickens with filtrates from a tumor he found in a Barrod Plymouth Rock hen (2). The tumor had been there for about two months before the fowl (1.5 years old) was brought to his laboratory for study. The virus responsible became known as the Rous sarcoma virus (RSV). In retrospect, however, the first actual retrovirus isolated was the equine infectious anemia virus, which in 1904, was shown by Vallee and Carre (3) to be a filterable agent which can induce autoimmune hemolytic anemia in susceptible horses. By 1912, several chicken tumors in Rous' laboratory and others' had yielded

TABLE 2A. DOGMAS IN RETROVIROLOGY

1. Viruses only cause tumors in avian species.

2. Mouse sarcoma viruses are <u>defective</u> in transforming cells. They require the help of an accompanying leukemia virus.

3. Viruses preferentially infect and replicate in cells of the species of origin.

4. RNA tumor viruses exist like episomes in infected cells.

5. Latent retrovirus infection involving a non-producer (NP) state exists only for sarcoma viruses.

6. There is no host reaction to endogenous retroviruses.

7. Retroviruses cause cancer by producing virus-specific transforming proteins.

8. Retrovirus-associated tumors are only caused by these viruses.

9. All retroviruses are transforming viruses.

10. There are no human retroviruses

TABLE 2B. CHANGES IN DOGMAS IN RETROVIROLOGY

1. Discovery of mouse leukemia virus (5)
2. MSV transforms rat cells by 1-hit kinetics. Defectiveness involves virus replication (12)
3. Xenotropic viruses (21).
4. Oncogene theory (23); Discovery of reverse transcriptase (29,30).
5. Identification of NP AKR mouse cells which can be activated to produce infectious retroviruses (37).
6. Antiviral binding antibodies found in mice (38); Anti-xenotropic virus neutralizing factor associated with mouse lipoproteins (41).
7. Kirsten sarcoma virus contains "normal" cellular rat genes (43); Copies of the RSV src gene can be found in uninfected avian and mammalian species (44).
8. Mouse leukemia and the Gross virus - The most proximal causative agent of AKR leukemia is the envelope recombinant virus (MCF) (26); Preleukemic cells can be found at birth in AKR bone marrow or embryonic liver (50); Pure ecotropic retroviruses can cause mouse thymic leukemias (51).

   Mouse mammary tumors and MMTV - An MMTV-negative mouse strain can be induced to develop mammary carcinomas (52).
9. Xenotropic virus; Caprine retrovirus (arthritis, encephalitis); Visna and mouse retroviruses (neurologic disease); Feline, mouse and human retroviruses (immune suppression); Equine infectious anemia virus (autoimmune disease); Retroviruses can be cytopathic, form syncytia, vacuoles (MSV, RSV, MCF, foamy viruses, Mason-Pfizer, AIDS lymphocytopathic retroviruses).
10. Exogenous - HTLV-I, (54,55); AIDS-associated lymphocytopathic retroviruses (56,57,58) Human foamy viruses (53).

    Endogenous - Retrovirus particles detected in human placentas (63).

filterable agents, and thus it was well established in the early 1900's that viruses could cause tumors in avian species.

DOGMA 1 - VIRUSES ONLY CAUSE TUMORS IN AVIAN SPECIES

These initial observations, however, were followed by over 35 years of frustrating research by individuals attempting to prove a similar viral etiology in mammalian species. Despite the isolation of mouse mammary tumor virus (MMTV) by Bittner in 1936, (4) the dogma that evolve was that "**viruses only cause tumors in avian species**". This tenet was finally reversed by the observation of Ludwik Gross in 1950 that mouse leukemia in the AKR strain developed by Furth could be passed by filtrates into susceptible mice (5). This discovery pointed out three aspects of retrovirus research which continue to have importance today.

1. The virus may be pathogenic for very young animals. The virus etiology of mouse leukemia was only discovered when newborn or very young animals were inoculated with filtered tumor extracts. Gross virus was not pathogenic in adult mice. Leukemia acceleration of disease only occurred in young animals. This latter observation has just recently been reused in the evaluation of the potential role of envelope recombinant viruses in AKR leukemia (see below).

2. The genetic make up of the host determines its sensitivity to virus-induced leukemias. C3H Bittner mice were susceptible to the Gross virus, whereas C3H/An mice were not (5).

3. Infectious virus production in tumors may be low. Only by using inbred strains and continual passage of tumor extracts (e.g. Gross passage A) can some retroviruses be obtained in high titer. We are reminded of the difficulties that Kaplan had in obtaining a virulent radiation leukemia virus (RadLV), since most of the tumors in C57Bl/6 mice yield such low titers of infectious virus

(6).

This first dogma that I have cited was certainly reversed permanently with the subsequent discovery of other leukemia viruses in mice (e.g. Friend, Moloney Rauscher) (6) and in other mammalian species, particularly the cat (7) and cow (8). The "four minute mile" in mammalian retrovirology had been broken by Ludwik Gross, and the race for the recognition of cancer viruses in many different animal hosts continued. The leukemia viruses were placed in the type C tumor virus group as classified morphologically by electron microscopy by Bernhard (6). Type C viruses have now been detected in animals from many taxonomic classes, including snakes and fish (see Table 1, Ref. 9).

But the discovery of mouse leukemia viruses led again to several years of difficulty as investigators attempted to grow these agents in tissue culture. Janet Hartley has commented that when she began research on the mouse viruses, many researchers believed that they could only be assayed in animals and thus could not be studied easily. Nevertheless, her work along with Rowe and Huebner led eventually to the development of complement fixation assays for detection of the chicken and mouse viruses in vitro (10) and ultimately to the tissue culture assays involving focus formation for the solid tumor producing viruses, or sarcoma viruses (11). When these latter agents were discovered in mice, it became apparent that the first recognized sarcoma virus, RSV, was an exception since it could transform and replicate in cells without the help of a non-transforming virus (6). Other sarcoma viruses, including all the mouse sarcoma viruses (MSV) (11), were found to be dependent on these helper viruses.

DOGMA 2 - MOUSE SARCOMA VIRUSES ARE DEFECTIVE IN TRANSFORMING CELLS AND REQUIRE THE HELP OF A LEUKEMIA VIRUS

The dogma that emerged from these early studies of

Hartley and Rowe (who showed 2-hit kinetics of MSV transformation of mouse embryo cells) was that helper viruses were necessary for MSV transformation of cells (11). Their tissue culture studies and those conducted in animals led to the tenet that I heard on arriving in their laboratory in 1967 that, **"mouse sarcoma viruses are defective in transforming cells and require the help of a leukemia virus"**.

It was two years later that Robertson Parkman, in Robert Ting's laboratory, and I studied MSV and found it was not different biologically from RSV. If rat cells were used as the assay cell monolayer, MSV transformed with 1-hit kinetics, but had a cytopathic effect on mouse embryo cells (12). The defectiveness of MSV was in replication and not in its ability to infect or transform a cell. Murine leukemia virus (MuLV) was needed to enable the spread of MSV to neighboring uninfected cells and thus recruit them into a recognizable focus of cell alteration. Our studies emphasized that the cell system used reflects the biologic effect of the virus, and that certain cells, like mouse embryo cells, once infected with a sarcoma virus may cease to divide. Other more specific cytopathic effects of MSV on mouse embryo cells, such as vacuolization, have also been described (13). These comments have relevance today with the recent discovery of human lymphocytopathic retroviruses (see below).

This effect of MSV on mouse embryo cells seemed universal until experiments were conducted with FBJ-MSV, the osteosarcoma virus discovered by Finkel, Biskis and Jenkins (14). Again, an exception was noted. This virus was found by us to infect mouse embryo cells without preventing their replication into a transformed focus (15). In other words, FBJ-MSV was not cytopathic for mouse embryo cells. The reason for these differences in biologic properties of MSV is still not known.

HOST RANGE DIFFERENCES At the time that the biologic functions of MSV were being evaluated in the laboratory, the "defectiveness" of mouse leukemia viruses was also being examined. For instance, it was found that mouse leukemia viruses did not cause disease in certain strains of mice considered immunologically resistant to the virus. Originally defined by Frank Lilly as a locus of resistance to Friend leukemia virus (16), this genetic resistance gene, Fv-1, was subsequently shown in tissue culture systems initially by Hartley, Rowe and Huebner and later with Ted Pincus to define a host cell: virus relationship in which N and B tropism was identified (17). For the first time, the ability of a virus to replicate in a cell of its host species was shown to be determined by certain genes within the host cell. It is also important to note the technologic advances that helped in these studies. Rowe adapted Vaclav Klement's observation of syncytia formation in cells, induced by mouse leukemia viruses into the very useful XC plaque assay (18). It greatly increased the facility to trace mouse leukemia viruses in culture, instead of using the complement-fixation (COMUL) test (10). Once again, however, nature provided exceptions and it was soon found that the XC plaque assay did not identify all mouse type C viruses. Mouse xenotropic and amphotropic viruses (see below) and some mouse-tropic (ecotropic) viruses do not induce XC plaque formation (9, 19).

DOGMA 3 - VIRUSES PREFERENTIALLY INFECT AND REPLICATE IN CELLS OF THE SPECIES OF ORIGIN

In discussing these host range differences of the mouse viruses, I have eluded to a third major dogma in retrovirology that also was eventually changed: **"viruses preferentially infect and relicate in cells of the species of origin".**

The reversal in this dogma was made possible by the use of the inbred New Zealand Black (NZB) mouse strain, established by Dr. Marianne Bielchowsky. Similar to Furth's valuable contribution to the discovery of the Gross murine leukemia virus, through studies of the AKR mouse, she derived a mouse strain with a hyperproduction of many factors including the mouse xenotropic virus.

This type C virus, first discovered in NZB mice in 1970 (20) and later in all house mice tested, is not able to reinfect mouse cells but can productively infect cells of many other animal species (9,21). Its identification opened up the possibility, that still remains, that similar endogenous viruses with this unusual selective host range would be present in other animal species, including man. The virus was called **xenotropic** because of its ability to infect only cells of animal species different from the host and these included those of a different taxonomic class (avian). The xenotropic virus was, therefore, distinguished from the endogenous mouse-tropic (**ecotropic**) viruses (22) such as the Gross leukemia virus and was universally detected in all strains of Mus musculus including wild house mice. Its identification explained the frequency of detection of MuLV proteins in mouse tissues, including embryos, in the absence of infectious viruses (9). It conclusively confirmed the vertical transmission of these viruses (the virogene hypothesis) (23). Similar endogenous viruses have since been identified in cats, baboons, mink, and other animals (9). The wide host range of xenotropic viruses enabled effective phenotypic mixing among both mouse and avian virus isolated, with the final observation that mouse and bird viruses could be enveloped in their respective different coats, which extended their host range substantially (24). I would like to add that, with the recognition that xenotropic viruses were not pathogenic but shared several antigens with mouse leukemia viruses, the abbreviation, MuLV, was redefined to include all mouse type C viruses.

A few years later, Rasheed et al. (25) and Hartley and Rowe (26) described mouse type C viruses in wild mice that constituted a third class of MuLV - **amphotropic** viruses. They had a differet envelope glycoprotein from the xenotropic and ecotropic viruses, but shared both host ranges - being able to infect mouse and a wide variety of heterologous cells. Finally, the observation that MMTV, once believed tissue and strain specific, can be replicated in cat and mink lung cells (27,28) underlined the possible expanded host range of some retroviruses.

DOGMA 4 - RNA TUMOR VIRUSES EXIST LIKE EPISOMES IN INFECTED CELLS

During the early experiences with the cicken and mouse viruses, the nature of their replicative cycle was frequently questioned. How did these agents establish infection in the host cells? It was evident that their infection did not generally lead to a lytic phase and many considered them present as small intracytoplasmatic RNA particles, like episomes, which replicated with the host cells.

This tenet was initially questioned by the oncogene hypothesis of Huebner and Todaro (23), who suggested that viral information was integrated in host cell DNA. The mechanism for this event awaited the dramatic discovery by Temin and Baltimore of reverse transcriptase (29,30). The concept of proviral copies in cellular DNA was soon further documented by the elegant transfection experiments with chicken DNA by Hill and Hillova (31). They demonstrated the integrated form of infectious RSV DNA in transformed cells. Finally, the extensive genetic studies of Rowe showed the existence of infectious viral genes as proviruses in the AKR mouse strain (32).

With the discovery of reverse transcriptase, retrovirology as a field became firmly defined and other viruses found to contain the enzyme were included in the classification (Table 3). The virus group was no longer limited to RNA tumor viruses as the first agents were originally called. Now it became apparent that retroviruses had properties aside from transformation and oncogenesis. Sub-groups, such as the spuma and lenti viruses, showed different cytopathic effects and morphologies by electron microscopy (33) (table 3).

TABLE 3 - ELECTRON MICROSCOPIC CLASSIFICATION OF RETROVIRUSES

Oncovirinae Type	Example	RT cation preference§
A	Double membrane particles (70 nm) no budding forms. Intracytoplasmic precursor for type B and type C viruses; intracisternal; cross react with *Mus cervicolor* endogenous virus genome.	Mn^{2+}/Mg^{2+}
B	Mouse mammary tumor virus; complete core forms during budding; eccentric nucleoid in mature particle.	Mg^{2+}
C.	Mouse leukemia virus; incomplete nucleoid during budding process; has immature and mature forms.	Mn^{2+}
D.	Mason-Pfizer monkey virus; complete nucleoid (42 nm) forms during budding;nucleoid has cylindrical form.	Mg^{2+}
Spumavirinae	Simian foamy virus; complete nucleoid forms during budding.	Mg^{2+}
Lentivirinae	Maedi-Visna; incomplete nucleoid during budding process; no electronlucent intermediate layer in virus particle.	Mg^{2+}

The first classification of tumor viruses by electron microscopy was done by Bernhard (Cancer Res. 20, 712, 1960) and included types A-C of the present retroviruses.

§ RT = reverse transcriptase. The general cation preference of the different subgroups of retroviruses is listed. Some type C viruses, such as the avian and human, prefer $Mg^{2+} > Mn^{2+}$ for the reaction with most template primers.

DOGMA 5 - LATENT RETROVIRUS INFECTION INVOLVING A NON-PRODUCER STATE ONLY EXISTS FOR SARCOMA VIRUSES

Our discussion thus far has demonstrated that by the early 1970's, a class of viruses originally found in birds could now be isolated from many animal species, although not yet man. Their biologic features included defects in replication, a variety of cytopathic effects, host range differences, and their universal ability to integrate into the host cell DNA. Transformation became linked to transforming proteins following the pioneer studies by Martin with temperature sensitive mutants of RSV (34). But, one dogma that continued to challenge investigators, particularly Rowe, was that, **"latent retrovirus infection involving a non-producer state only exists for sarcoma viruses".** Wally used to say in the laboratory that a powerful insight into how these viruses function would come from the identification of the non-producer state for leukemia viruses. Certainly, recovery of these viruses from mice at different periods of their life suggested they could remain latent in the host. The first indication of this possibility came from the observation of Aaronson, et al. (35) that clones of mouse 3T3 cells, after growth in tissue culture, spontaneously produced viral antigen in culture. The real turning point in our understanding of latent type C virus infection, however, came when Rowe and co-workers demonstrated that AKR mouse embryo cells could be derived which did not spontaneously release virus (36,37). By using this non-producer system, Rowe was the first to recognize that a variety of inducing agents can activate viruses from a latent state in cells (see Table 10 of ref. 9).

DOGMA 6 - THERE IS NO HOST REACTION TO ENDOGENOUS RETROVIRUSES

We have been discussing various dogmas surrounding the discovery and life cycle of retroviruses. Some basic tenets also dealt with the interaction of the host with its endogenous viruses. One emerged following the observation that MuLV antigens were expressed in mouse embryos (9) and that antiviral neutralizing antibodies could not be found in mouse sera. It was assumed that as embryonic antigens, these viral proteins induced tolerance in the host. With the adaption of radio-immunoassays to retrovirus research, Hanna, Ihle and associates demonstrated in the early 1970's that there are binding, but not effective, neutralizing antibodies to mouse ecotropic viruses (38,39). Recently the studies of Sarma and Rowe (40) uncovered the presence of complement mediated anti-AKR virus neutralizing antibodies in some strains of mice. It is noteworthy that these antibodies first appear with the earliest expression of infectious ecotropic virus in the host.

With the endogenous xenotropic viruses, however, immunologic tolerance still appears to be the rule. Yet, shortly after the discovery of this virus group, neutralizing activity in mouse serum was noted and initially considered to represent antibodies to the virus. Our group, believing it difficult to explain the presence of antibody to a class of inherited viruses expressed during embryonic life, set out to identify the responsible factor. We discovered that it was associated with mouse lipoproteins and was mediated by an apolipoprotein found on the VLDL and HDL sub-classes of these lipid containing particles (9,41,42). This neutralizing factor, still to be fully characterized, is a unique non-immunoglobulin factor with specific antiviral activity. Its role in the mouse is unknown, but we would predict that it probably functions by modulating immune responses by cells activated to express xenotropic virus (9).

DOGMA 7 - RETROVIRUSES CAUSE CANCER BY PRODUCING VIRUS-SPECIFIC TRANSFORMING PROTEINS

The last four dogmas that I would like to consider

today deal with retroviruses as pathogenic agents. Dogma 7, **"that retroviruses cause cancer by producing virus-specific transforming proteins"** was initially questioned by two observations. First, Scolnick and his co-workers found that the Kirsten strain of MSV, and later the Harvey strain, contained normal rat cellular sequences (43). While definite proof that this DNA was associated with transforming properties was not provided, their data introduced the concept that these retroviruses could transduce normal cellular information into cells. The second observation, made by Stehelin, et al. (44) linked these cellular sequences to oncogenes. They demonstrated that the region of the Rous sarcoma virus genome not found in avian leukosis viruses (45) which they called src, was the gene responsible for transformation. They showed that this gene was represented by similar sequences in cells from normal avian and mammalian species. Their observation led to the recognition of "oncogenes" with cellular counterparts in human cells and to new speculations on the function of these genes in cancer. Many other oncogenes with cellular protooncogene counterparts have since been uncovered (46). All these data indicate that what were considered previously virus-specific genes were really modified versions of genes already located in normal cells. The function of these oncogenes and their relationship to cancer appears partially explained by their coding for "normal" cellular enzymes such as protein kinase, DNA binding proteins, or growth promoting factors. Other mechanisms for oncogenesis, besides transduced oncogenes, have now been suggested by recent research: an insertion-promotion model (47) and trans-acting proteins (48) that involve viral activation or promotion of cellular protoncogenes with transforming potential (Table 4).

DOGMA 8 - RETROVIRUS-ASSOCIATED TUMORS ARE ONLY CAUSED BY THOSE VIRUSES

TABLE 4. MECHANISM FOR INDUCTION OF MALIGNANCY BY RETROVIRUSES

1.	Oncogenes Translation of virus-transduced oncogenes which resemble normal cellular genes. The products have protein kinase activity, bind to cellular DNA, or act as growth promotors.
2.	Insertion - Promotion Virus integrates near proto-oncogene and promotes induction of its product.
3.	Trans-acting Proteins Viral product acts distant to virus insertion site and activates cellular proto-oncogene with transforming properties

TABLE 5. PRESENT-DAY DOGMAS

1.	Oncogene-related normal cellular genes have oncogenic potential.
2.	Retroviruses need to be present in the cell to maintain transformation.
3.	There are no endogenous human retroviruses.
4.	Retroviruses have no role in normal life processes.
5.	Retroviruses have evolved from extracellular genetic material.

Dogma 8 deals with the recurrent questioning of the tenet, "**that retrovirus-associated tumors are only caused by those viruses**". With mouse leukemia, for instance, the direct role of Gross virus itself in the disease has been challenged. Hartley and her co-workers discovered in AKR mice, envelope recombinant viruses which appear just prior to the development of leukemia. Some of them, termed MCF, cause lytic changes in mink lung cells (49). Because of their late appearance in AKR mice, these viruses, with both ecotropic and xenotropic host ranges, have been considered the proximal cause of the disease. Nevertheless, two other more recent observations have challenged this view. First, research by Haran-Ghera (50) showed that preleukemic cells already exist in the bone marrow and embryonic liver of AKR mice at birth before leukemia viruses can be detected, and they require a set period of time in the host to develop into frank leukemia. The transfer of these cells to irradiated F_1 hybrids led eventually to the development of leukemia of donor cell type (50). Thus, these cells appear programmed by genetic changes to develop into leukemic cells and co-factors, such as MCF, help them acquire this autonomous state. Recent work by Hara-Ghera and our group has indicated that the envelope recombinants may indeed be promotors in the disease process, since they have the ability to immunosuppress the mouse. The importance of the envelope recombinant viruses has also been questioned by the recent studies of Haseltine and his co-workers, who have shown that ecotropic viruses, such as SL3-3, cloned by molecular techniques, can induce leukemia in mouse strains without the activation or help of envelope recombinants (51). Thus, with this important animal model which reversed the first dogma that we discussed, some basic tenets continue to be challenged. Are dual-tropic or ecotropic viruses involved? Are viruses the proximal cause of leukemia? One could add as well, for instance, that leukemia in NZB, 129, and NIH Swiss mice develops in the absence of infectious ecotropic virus or envelope recombinants. Thus, other factors besides virus may be directly involved in the development of this cancer.

The second example deals with the primary role of MMTV in mammary tumors of mice (4). It has been challenged by the studies of Murray Gardner and his co-workers who derived an MMTV-free mouse that develops mammary tumors in the absence of MMTV (52). In summary, all these observations indicate that certain tumor viruses may be promotors and not initiators of cancer.

DOGMA 9 - ALL RETROVIRUSES ARE TRANSFORMING AGENTS

Dogma 9, "**that all retroviruses are transforming agents**," also needs clarification. Xenotropic viruses do not appear to have any pathogenic role in the host, and other retroviruses can produce diseases such as arthritis, encephalitis, pneumonia, paralysis, immune suppression, and autoimmunity. Moreover, as noted before, in cell culture systems, retroviruses are not only transforming viruses but can be cytopathic and form syncytia, vacuoles, or lytic lesions (9,13,18,33,54-59).

DOGMA 10 - NO HUMAN RETROVIRUS EXISTS

I shall conclude with the most exciting recent reversal of a dogma, i.e. that "**no human retrovirus exists**". Its history goes back just a few years ago to 1980. The initial discovery of these human viruses reflects the perserverance of Bob Gallo and his associates, who never gave up the challenge of finding a human retrovirus. They found, as early observations in animals had shown (9), that virus expression may be at such low levels in some cancers that their detection can be very difficult. The identification of the human T cell leukemia virus I (HTLV-I) (54) and the subsequent recognition by Hinuma and associates in Japan of a similar type C virus, ATLV, in Japanese leukemic patients (55), has defined a retrovirus associated with human malignancy.

Now the important discovery last year of the lymphocytopathic retroviruses associated with AIDS by Barre-Sinoussi, Chermann, Montagnier, et al. (56) has demonstrated to the world that other retroviruses can be found in the human population. These viruses, in contrast to HTLV-I have a type D morphology by electron microscopy and replicate to high levels in human cells. However, they pose other difficulties because of their cytopathic effects on the susceptible T cells. Similar retroviruses have since been isolated by Gallo, et al. (57) and by us (58). It is more than ironic that a type D retrovirus closely resembling the Mason-Pfizer virus has also been found associated with immune suppression in macaque monkeys (59). Recognition of the role of retroviruses in two human diseases, T cell leukemias and AIDS, should encourage pursuit of finding viruses involved in other still unsolved human problems such as autoimmune disease and other cancers. I should add, moreover, that since spumavirinae are retroviruses, the human foamy virus, isolated by Achong, et al. in 1971, should be considered the first human retrovirus identified.

From this quick review of selected dogmas in retrovirology, I have attempted to indicate how scientific minds locked into an accepted belief may be reluctant at times to recognize important exceptions. Eventually, however, research by inquisitive individuals will cause the necessary changes in thinking to take place. We once accepted as another dogma, for instance, that sarcoma viruses could only be recovered from animal tumors. Rasheed et al. (60) clearly indicated this need not be the case when they derived the rat sarcoma viruses through the rescue of oncogenes from cultured rat cells. Today, as always, we must continue to question tenets which appear to be modern day dogmas (Table 5).

1. The oncogene related cellular oncogenes may not have oncogenic potential in normal cells. The multiple base changes and permutations which distinguish cellular protoncogenes from viral oncogenes need to be explained

(61).

2. The retrovirus may not need to be present to maintain transformation. The provocative studies of Risser and his colleagues (62) have shown that Abelson virus may induce transformation of mouse B cells but their maintenance as leukemic cells occurs even after the disappearance of the Abelson genome.

3. Endogenous human retroviruses may exist. The initial observation by Kalter, et al. (63) of virus-like particles in human placentas, the detection by Nelson et al.of specific viral reverse transcriptase activity in this human tissue (64), and the recent studies by several investigators showing viral forms in human embryos (65,66) and teratocarcinomas (67) certainly suggest that endogenous human retroviruses await cultivation in the laboratory.

4. Retroviruses may have a role in normal life processes. This concept is becoming more and more acceptable, particularly with the identification of viruses such as the xenotropic viruses in developing mouse embryos, in immune cells during activation, and in human and mouse placentas (9,63,64,68).

5. Finally, the protovirus hypothesis presented by Temin (69), that retroviruses evolved from normal cellular genes, may prove to be correct. It is finding more support as research on retroviruses continues. Absolute proof of RNA-directed polymerase in uninfected tissues of normal organisms is not yet available; however, the recognition that portions of viral genes are represented throughout animal host genomes certainly suggests that retroviruses could have evolved by rearrangements, recombinations and permutations from normal cellular genes. Within the next decade, perhaps all or most of these challenges to present day dogmas will be accepted as truths.

In conclusion, I want to thank the chairman, Dr. Varnier, for giving me this challenging responsibility of honoring Dr. Wallace Rowe, and of discussing the progress

TABLE 6. CHANGES IN DOGMAS IN RETROVIROLOGY (1950-1984)

A. **Retroviruses as infectious agents:**

1. Retroviruses can be recovered from many animal species, including man.
2. Retroviruses are both endogenous and exogenous to the species.
3. Retroviruses integrate into the genome of host cell via reverse transcription.
4. Retroviruses can remain latent in host cells.
5. Sarcoma viruses are defective in their replicative properties.
6. Retroviruses can show specific (N and B tropism), selective (xenotropism, thymotropism), and extensive (amphotropism, dual-tropism) host range.

B. **Host response to endogenous retroviruses:**

1. Binding and neutralizing antibodies.
2. Antiviral non-immunoglobulin factors (mouse lipoproteins).

C. **Retroviruses as pathogenic agents:**

1. Retroviruses cause cancer by transducing modified normal cellular genes.
2. Retroviruses cause neurologic diseases.
3. Retroviruses cause arthritis and pneumonia.
4. Retroviruses cause immune suppression.
5. Retroviruses can be promotors of malignant processes.
6. Retroviruses cause a variety of cytopathic changes in cells.
7. Some retroviruses have no known pathogenic role.

---

made in retrovirology. I hope by reviewing the past seven decades, and in particular the last three decades, we can all recognize the great speed at which new discoveries, changes and redefinitions of dogmas are taking place (Table 6). As Sandra Panem reminded me, it is important to avoid the conclusions too often made by researchers, that, "what we don't know, doesn't exist", and "what we find, is a new discovery". Only by questioning present day tenets can we expect to uncover the real truth. The progress achieved is what makes science interesting, and research in the laboratory such an enlightening, provocative and exciting adventure.

REFERENCES

1. Ellerman, V. & Bang, O. (1908) Centralbl. f. Bakt. 46, 595-602.
2. Rous, P. (1911) J. Exp. Med. 13, 397-411.
3. Vallee, H. & Carre H. (1904) C.R. Acad. Sci. 139, 331-333.
4. Bittner, J.J. (1936) Science 84, 162.
5. Gross, L. (1951) Proc. Soc. Exp. Biol. & Med. 76, 27-32.
6. Gross, L. (70) Oncogenic Viruses, Second Edition, Pergamon Press, London.
7. Jarrett, W., Jarrett, P., Mackey, L., Laird, H., Hardy, W., Jr., & Essex, M. (1973) J. Natl. Cancer Inst. 51, 833-841.
8. Ferrer, J.F., Stock, N.D., & Lin, P. (1971) J. Nat. Cancer. Inst. 47, 613-621.
9. Levy, J.A. (1978) Curr. Top. Microbiol. Immunol. 79, 111-213.
10. Hartley, J.W., Rowe, W.P., Capps, W.I., & Hebner, R.J. (1965) Proc. Natl. Acad. Sci. 53, 931-938.
11. Hartley, J.W. & Rowe W.P. (1966) Proc. Natl. Aad. Sci. 55, 780-786.
12. Parkman, R., Levy, J.A. & Ting, R.C. (1970) Science 168, 387-389.

13. Levy, J.A. (1971) J. Nat. Cancer Inst. 46, 1001-1007.
14. Finkel, M.P., Biskis, B.O. & Jenkins, P.B. 1966 Science 151, 698.
15. Levy, J.A., Hartley, J.W., Rowe, W.P. & Huebner, F.J. (1973) J. Natl. Cancer Inst. 51, 525-539.
16. Lilly, F. (1967) Science 155, 461-462.
17. Hartley, J.W., Rowe W.P. & Huebner, R.J. (1970) J. Virol. 5, 221-225.; Pincus, T., Hartley, J.W. & Rowe, W.P. (1971) J. Exp. Med. 133, 1219-1233.
18. Rowe, W.P., Pugh, W.E. & Hartley, J.W. (1970) Virology 42, 1136-1139.
19. Hays, E.F. & Vredevoe, D.L. (1977) Cancer Research 37, 726-730.
20. Levy J.A. & Pincus, R. (1970) Science 170, 326-327.
21. Levy, J.A. (1973) Science 132, 1151-1153.
22. Levy, J.A. (1974) Amer. J. Clin.Pathol. 62, 258-280.
23. Huebner, R.J. & Todaro, G.J. (1969) Proc. Natl. Acad. Sci. 64, 1087-1094.
24. Levy, J.A. (1977) Virology, 77, 811-825.
25. Rasheed, S., Gardner, M.B. & Chan, E. (1976) J. Virol. 19,413-18.
26. Hartley, J.W., & Rowe, W.P. (1976) J. Virol. 19, 19-25.
27. Lasfargues, E.Y., Lasfargues, J.C., Dion, A.S., Green, A.E. & Moore, D.H. (1976) Cancer Research 36, 67-72.
28. Howard, D.K., Colcher, D., Teramoto, Y.A., Young, J.M. & Schlom, J. (1977) Cancer Research 37, 2696-2704.
29. Temin, J.M. & Mizutani, S. (1970) Nature 226, 1211-1213.
30. Baltimore, D. (1970) Nature 226, 1209-1211.
31. Hill, M. & Hillova, J. (1972) Nature New Biology 237, 35-39.
32. Rowe, W.P. (1973) Cancer Research 33, 3061-3068.
33. Bouillant, A.M.T. & Becker, S.A.W.E. (1984) J. Nat. Cancer Inst. 72, 1075-1084.
34 Martin, G.S. (1970) Nature 227, 1021.
35. Aaronson, S.A., Hartley, J.W., & Todaro, G.J. (1969) Proc. Natl. Acad. Sci. 64, 87-94.
36. Lowy, D.R., Rowe, W.P., Teich, N. & Hartley J.W.

(1971) Science 174, 155-156.
37. Rowe, W.P., Hartley, J.W., Lander, M.R., Pugh, W.E. & Teich, N. (1971) Virology 46, 866-876.
38 .Hanna, M.G., Jr., Tennant, R.W., Yuhas, J.M., Clapp, N.K., Batzing, B.L. & Snodgrass, M.J. (1972) Cancer Res. 32, 2226.
39. Ihle, J.N., Hanna, Jr., M.G., Roberson & Kenney, F.T. (1974) J. Exp. Med. 139, 1568-1581.
40. Sarma, P.S. & Rowe, W.P. (1983) J. Virol. 45, 956-960.
41. Levy, J..A, Ihle, J.N., Oleszko, O. & Barnes, R.D. (1975) Proc. Natl. Acad. Sci., 72, 5071-5075.
42. Kane, J.P., Hardman, D.A., Dimpfl, J.C. & Levy, J.A. (1979) Proc. Natl. Acad. Sci., 76, 5957-5961.
43. Scolnick, E.M., Rands, E., Williams, D. & Parks, W.P. (1973) J. Virol. 12, 458-463.
44. Stehelin D., Varmus, H.E., & Bishop, J.M., (1976) Nature 260, 170-173.
45. Duesberg, P.H. & Vogt, P.K. (1970) Proc. Natl. Acad. Sci. 76, 1633.
46. Slamon, D.J., deKernion J.B., Verma, I.M. & Cline M.J. (1984) Science 224, 256-262.
47. Hayward, W.S., Neel, B.G., & Astrin, S.M. (1981) Nature 290, 475-480.
48. Sodroski, J., Trus, M., Perkins, D., Patarca, R., Wong-Staal, F., Gelmann, E., Gallo, R.C. & Haseltine, W.A. (1984) Proc. Natl. Acad. Sci., 81, 4617-4621.
49. Hartley, J.W., Wolford, N.D., Old, L.J., & Rowe, W.P. (1977) Proc. Natl. Acad. Sci. 74, 789-792.
50. Haran-Ghera, N. (1980) Proc. Natl. Acad. Sci 77, 2923-2926.
51. Lenz, J., Crowther, R., Klimenko, S., & Haseltine, W. (1982) J. Virol. 43, 943-951.
52. Cohen, J.C., Traina, V.L., Breznik, T. & Gardner, M. (1982) J. Virol. 44, 882-885.
53. Achong, B.G., Mansell, P.W.A., Epstein, M.A., & Clifford, P. (1971) J. Nat. Can. Inst. 46, 299-320.
54. Poiesz, B.J., Ruscetti, R.W., Gazdar, A.F., Bunn, P.A., Minna, J.D., & Gallo, R.C. (1980 Proc. Natl. Acad. Sci. 77, 7415-7519.

55. Hinuma, Y., Nagata, K., Hanaoka, M., Nakai, M., Matsumota, T., Knowhita, K., Shirakawa, S. & Miyoshi, I. (1981) Proc. Natl. Acad. Sci. 78, 6476-6480.

56. Barre-Sinoussi, F., Chermann, J.C., Rey F., Nugeyre, T., Chamaret, S., Gruest, J., Dauget, C., Axler-Blin, C. Vezinet-Brun, F., Rouzioux, C., Rozenbaum, W. & Montagnier, L. (1983) Science 224, 500-503.

57. Gallo, R.C., Salahuddin, S.Z., Papovic, M., Shearer, G.M., Kaplan M., Haynes, B.F., Palker, T.J., Redfield, R., Oleske, J., Safai, B., White G., Foster, P. & Markham P.D. (1984) Science 224, 500-503.

58. Levy, J.A., Hoffman, A.D., Krame, S., Landis, J.A., & Shiukuro, J.M. (1984) Science, 225, 840-842.

59. Marx, P.A., Maul, D.H., Osborn, K.G., Lerche, N.W., Moody, P., Lowenstein, L.J., Hendrickson, R.V., Arthur, L.O., Gilden, R.V., Gravell, M., London, W.T., Sever, J.L., Levy, J.A., Munn, R.J. & Gardner, M.B. (1984) Science 223, 1083-1085.

60. Rasheed, S., Gardner, M.B. & Huebner, R.J. (1978) Proc. Natl. Acad. Sci. 75:6, 2972-2976.

61. Duesberg, P.H. (1983) Nature 304, 219-226.

62. Grunwald, D.J., Dale, B., Dudley, J., Lamph, W., Sugden, B., Ozanne, B. & Risser, R. (1982) J. Virol. 43, 92-103.

63. Kalter, S.S., Helmke, R.J. Heberling, R.L., Panigel, M., Fowler, A.K. Strickland, J.E. & Helleman, A. (1973) J. Nat. Can. Inst. 50, 1081-1084.

64. Nelson, J., Leong, J. & Levy, J.A. (1978) Proc. Natl. Acad. Sci. 75, 6263-6267.

65. Larsson, E., Nilsson, B., Sundstrom, P. & Widehn, S. (1981) Int. J. Cancer 28, 551-557.

66. Mondal, H? Hofschneider, P.H. (1982) Int. J. Cancer 30, 281-287.

67. Boller, K., Frak, H., Lower, j., Lower R. & Kurth, R. (1983) J. Gen. Virol. 64, 2349-2559.

68. Levy, J.A. (1977) Cancer Research 37, 2957-2968.

69. Temin, H.M. (1971) J. Nat. Can. Inst. 46, iii-vii.

1. Retroviruses and the Murine Model System

THE BIOLOGY OF ENDOGENOUS LEUKEMIA VIRUSES: A STUDY OF THE DBA/2 MOUSE

B. A. Nexø

The Fibiger Institute, 70 Ndr. Frihavnsgade, DK 2100 Copenhagen, Denmark
Current address: Novo Research Institute, DK 2880 Bagsvaerd, Denmark

Endogenous C-type retroviruses are present as elements of DNA in the chromosomes of many vertebrate species. The endogenous viruses could generally be important determinants in disease and survival of their hosts, and in one situation, the high-leukemia mouse strains, a pathogenic role of the viruses is commonly accepted. To evaluate the role of the endogenous viruses in a system which has not been preselected for a specific oncogenic response, we have studied the C-type retroviruses of the low-leukemia mouse strain DBA/2.

DBA/2 mice harbor only one known locus, Emv-3, encoding a virus of the ecotropic host-range, which mediates efficient replication in mice. Our results indicate that this locus carries a defect in the gag gene. Compensation of the defect seems to occur either by mutation or recombination, and the viruses obtained as a result are structurally polymorphic. They largely form three groups: E_a viruses appear relatively inocuous, while E_b and E_c viruses cause viremia and a moderate incidence of late leukemias. The two latter groups of virus also cause an appreciable number of early deaths without signs of malignancy.

To study the pathogenicity of the viruses in the

original host, we matched occurrence of spontaneous viremia in individual untreatd adult mice with later appearance of disease and overall survival. The results indicate that viremia is associated with reduced lifespan. Thus, the viruses exert a significant physical stress on the animals. This is the first demonstration that endogenous leukemia viruses are pathogenic in a host which was not preselected for an extreme disease incidence.

The documentation of pathogenicity of endogenous C-type retroviruses stems almost exclusively from studies of a few inbred strains of mice such as AKR, C58, and BALB/Mo, that have exceptionally high incidences of leukemia (1,2). In these animals, an endogenous ecotropic virus replicates extensively in a variety of organs and produces lifelong viremia (3,4). The viral replication appears to be a prerequisite for disease, since genetic and immunological manipulations that eliminate replication also repress leukemia (5,6,7,8). Consistent with a viral involvement in disease is the appearance in the preleukemic period of variants of the endogenous virus that are highly oncogenic when injected into animals (9,10), and the presence of proviral copies of such variants clonally integrated in the cells of the spontaneously arising leukemias (11,12).These findings have led to a general acceptance that the endogenous viruses and their derivatives are instrumental in the oncogenesis in high leukemia strains. However, extrapolation from these strains to other animals is controversial because AKR and C58 mice are specificaly bred for high incidences of leukemia, and BALB/Mo are a laboratory construction in which a highly oncogenic virus was deliberately introduced into the germline (13).

The pathogenicity of endogenous viruses in other strains of mice is less well known. Many mouse strains contain gene(s) coding for virus resembling the AKR-virus (14,15), and spontaneous activation occurs in some adult animals, although rarely to the extent observed in the AKR strain. In some strains a genetic restriction appears to limit viral replication in the host while in others spontaneous formation of antibodies offers plausible explanations for the lower disease incidence. These observations, however, provide inadequate information on the origin of the sporadic leukemias that do occur. It is also known that highly oncogenic viruses can be derived by cell free passage from tumors of low leukemic strains of mice (16), but such viruses do not appear to be regularly present, and could actually be generated by the severe selective pressure of the passage procedure.

One additional limitation in present data on the pathogenicity of endogenous viruses must be mentioned. The prominent role of high-leukemia mouse strains in experimental studies has led to a focus of interest on oncogenicity. However, analogous horizontally transmitted retroviruses often demonstrate a much broader spectrum of pathogenic effects (17,18,19,13) and there is little reason a priori to expect endogenous viruses to be different.

For these reasons we felt that a general evaluation of the replicational activity, biological properties and pathogenicity of the viruses which result from the endogenous proviral loci of a single low-leukemia mouse strain would provide valuable new information.

We chose to study the DBA/2 mice. Nucleic acid hybridization data indicate that this strain carries one ecotropic provirus, Emv-3, whose structure resembles that of the prototype virus from AKR mice (14,15). Weanling DBA/2 mice appear to be virus-negative while some adult mice become virus-positive and accumulate detectable amounts of viral protein in the blood (3,4,20). Studies of spontaneous mortality of our substrain indicate an overall rate of lymphoreticular malignancies of 17 per cent which typically occur late, i.e. around 2 years of age.

VIRUSES ISOLATED FROM DBA/2 MICE

When splenocytes of adult DBA/2 mice are cocultivated with fibroblasts suitable for the propagation of mouse retroviruses, approximatey one third of the animals will give rise to infectious ecotropic viruses and the majority of animals to xenotropic viruses. No polytropic viruses have yet been obtained from DBA/2. The proportion of ecotropic positive individuals can be dramatically increased by prior exposure to the carcinogen dimethylbenzanthracene (20).

Viruses obtained by the cocultivations are polymorphic and largely form four groups, three ecotropic and one xenotropic in host-range. We have called the ecotropic groups E_a, E_b, and E_c (21). The polymporphism is reflected in structural differences in the proteins as well as in tropism and replicative behaviour. E_a and E_b viruses are N-tropic and resemble the prototype endogenous virus of AKR-mice, they differ in the fine structure of the gag-proteins. E_c viruses are NB-tropic, more related to FMR-viruses and differ from the other groups in gag as well as env proteins. The xenotropic viruses, as expected, have envelope glycoproteins substantially different from the other types of viruses. Two viral isolates, D2E7 and ND2, do not directly fit the grouping. They resemble E_b viruses, but differ from those in one protein p15.

Analysis of viruses derived by transfection of the molecularly cloned ecotropic locus <u>Emv-3</u> has in part provided an explanation for the polymorphism (22). The endogenous provirus appears to carry a defect in the 5' portion of the gag gene which can be complemented either by mutation or recombination. E_b viruses are virtually indistinguishable from the transfection-derived isolates by peptide mapping of the proteins. They are probably derived directly from the endogenous locus, possibly by a mutational event. This would fit the observation that E_b viruses are the predominant type of virus isolated after carcinogen-treatment of DBA/2 mice (23). E_a viruses have env proteins that resemble those of <u>Emv-3</u> derived viruses,

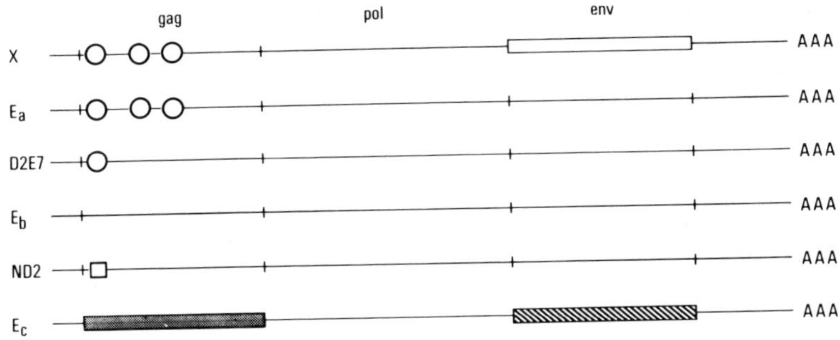

Figure 1. Schematic representation of gag and env differences among DBA/2 virus isolates. The viral genomic RNAs are depicted with the 5'end to the left and the 3' polyadenylated tail to the right. X, xenotropic DBA/2 virus; E_a, E_b and E_c, groups of ecotropic DBA/2 viruses as detailed in Nexo and Ulrich (1983). D2E7 and ND2, unique DBA/2 isolates. O, □, single peptide differences as detected by peptide mapping. ▭, ▨, ▬, extensive peptide differences within the region. The ecotropic viruses derived from endogenous locus Emv-3 by transfection are E_b. The figure illustrates the high variability of the 5' part of gag including p15 among ecotropic viruses., the homology of E_a and xenotropic viruses in this region and the unique character of E_c viruses.

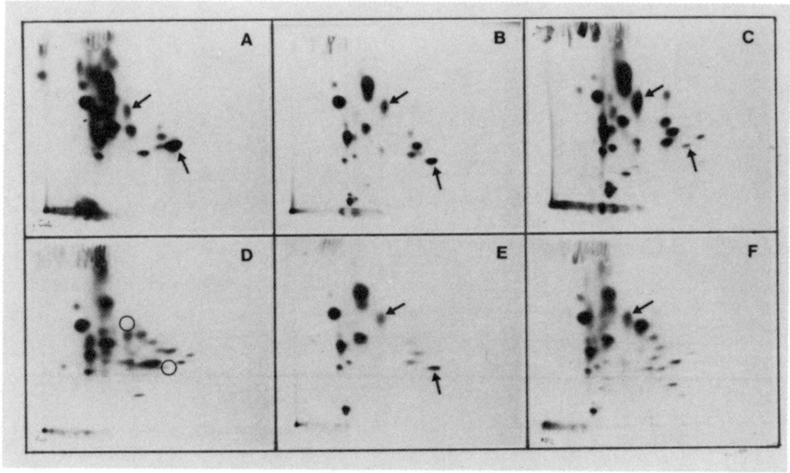

Figure 2. Search for homology between gp70s of ecotropic DBA/2 viruses and gp70s derived from DBA/2 organs. The envelope glycoproteins were purified from tissue culture supernatants or organ extracts by affinity chromatography, radioiodinated and purified by SDS-electrophoresis. They were then analyzed by tryptic peptide mapping. A, E_c virus gp70; B, seminal fluid gp70; C, kidney gp70; D, E_a virus gp70; E, epididymis gp70; F, serum gp70. The arrows point to two iodopeptides that are shared by gp70 from E_c viruses and from solid organs, but absent in gp70 from E_a virus. One of the peptides is also recognizable in gp70 from serum. The circles in frame D indicate where the peptides should have been located.

whereas the gag-proteins closely resemble those of infectious xenotropic isolates. These viruses have apparently compensated for the original defect in the ecotropic provirus by recombination with xenotropic sequences. It is quite likely that the unique isolate D2E7 also belongs to this category of recombinant viruses, but acquired a more limited part of the gag gene. The only peptide recognizably foreign to Emv-3, occurs in p15 and resembles that of E_a and xenotropic viruses. Figure 1 summarizes the homologies of the various isolates.

While these findings provide a plausible model for the origin of the AKR-virus-like isolates, the third group of ecotropic isolates, E_c, remains an enigma. The protein structure and biological properties differ so much from the Emv-3 derived and from the infectious xenotropic isolates, that a major portion of the genome must have an independent origin. A specific homology to xenotropic isolates from other mouse strains such as C57L and NZB, that could be present in DBA/2 but normally remain unexpressed is also not apparent (24).

We have also searched for homology between E_c viruses gp70 and the gp70-like molecules constitutively expressed in considerable amounts in some organs of DBA/2 mice, using peptide mapping as our primary tool. The proteins were purified from organs and tissue culture supernatants of infected cells by affinity chromatography on columns containing polyvalent antibodies to gp70, radioiodinated in vitro and analysed (25, 16, 27). A set of maps of ^{125}I-peptides is depicted in Fig. 2. The maps document a general homology between all gp70 molecules, as would be expected. A search for peptides shared by E_c and organ-derived gp70 that are not also present in the E_a protein reveals only two candidates. The peptides are indicated with an arrow on the maps. This is in my opinion insufficient to document a parental role of the corresponding genes in a recombination generating the E_c viruses. A satisfactory elucidation of the origin of the E_c viruses must await the development of specific nucleic acid probes and rigorous analysis of all sequences endogenous to the DBA/2 genome.

PATHOGENICITY OF DBA/2 VIRUSES

To evaluate the pathogenicity of the various viral

isolates, supernatants of infected tissue cultures were injected into mice of the strain C3H (23). The ability of the viruses to establish an infection in the animals was evaluated as the level of the core protein p30 in their blood when young adults, and the animals were monitored for survival and appearance of tumors. Figure 3A illustrates some important aspects of the results. For each virus isolate the median value of p30 in the blood of infected C3H animals is depicted against their median survival. The three groups of isolates, E_a, E_b and E_c form separate clusters. This demonstrates that the classification, which originally was developed on the basis of structure, is biologically important and reflects virulence in vivo. E_a viruses have little if any effect on the animals, E_b viruses cause moderate viremias and a reduction of approximatey one half year in average survival, while E_c viruses are more potent and cause higher levels of viremia and reduce average lifespan by more than a year. Moreover, there is a simple monotonous relationship between viremia and lifespan, which suggests that the one overridingly important determinant of pathogenicity of these viruses is related to their replication. E_b and E_c viruses increased the frequency of leukemia substantially and were thus clearly oncogenic. Equally interesting, however, a large number of the animals died early without signs of a malignant disease. Thus, the viruses clearly also had other pathogenic effects. The phenomenon is reminiscent of the spontaneous virus-related mortality in DBA/2 mice described below.

Since experimental inoculations were designed to detect viral pathogenic effects as efficiently as possible, they provide information about the viral pathogenic potential of the viruses, rather than their actual role in the original host. We, therefore, also evaluated the importance of endogenous viruses in DBA/2 mice more directly, taking advantage of the fact that some adult animals become spontaneously viremic, and have increased levels of the core protein p30 in their blood (23). By measuring blood p30 levels radioimmunologically

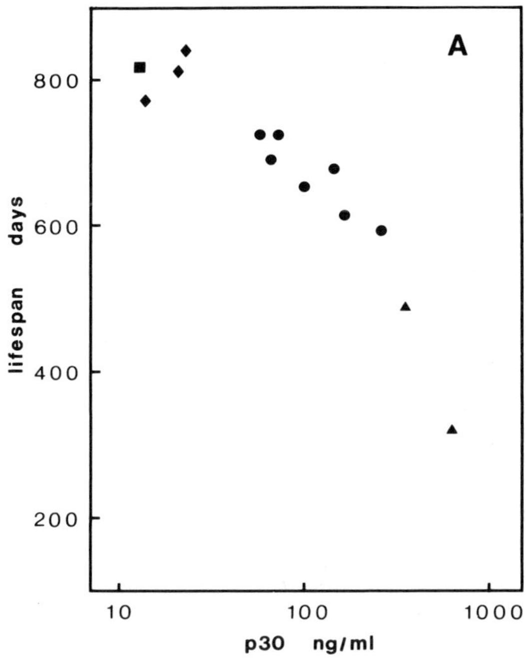

Figure 3. Pathogenicity of DBA/2 virus isolates inoculated into C3H mice. Groups of 6 to 14 C3H mice were infected as newborn with individual ecotropic isolates from DBA/2 mice. The figure depicts the median level of p30 in the blood as young adults and the median lifespan for each group. Thus, each spot represents a viral isolate. ■, no virus; ♦, E_a viruses; ●, E_b viruses; ▲, E_c viruses.

and relating the results to disease and survival, we could search directly for an association. The results obtained with male mice is depicted in Figure 3. Roughly similar results were obtained with the female mice. The inverse relation between p30 expression is statistically significant (P 0.01). Thus, the results demonstrate that animals with viremia indeed tend to die early, as would be expected if the viruses are pathogenic in their original host. Most of the early deaths occurred without macroscopic signs of a malignancy, and association between virus expression and leukemia could not be proven statistically.

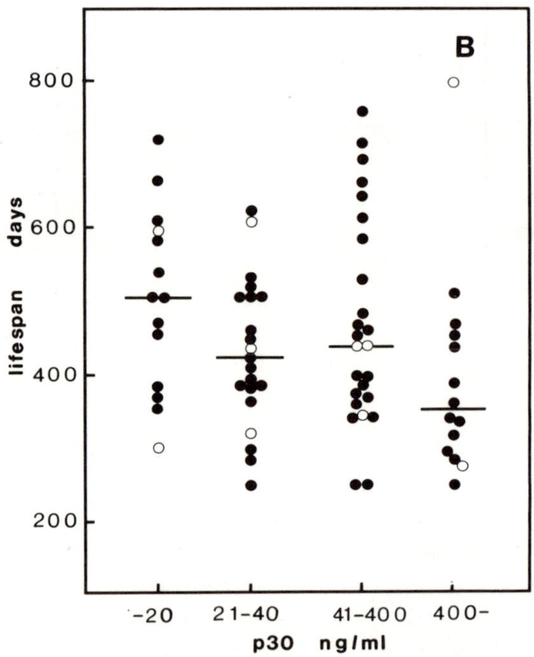

Figure 4. Lifespan of male DBA/2 mice in relation to their content of p30 in blood at 204 days of age. O, animals which died with malignancies; ●, animals which died without signs of malignancies.

We have not yet been able to identify the specific causes of death. Certain exogenous retroviruses, however, can cause nonmalignant diseases, typically of tissue-destructive or autoimmune character (13). Some of those diseases, such as osteopetrosis or neural degeneration cause obvious macroscopic or behavioral abnormalities and would probably have been detected in DBA/2 if common. Others, particularly immune suppression and anemia, with secondary opportunistic infections as the immediate causes of death would not have been easily recognized in post mortem examinations, and are the primary candidates for viremia-associated disease in DBA/2.

Whatever the mechanism, the strain on the animals exerted by the viruses appears to be of some magnitude. Half of the male mice with the lowest p30 levels lived for more than 505 days. Fourteen of the males with higher levels of viremia also lived past that age. If viremia was inconsequential, the viremic group should have totalled 28. The actual number is 57. The difference, 29, is unexplained early viremia-associated deaths. Out of a total of 74 animals, this corresponds to 40 percent. A similar calculation on the female mice indicates approximately 60% early viremia-associated deaths. Thus approximately half of all deaths among DBA/2 mice are caused by or at least accelerated by the viral replication.

PERSPECTIVES

An important lesson from our study is that the defective provirus Emv-3, not only is a remnant of a past infection, but also an active reservoir of viral information. Tha main result of defectiveness is a delayed appearance of virus. Thus, the defect largely serves as a means to achieve latency. Apparently, so many cells are present in an animal that compensation of a defect by mutation or recombination is probably within the normal lifespan.

Perhaps the relevant determinant of infectivity is not the individual locus, but the entire repertoire of proviral sequences.

It is clear that some of the infectious viruses appearing in the course of life in DBA/2 mice have a significant pathogenic potential. It is also clear that spontaneous viremia in DBA/2 mice is associated with reduced lifespan. As far as I am aware, this is the first direct evidence that endogenous C-type viruses contribute signicantly to the mortality of animals that have not been bred specifically for disease. The relatively few other experiments that have attempted to correlate viral activity and disease in the original host have failed (28,29,30). However, a pathogenic potential of several other endogenous viruses is beyond doubt (31,32).

Endogenous viruses could well be generally important determinants in disease and survival of their hosts. C-type retroviral sequences are present as repetitive elements in the chromosomes of many vertebrate species. In man, for example, two classes of proviruses have recently been identified (33,34) both of which occur in multiple copies. Some of these appear grossly defective by restriction enzyme analysis, while others seem structurally intact.

It would be very time consuming and require large resources to repeat a prospective study, such as ours, in an outbred population, where multiple viral loci and host resistance genes are randomly distributed, especially if the species is as long-lived as man. What will be needed are tests that can directly evaluate if viral activity has induced disease in an individual. A continued effort to elucidate the specific pathogenic mechanisms of the viruses is therefore of paramount importance.

ACKNOWLEDGEMENTS

This work was supported by the Danish Cancer Society and the Danish Medical Research Council.

REFERENCES

1. Gross, L. (1951) Proc. Soc. Exp. Biol. Med. 76, 27-32.
2. Jaenisch, R. (1976) Proc. Natl. Acad. Sci. USA 73, 1260-1264.
3. Hartley, J.W., Rowe, W.P., Capps, W.I., & Huebner, R.J. J. Virol. 3, 126-132.
4. Nexø, B.A., & Krog, H.H. (1977). Infect. Immun. 15, 276-381.
5. Lilly, F., Duran-Reynals, M.L., & Rowe, W.P. (1975) J. Exp. Med. 141, 882-889.
6. Huebner, R.J., Gilden, R.V., Toni R., Hill, R.W., Trimmer, R.W., Fish, D.C. & Sass, B. (1976) Proc. Natl. Acad. Sci. USA 73, 4633-4635.
7. Schwarz, H., Ihle, J.N., Wecker, E., Fischinger, R.J., Thiel, H.-J. Bolognesi, D.P., & Schafer, W. (1981) Virology 111, 568-578.
8. Nobis, P., & Jaenisch, R. (1980) Proc. Natl. Acad. Sci. USA 77, 3677-3681.
9. Hartley, J.W., Wolford, N.K., Old, L.J., & Rowe, W.P. (1977) Proc. Natl. Acad. Sci. USA 74, 789-792.
10. Cloyd, M.W., Hartley, J.W., & Rowe, W.P. (1980) J. Exp. Med. 151, 542-552.
11. Quint, W., Quax, W., Putten, H., & Berns, A. (1981) J. Virol. 39, 1-10.
12. Chattopadhyay, S.L., Cloyd, M.W., Linemeyer, D.L., Lander, M.R., Rands, E., & Lowy, D.R. (1982).Nature 295, 25-31.
13. Weiss, R., Teich, N., Varmus, H., & Coffin, J. (eds.) (1982) RNA Tumor Viruses. Cold Spring Harbor Monographs, 10C. Cold Spring Harbor, New York.
14. Chattopadhyay, S.K., Lowy, D.R., Teich, N.M., Levine, A.S. & Rowe, W.P. (1974) Cold Spring Harbor Symp. Quart. Biol. 39, 1085-1101.
15. Jenkins, N.A., Copeland, N.G., Taylor, B.A., & Lee, B.K., J. Virol. 43, 26-36.
16. Kaplan, H.S. (1967) Cancer Res. 27, 1325-1340.
17. Gardner, M.B., Henderson, B.E., Estes, J.D., Rongey, R.W., Casagrade, J., Pike, M. & Huebner, R.J. (1976).

Cancer Res. 38, 729-735.

18. Hardy, W.D., Hess, P., MacEwen, E.G., McClelland, A.J., Zuckerman, E.E., Essex, M., Cotter; S.M., & Jarrett, O. (1976). Cancer Res. 36,582-588.
19. Jarrett, O., (1980) Cold Spring Harbor Conf. Cell Proliferation 7, 603-611.
20. Nexo, B.A. & Ulrich, K. (1978) Cancer Res. 38, 729-735.
21. Nexø, B.A. & Ulrich; K. (1983) Virology 125, 454-467.
22. Jenkins, N.A., Bedigan, H.G., Thomas, C.Y., & Copeland, N.G. (1984) J. Virol. 49, 437-444.
23. Ulrich, K. & Nexo, B. (1984) in press.
24. Varnier, O.E., Hoffman, A.D., Nexø, B.A., & Levy, J.A. (1984) Virology, 132, 79-94.
25. Gibson, W., & Verma, I.M. (1974) Proc. Natl. Acad. Sci. USA 71, 4991-4994.
26. Elder, J.H., Jensen, F.C., Bryant, M.L., & Lerner, R.A. (1977) Nature 267, 23-28.
27. Nexø, B.A., & Nexø, E. (1982) Biochem. Biophys. Acta, 708, 178-184.
28. De Rossi, A., D'Andrea, E., Colombatti, A., Fischinger, P.J., & Chieco-Bianchi, L. (1981) J. Natl. Cancer Inst. 67, 1241-1250.
29. Motta, J.V., Crittendon, L.B., Purchase, H.G., Stone, H.A., & Witter, R.L. (1975) J. Natl. Cancer Inst. 55, 685-689.
30. Crittenden, L.B., Witter, R.L., Okazaki, W., & Neiman, P.E. (1979) J. Natl. Cancer Inst. 63, 191-200.
31. Greenberger, J.S., Stephenson, J.R., Moloney, W.C., & Aaronson, S.A. (1975) Cancer Res. 35, 245-252.
32. Weiss, R.A., & Frisby, D.A. (1982) in Yohn, D.A., & Blakeslee, J.A. (eds.) Advances in Comparative Leukemia Research 1981. Elsevier North Holland Inc.
33. Martin, M.A., Bryan, T., Rasheed, S., & Khan, A.S. (1981) Proc. Natl. Acad. Sci. USA, 78, 4892-4896.
34. Bonner, T.I., O'Connell, C.O., & Cohen, M. (1982) Proc. Natl. Acad. Sci. USA 79, 4709-4713.

MURINE XENOTROPIC RETROVIRUSES: IN THE COMPUTER AGE

O.E. Varnier

Institute of Microbiology, School of Medicine
V.le Benedetto XV, 10 - 16132 Genova, Italy

> The "C-type" particles in NZB mice, therefore, have biologic activity similar to other murine leukemia viruses (Science 170, 326-327, 1970)
>
> This NZB type virus is endogenous in other strains of mice and is xenotropic; that is, it grows only in cells foreign to the host. (Science 182, 1151-1153, 1973)

The xenotropic retrovirus is endogenous to most if not all mouse strains and its simple genome seems to be dedicated to only essential biological functions, since it lacks any known oncogene. Host range analyses clearly showed that heterogeneity is the rule in the xenotropic class. A computer program was developed to compare one virus to all others yielding values for homologies for the core and envelope protein peptides. While the env peptides separate the ecotropic from the xenotropic viruses, the gag peptides distinguish the NZBs from the non-NZB isolates and confirm that the latter are less divergent from the ecotropic viruses. Among the ten xenotropic viruses tested, only two DBA/2 viruses are identical.

The mouse has been the animal of choice for virologists ever since retroviruses and their stigmata were recognized as a common murine feature which had resisted to natural selection. In the last thirty years several different retroviruses have been isolated from mice. This abundance of retroisolates and retrogenomes, first accepted as a species curiosity (1), led to the finding that type C viruses are present in most animal species (Table 1). As data accumulated, researchers have defined, challenged and redefined the dogmas in retrovirology. These dogmas are reviewed by J.A. Levy in this volume.

Only after twenty years of studies on murine sarcoma (MSV) and leukemia viruses (MLV) (2), was the most common endogenous class of murine retroviruses isolated in the New Zealand Black (NZB) mouse (3). This retrovirus was termed **XENOTROPIC** because of its unique relationship with its natural host (4,5). As R. Dulbecco has aptly pointed out above, this virus is prisoner of its cellular host, unable to infect neighboring cells. Escape is possible only through experimental exposure to heterologous cells in which these retroviruses are able to replicate. The peculiar xenotropism is due to at least two different blocks in the infection cycle: one within the cell (5) and one associated with the virion envelope glycoprotein complex (Nexo and Varnier, in preparation). The xenotropic retrovirus is endogenous to most if not all mouse strains including those phylogenetically distant (6), and its simple genome seems to be dedicated solely to the essential biological functions.

In the past, several systems have been proposed to classify the murine xenotropic retroviruses into Class II and Class III (7), or X-alfa and X-beta subclasses (8). Further investigations have demonstrated other distinguishing properties (9,10,11), which suggested a greater degree of heterogeneity. This heterogeneity raises several intriguing questions:

1. How many murine xenotropic retroviruses exist in the mouse?

2. Do the six to nine proviral copies present in the mouse DNA code for the same or different xenotropic retroviruses?
3. Do xenotropic retroviruses exist that are specific to a particular mouse strain, organ or type of tissue?

Initially we selected the NZB strain as our experimental model, because in these mice, from embryo to adulthood, cells spontaneously release substantial amounts of xenotropic retroviruses (12). To select representative isolates from this heterogenous viral population, we performed long term cocultivation of NZB kidney culture with heterologous cell lines (13), in which high titering isolates were subsequently biologically cloned (14).

Table 1. Major animal vertebrate species in which retroviruses have been detected

Mammalian	Aves	Primates	Pisces	Reptilia
Cat	Chicken	Baboon	Fish	Viper
Cow	Duck	Chimpanzee		
Deer	Pheasant	Gibbon		
Dog	Quail	**HUMAN**		
Guinea pig	Turkey	Marmoset		
Hamster		Monkey		
Horse				
Mouse				
Pig				
Rabbit				
Rat				
Sheep				

Table 2. Detection of xenotropic retroviruses.

Retrovirus	S+L-Ml	S+L-Cat	Polymerase activity
X-NZB/K-MLc	6.3	6.9	278,360
X-C57L/T-Mlc	5.5	nd	182,797
X-NZB/E-Mlc	5.3	5.5	221,665
X-NZB/Br-Ml	5.1	nd	262,740
X-NZB/S-Mlc1	4.9	5.6	210,634
X-NZB/K-Dgc	4.8	5.3	nd
X-AKR/T-Mlc	4.7	2.6	139,903
X-NZB/S-Huc	4.6	5.7	211,034
X-DBA2/Ei-Ml	4.4	nd	98,381
X-NZB/K-Huc	4.0	5.8	293,490
X-NZB/S-Ml	3.9	nd	168,317
X-NZB/E-Ml6	3.9	5.0	136,530
X-NFS/T-Mlc	3.8	nd	63,994
X-NZB/T-Ml	3.5	3.8	181,923
X-NZB/S-Mlc2	3.4	3.2	150,991
X-NZB/K-Rbc	3.4	4.3	29,650
X-NZB/Bm-Ml	3.4	nd	138,464
X-NZB/ i-Mlz	3.1	2.4	70,863
X-NZB/Esp	1.6	2.2	nd
X-NZB/Ksp	-	1.2	nd
X-C57L/T-Hu	-	nd	1,064
X-C57L/T-Dgc	-	nd	171,713
X-NZB/Ei-Ml	-	nd	6,468

Viral titers are expressed either by foci of cell transformation in S+L- mink and cat cells (15) or by reverse transcriptase activity in culture supernatant.

For the first time we have shown that at least three different xenotropic retroviruses can be expressed by one mouse organ (16).

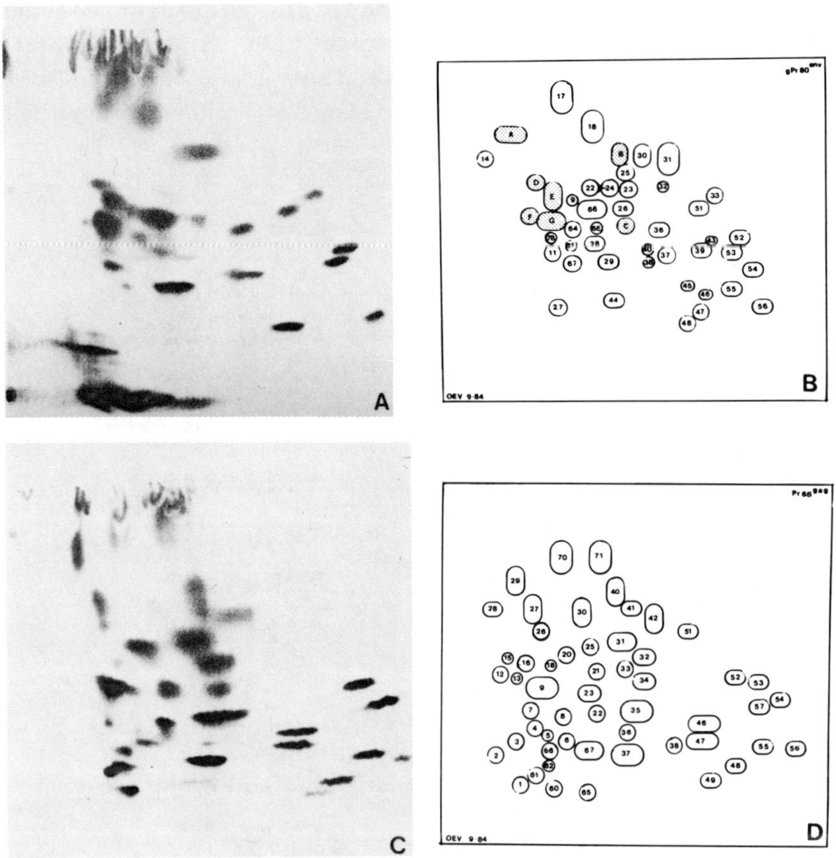

Figure 1. Tryptic peptide maps of 3H-leucine labeled proteins of X-NZB/K-Huc isolates. Precursors gPr80^{env} and Pr68^{gag} were immunoprecipitated from infected cells, purified electrophoretically and mapped, as previously described (16). A = gPr80^{env}; C = Pr68^{gag}; B and C = schematic representation of the maps. Shaded spots represent overlapping of gp70 and p15E peptides

Further studies on host range and replication properties have been extended to include twenty-three different xenotropic isolates, originally obtained from six different mouse strains (C57L, NIH, NFS, AKR, DBA/2 and seventeen from the NZB mouse), six different tissues and propagated in four heterologous cell lines. The data obtained so far clearly indicate that among the isolates tested there is great variability in infectivity and replication properties (Table 2).

```
** VIRUS CARD **

Virus    -> X-NZB/K-Huc
Species  -> MURINE
Strain   -> NZB
Tropism  -> X
Organ    -> K
Cells    -> Hu
Clone    -> Y

GAG protein peptides
 1 ->    2 ->    3 ->0   4 ->1   5 ->0   6 ->1   7 ->0   8 ->1   9 ->1  10 ->
11 ->   12 ->0  13 ->0  14 ->   15 ->0  16 ->0  17 ->   18 ->1  19 ->1  20 ->1
21 ->1  22 ->1  23 ->1  24 ->1  25 ->1  26 ->1  27 ->1  28 ->1  29 ->1  30 ->1
31 ->1  32 ->1  33 ->0  34 ->1  35 ->1  36 ->1  37 ->1  38 ->1  39 ->   40 ->1
41 ->1  42 ->1  43 ->   44 ->   45 ->   46 ->1  47 ->1  48 ->1  49 ->1  50 ->0
51 ->1  52 ->0  53 ->1  54 ->1  55 ->1  56 ->1  57 ->1  58 ->   59 ->   60 ->1
61 ->1  62 ->1  63 ->   64 ->   65 ->1  66 ->1  67 ->0  68 ->   69 ->   70 ->1
71 ->1

ENV protein peptides
 1 ->    2 ->    3 ->    4 ->    5 ->    6 ->3   7 ->5   8 ->5   9 ->5  10 ->5
11 ->5  12 ->6  13 ->   14 ->5  15 ->3  16 ->3  17 ->5  18 ->5  19 ->3  20 ->5
21 ->   22 ->3  23 ->4  24 ->4  25 ->4  26 ->3  27 ->6  28 ->3  29 ->5  30 ->5
31 ->4  32 ->5  33 ->5  34 ->5  35 ->   36 ->3  37 ->5  38 ->3  39 ->   40 ->4
41 ->   42 ->   43 ->6  44 ->6  45 ->6  46 ->5  47 ->4  48 ->4  49 ->   50 ->
51 ->3  52 ->5  53 ->3  54 ->4  55 ->4  56 ->5  57 ->   58 ->   59 ->   60 ->
61 ->3  62 ->3  63 ->3  64 ->   65 ->3  66 ->3  67 ->4  68 ->3  69 ->1  70 ->
71 ->   72 ->   73 ->   74 ->   75 ->   76 ->   77 ->5  78 ->   79 ->6
```

Figure 2.Computer virus card of the X-NZB/K-Huc isolate

Two years ago we began a new approach to study the intracellular gag and env coded proteins of the xenotropic isolates in collaboration with B.A. Nexo.

Chronically infected cell cultures were metabolically labelled with ^{3}H-leucine. After two hours, cell extracts were obtained with various detergents, immunoprecipitated and run on gel electrophoresis. Protein bands, recovered from dried gels, were treated with trypsin and the peptides separated by thin-layer electrophoresis and ascending chromatography (18,19).

The structural protein profile of the xenotropic isolates tested shows differences in the gag-coded intermediates, while the envelope proteins are similar, with one prominent exception. The envelope associated protein p15E of the X-NZB/K-Mlc isolate has a higher mobility corresponding to a lower molecular weight (16).

We obtained tryptic peptide maps of gag and env protein precursors ($Pr68^{gag}$ and $gPr80^{env}$, respectively). To facilitate comparison of the different peptide maps, we designed diagrams representing all the major distinct peptides of the two precursors (Fig. 1).

As our studies expanded, we became aware of the impossibility of comparing all the peptides from the evergrowing list of viruses. The solution to this problem was obtained by developing a suitable computer program (Tarantola et al., in preparation). Each virus is coded in the computer using a nomenclature which specifies the tropism, strain, organ and cells used for virus propagation. The presence and absence of protein peptides is indicated by a numerical code (Fig. 2). With this program comparison of one virus to all others tested yield values for homologies and divergences (absolute and relative percentages) for the core and envelope (Fig.3).

As indicated in Fig.3, the NZB xenotropic prototype X-NZB/K-Huc is not identical to any of the other isolates; gag homology with the other NZB viruses is very high with only one exception, the X-NZB/S-Mlc1; non-NZB xenotropic and the ecotropic AKR virus diverge to almost the same extent (37-40%). The env peptides are identical to those of the X-NZB/K-Dgc isolate, and are highly homologous to all the other xenotropic peptides, but quite distinct from those of the ecotropic AKR retrovirus. The total homology identifies three groups: the NZBs, the non-NZBs and the ecotropic virus. The non-NZB xenotropic subgroup is more closely related to the ecotropic retroviruses than the NZBs.

HOMOLOGY OF THE VIRUS X-NZB/K-Huc

	GAG Protein Peptide Homology	GAG Protein Peptide Divergence
X-NZB/K-Dgc	96	4
X-NZB/E-M1	96	4
X-NZB/S-M1c2	96	4
X-NZB/K-M1c	94	6
X-NZB/S-M1c1	87	13
X-AKR/T-M1c	63	37
E-AKR	60	40
X-DBA/E-M1	60	40
X-DBA/S-Rb	60	40
X-C57L/T-M1c	60	40

	ENV Protein Peptide Homology	ENV Protein Peptide Divergence
X-NZB/K-Dgc	100	0
X-NZB/S-M1c2	96	4
X-NZB/K-M1c	96	4
X-DBA/E-M1	94	6
X-DBA/S-Rb	94	6
X-NZB/E-M1	94	6
X-AKR/T-M1c	92	8
X-C57L/T-M1c	92	8
X-NZB/S-M1c1	90	10
E-AKR	52	48

	TOTAL HOMOLOGY	TOTAL DIVERGENCE
X-NZB/K-Dgc	98	2
X-NZB/S-M1c2	96	4
X-NZB/E-M1	95	5
X-NZB/K-M1c	95	5
X-NZB/S-M1c1	88	12
X-AKR/T-M1c	77	23
X-DBA/E-M1	76	24
X-DBA/S-Rb	76	24
X-C57L/T-M1c	75	25
E-AKR	56	44

Figure 3. Homology of the X-NZB/K-Huc virus

In conclusion, heterogeneity is a frequent occurrence in nature and distinguishing characteristics in a given population are often associated with specific functions: fat and fur in cold regions or salivary glands and melanin in warm countries. Life is individualism and evolution selects individuals in a species for survival. In virology differences exist between the various families, genera, classes, groups and types. In retrovirology, and especially the xenotropic class, heterogeneity is the rule. In fact among the ten xenotropic viruses tested only the two DBA/2 viruses are identical. While the env protein peptides separate the ecotropic from the xenotropic viruses, the gag peptides distinguish the NZBs from the non-NZB isolates and confirm that the latter are less divergent from the ecotropic viruses (8).

The extension of these studies to include a large number of representative isolates (other NZB and non-NZB xenotropic, ecotropic, amphotropic and recombinant isolates), together with sequencing analysis of the coding and non-coding regions, will give insight into the process of recombination, which gives rise to the pathogenic oncogene-free recombinants.

ACKNOWLEDGMENTS

The research described in this paper was supported by grants from CNR N. 84.0841, 84.00838 and 84.02327 and by NATO grant N. 137.80.

I would like to thank Drs. J.W. Hartley, A.D. Hoffman, J.A. Levy, B.A. Nexo, S.P. Raffanti and S. Rasheed for their collaborative help.

REFERENCES

1. Lieber, M.M., Benveniste, R.E., Livingston, D.M. & Todaro, G.J. (1973) Science 182, 56-59.
2. Gross, L. (1970) In Oncogenic viruses. Pergamon Press,

Oxford
3. Levy, J.A. (1970) Science 170, 326-327.
4. Levy, J.A. (1973) Science 182,1151-1151.
5. Levy, J.A. (1978) Curr. Top. Microbiol. Immunol. 79, 111-213.
6. Lieber, M.M., Sherr, C., Potter, M. & Todaro, G.J. (1975) Int. J. Cancer 15, 211-220.
7. Stephenson, J.R., Aaronson, S.A., Arstein, P., Huebner, R.J. & Tronick, S.R. (1974) Virology 61, 56-63.
8. Callahan, R., Lieber, M.M. & Todaro, G.J. _1975) J. Virol. 15, 1378-1384.
9. Gazdar, A.F., Oie, O.H.K., Russel, E.K. & Minna, J.D. (1976) Bibl. Haematol. 43, 154-157.
10. Gautsch, J.W., Elder, J.H., Schindler, J., Jensen, F.C. & Lerner, R.A. (1978) Proc. Natl. Acad. Sci. USA 75, 4170-4174.
11. Bosselman, R.A., Van Griensven, L.J., Vogt, M. & Verma I.M. (1979) J. Virol. 32, 968-978.
12. Levy, J.A., Kazan, P., Varnier, O.E. & Kleiman, H. (1975) J. Virol. 16, 844-853.
13. Varnier, O.E., Repetto C.M., Raffanti, S.P., Alama, A. & Levy, J.A. (1983) J. gen. Virol. 64, 425-428.
14. Varnier, O.E., Melioli, G., Repetto, C.M. & Raffanti, S.P. (1983) Intervirology 20, 159-163.
15. Varnier, O.E., Hoffman, A.D., Nexø, B.A. & Levy, J.A. (1984) Virology, 132, 79-94.
16. Varnier, O.E. & Levy, J.A. (1979) Virology 96, 604-610.
17. Rasheed, S., Gardner, M.B., Rongey, R.W., Nelson-Rees, W.A. & Arnstein, P. (1977) J. Natl. Cancer Inst. 58, 881-890.
18. Nexø, B.A. & Nexo, E. (1982) Bioch. Bioph. Acta 708, 178-184.
19. Nexø, B.A. & Ulrich, K. (1983) Virology 125, 454-467.

VIRAL AND NONVIRAL MAMMARY TUMORIGENESIS

J. Hilgers and A. Sonnenberg

Division of Tumor Biology, The Netherlands Cancer Institute, Antoni van Leeuwenhoek Huis, Plesmanlaan 121, 1066CX, Amsterdam

Mammary tumors in the mouse are of very different histological types and histogenesis. Etiological agents include the mammary tumor virus, excessive hypophyseal and steroid hormone stimulation, chemical carcinogens and unknown factors, such as in mice after reproductive age.

Mammary tumors in man are mainly of one histological type, called invasive ductal carcinoma, its histogenesis being unique and different from all types of murine mammary cancer. The etiological agent is unknown and most likely not a virus.

HISTOPATHOGENESIS

Mammary tumors occurring in inbred mouse strains may be of different histological types and their histogenesis seems to proceed along different paths occurring in different cell types in the normal gland. To some extent the etiological factor involved seems to determine the peculiar histogenetic path of the induced tumor in mammary gland epithelium. For extensive reviews, see Hilgers and Sluyser (1).

The mammary tumor virus, such as the milkfactor in the C3H mouse strain, induces adenocarcinomas, tumors in which the epithelial and stromal components of mammary tissue seem to grow equally well and in which normal orientation of the tissue and its cell types, together with an intact basement membrane prevail at least for some time. Progression through several distinct stages is a well known phenomenon in these tumors, starting with hyperplastic nodules (2), proceeding via adenocarcinomas of different types (3) to sarcomatoid carcinomas, at least in some cases. The last step involves complete loss of orientation of the various cellular components of the tumor tissue, destruction of the barrier between epithelium and mesenchyme (basement membrane) and invasiveness combined with metastatic properties. The last process is, however, rare in all murine tumors and usually only occurs to the lungs (4).

The inherited mammary tumor virus in the GR mouse strain, at the Mtv-2 locus on chromosome 18, induces a different type of tumor in the mouse mammary gland, the so-called type P tumor (5), a tumor with an organoid character, somewhat resembling yet another tumortype induced by the mammary tumor virus, the so-called "plaque" (6). These lesions progress easily towards less organized tissue structures and can become hormone-independent in their growth during the process (7).

Hormonally induced mammary tumors, for example by hypophyseal isografts in estrogen-producing female mice, are often called adenocarcinomas, but they may show squamous features and are sometimes referred to as papillary tumors, to distinguish them from the virus-induced adenocarcinomas (for review, see 8). These tumors do not seem to have clearly distinct preneoplastic stages and do not seem to progress into sarcomatoid carcinomas.

Chemically-induced tumors, e.g. by urethane (9) or methylcholanthrene (10), are usually squamous cell tumors and may exhibit so-called keratinized nodules. These nodules, in contrast to so-called hyperplastic alveolar nodules appear in lobular regions of the gland and show heavy infiltration with lymphocytes. It is unknown whether they are "preneoplastic" in the sense that they can progress focally towards the squamous cell tumor, such as is the case for the hyperplastic alveolar nodule progressing towards an adenocarcinoma (9).

Spontaneous mammary cancer occurs in some mouse strains fairly regularly after reproductive age. The BALB/c mouse strain has in fact a spontaneous tumor incidence of over 30% and although the mammary tumors may be of different histological types, they are usually quite squamous in appearance. A strain which gets an appreciable incidence of spontaneous adenocarcinomas, of slightly unique histological type, is the 020. In this strain tumors occur mainly in older females after so-called forced-breeding (11).

The question whether the types of prevalent mammary tumors in mice and their histogenesis are similar to tumors and histogenesis in the human mammary gland should be answered in the negative. The prevalent type of tumor in women is the so-called ductal carcinoma, proceeding from a hyperplastic-like stage within ducts, having their basement membrane intact, towards a invasive neoplastic stage outside ducts and without a basement membrane separating epithelium from mesenchyme and stromal cells. The human tumor called invasive ductal carcinoma shows an extreme capacity to invade not only stromal and fatty tissues, but also lymphnode and blood vessels and an even more extreme capacity to metastasize to very many different tissues of the body. The later feature distinguishes the prevalent human tumor very much from all kinds of mouse and rat tumors and is only found in cases of cat mammary tumors.

There are of course a wide variety of mammary tumor types in the human mammary gland also and with widely divergent histogenesis, but all these tumors taken together constitute only 10-20% of human mammary gland cancers. Some of these may be similar to tumors in mice, but this should be studied carefully using differentiation markers for stages of normal differentiation of the gland.

DIFFERENTIATION OF THE NORMAL GLAND

The development of the mouse mammary gland is characterized by the growth of a system of branching ducts in the mammary fat pad. The tip of the ducts shows club-shaped structures, commonly referred to as endbuds. These structures are numerous and large at about three weeks of age, when under the influence of sex and hypophyseal hormones, the ductal system of the mammary gland develops. Endbuds disappear after the mammary fat pad has been filled with ducts, and hormones produced by the ovaries during pregnancy induce a new cycle of events. Buds appear laterally along ducts and alveolar buds emerge from lateral buds. They represent the precursor stage of the functional alveoli fully developed during lactation.

Within the gland two main epithelial cell types are recognized: lumenal and myoepithelial cells. They both develop from a common precursor cell, a stem cell, present in the terminal endbud and most likely also in the developing ducts.

We have recently studied the various cell types of the mammary gland in more detail, using immunoperoxidase tests on frozen sections of the developing and mature gland with a variety of monoclonal antibodies and polyvalent antisera against cell surface, cytoskeletal and basement membrane proteins (12). Our conclusion is that at last five different cell types can be distinguished: one basal, one myoepithelial and three lumenal types. Each cell type was characterized by a specific set of cell markers.

Basal cells express primitive markers not present in myoepithelial and lumenal cells. These cells are present in endbuds and ducts and believed to be stem cells capable of producing myoepithelial as well as lumenal epithelial cells. In the tip of the endbud, where the basement membrane is not yet visible by light microscopy, a basement membrane protein (laminin) appears in the cytoplasm of basal cells. Basal and myoepithelial cells in differentiated structures, including the alveolar buds, do not exhibit cytoplasmic staining for laminin. These structures are surrounded by a basement membrane, separating epithelial from mesenchymal cells. Basal and myoepithelial cells in differentiated structures, including the alveola buds, do not exhibit cytoplasmic staining for laminin. These structures are surrounded by a basement membrane, separating epithelial from mesenchymal cells.

The differentiation process of lumenal cells is characterized by a successive loss of various cell markers and by a polarization process of certain cell markers within cells, some of which redistribute towards the basolateral membranes, while others localize at the apical region of lumenal cells. We could distinguish three types of lumenal cells, two types in the ducts, a keratin-poor and a keratin-rich type, and one type in the alveoli.

These studies on the evolution of various cell types in mammary gland epithelium of the mouse were preceded by similar studies in the rat (13,14), but have not yet been carried out in detail for the human mammary gland. Such studies are, however, necessary to understand the precise histogenesis of the various types of mammary cancer developing in the epithelium. They will eventually lead to identification of the cell type which gets transformed by the various etiological agents, be it the basal or stem cell or a cell type already differentiated to some extent. This problem is, however, very difficult to solve because after transforming events and progression, differentiating capacity still is retained at least to some extent.

SUSCEPTIBILITY GENES AND ONCOGENES

The role of genetic factors in mammary carcinogenesis was suspected already in the beginning of the century. Great differences in the frequency of tumors were found in various mouse stocks and in attempts to determine quickly the susceptibility to cancer by transplanting mammary carcinomas like the Jensen and Ehrlich tumors; the laws governing transplantation immunity, i.e.

histocompatibility, were accidentally discovered by Little and Tyzzer (15). The subsequent development of highly inbred strains by sibmating, initiated by Little has led to fixation of susceptibility and resistance to spontaneous mammary cancer and the discovery of the mammary tumor virus by Bittner and Korteweg (16, 17).

When mice develop a mammary carcinoma before one year of life, a virus is almost always involved in the causation of the tumor. In general this virus is transmitted via the milk from mother to offspring, but occasionally the virus is transmitted with the seminal fluid or by yet other alternative routes (for review, see 18). Only in two instances is a virulent mammary tumor virus efficiently transmitted by the male, in the GR and SHN mouse strains (19, 20). Such a mode of transmission has proven to be genetic (21).

Most mouse strains tested thus far contain in their normal cellular DNA some proviral copies of the genome of the mammary tumor virus (22). There is evidence that some of these proviruses, when they become expressed and produce virions, also play a role in late-appearing mammary carcinomas of some mouse strains, such as the C3Hf (23).

Host genes interfering with viral replication or infection of the target mammary gland cell for tumorigenesis can modify susceptibility for the virus and are as such indirect susceptibility genes for tumorigenesis (24, 25, for reviews). None of these gene systems have been located in the genome and their action is hardly known.

Great interest in this virus has been aroused by the observed potentiation of proviral transcription by glucocorticoids (26, 27), due to the presence of a nucleotide sequence in the virus which binds the glucocorticoid-receptor complex, leading to enhanced transcription of the whole viral genome (28). The enhancement of viral replication is correlated strongly with an increased risk for mammary tumors (29).

Current thinking about this virus in its role in

mammary tumorigenesis holds that the viral genes are responsible for so-called insertional mutagenesis, being responsible for expression of normal cellular genes apparently involved in growth promotion of epithelial cells. Such normal genes, or putative oncogenes, would be present at preferred sites of integration for the viral genome in chromosome 15 and 7, at the respective Int-1 and Int-2 gene locations (30, 31). These genes are expressed in virally-induced mammary tumors and they are unique among the increasingly larger family of so-called oncogenes. Their nature and mode of action is not yet known, but is being intensely studied. Whether these genes are also involved in nonviral mammary tumorigenesis in mice and men remains to be determined.

It would not be very surprising that activation of an oncogene like H-ras-1, found to occur in chemically induced rat mammary tumors (32), is a prequisite also for mouse mammary gland carcinogenesis, and that genes at the Int-1 or Int-2 locus are not at all involved in the squamous cell cancers induced by chemicals such as urethane and methylcholanthrene, etc.

It would also not be very surprising that activation of yet other oncogenes are needed to obtain hormonally induced mammary cancer, with their own unique type of histogenesis. And this can also be safely stated for different tumor types of the mammary gland occurring spontaneously.

Although different oncogenes may be involved in different types of mammary tumorigenesis, and more than one per tumor system, especially where progression of stages occurs, it seems that all tumors have one genetic defect in common, i.e. trisomy of chromosome 13 (33). This constant chromosomal aberration may be necessary to promote action of genes on chromosome 13, which is necessary for uncontrolled epithelial cell growth of the mammary gland. No oncogenes have been found, however, so far on that mouse chromosome, and the nature of the gene and even its precise location is unknown.

Invasive ductal carcinomas of the human mammary gland

with their unique histogenesis and their aggressive invasiveness and high metastatic properties have not yet been understood in terms of involved oncogenes. In fact there is virtually no evidence for involvement of any of the known oncogenes. There may be some myc genes amplified in cell lines capable of transforming NIH 3T3 cells (35). Int-1 may be involved because it is highly conserved in human DNA (36). Members of the ras-gene family may be involved because they are involved in tumors of other epithelia (37).

It seems likely that in the near future, oncogenes will be implicated in this major tumor type in women, but for the time being it is a riddle whether they will be the ones also involved in viral tumorigenesis in the mouse, or those of chemical tumorigenesis in the rat, or none of these.

Whether constant chromosomal aberrations play a role in human mammary tumorigenesis is not known. Chromosome 1 has sometimes been implicated but good karyology of primary mammary cancers is extremely difficult. One clearly needs also for oncogene work a method by which to culture each biopsy specimen with ease and high frequency of success, before one can study human tumorigenesis in the same detail as one can now do in the mouse and the rat systems.

REFERENCES

1. Hilgers, J. and Sluyser, M., Eds. (1981) in Mammary Tumours in the Mouse, (Elsevier/North-Holland Biomedical Press, Amsterdam), pp. 1-691.
2. Medina, D. (1973) Meth. Cancer Res. 7, 3-51.
3. Dunn, T.B., (1958) in The Physiopathology of Cancer, ed. Homburger, F. (Hoeber Inc. New York), pp. 38-84.
4. Van der Valk, M. (1981) in Mammary Tumours in the Mouse, eds. Hilgers, J. and Sluyser, M. (Elsevier/North-Holland Biomedical Press, Amsterdam), pp. 45-116.

5. Van Nie, R., and Dux, A. (1971) J. Natl. Cancer Inst. 46, 885-897.
6. Foulds, L. (1956) J. Natl. Cancer Inst. 17, 755-781.
7. Squartini, F. (1962) J. Natl. Cancer Inst. 28, 911-926.
8. Boot, L.M., Kwa, H.G., and Ropcke, G. (1981) in Mammary Tumours in the Mouse, eds. Hilgers, J. and Sluyser, M. (Elsevier/North-Holland Biomedical Press, Amsterdam), pp. 117-200.
9. Imai, S., Tsubura, Y. and Hilgers, J. (in press) Urethane-induced mammary tumorigenesis in a mammary tumor virus (MuMTV)-positive mouse strain: evidence for a keratinized nodule as an MuMTV-negative precursor lesion for squamous cell tumors. J. Natl. Cancer Inst.
10. Kirschbaum, A., Williams, W.L. and Bittner, J.J. (1946) Cancer Res. 6, 354-362.
11. Muhlbock, O. and Dux, A. (1981) in Mammary Tumours in the Mouse, eds. Hilgers, J. and Sluyser, M. (Elsevier/North-Holland Biomedical Press, Amsterdam), pp. 545-572.
12. Sonnenberg, A., Daams, J., Van der Valk, M.A., Hilkens, J. and Hilgers, J. (submitted) Development of the mouse mammary gland; identification of stages in the differentiation of lumenal and myoepithelial cells using monoclonal antibodies and polyvalent antiserum against differentiation antigens.
13. Dulbecco, R., Henhan, M. and Armstrong, B. (1982) Proc. Natl. Acad. Sci. USA 79, 7346-7350.
14. Warburton, M.J., Mitchell, D., Ormerod, E.J., and Rudland, P. (1982) J. Histochem. Cytochem. 30, 667-676.
15. Little, C.C. and Tyzzer, E.E. (1916) J. Exp. Med. 33, 393-453.
16. Staff of the Roscoe B. Jackson Memorial Laboratory (1933) Science 78, 465-466.
17. Korteweg, R. (1934) Ned. Tijdschr. Geneeskd. 78, 240-245.
18. Hilgers, J. and Bentvelzen, P. (1978) Adv. Cancer Res.

26, 143-195.

19. Muhlbock, O. (1965) Eur. J. Cancer 1, 123-124.
20. Imai, S., Tsubura, Y., Hilgers, J. and Michalides, R. (1983) J. Natl. Cancer Inst. 71, 517-521.
21. Bentvelzen, P. (1968) in Genetical Control of the Vertical Transmission of the Muhlbock Mammary Tumor Virus in the GR Mouse Strain (Hollandia, Amsterdam).
22. Varmus, H.E., Bishop, J.M., Nowinski, R.C. and Sarkar, N.H. (1972) Nat. New Biol. 238, 189-190.
23. Van Nie, R. and Verstraeten, A.A. (1975) Int. J. Cancer 16, 922-932.
24. Verstraeten, A.A., Van Nie, R. and Bentvelzen, P. (1981) in Mammary Tumours in the Mouse, eds. Hilgers, J. and Sluyser, M. (Elsevier/Norh Holland Biomedical Press, Amsterdam), pp. 505-514.
25. Hageman, Ph. C., Calafat, J. and Hilgers, J. (1981) in Mammary Tumours in the Mouse, eds. Hilgers, J. and Sluyser, M. (Elsevier/North Holland Biomedical Press, Amsterdam), pp. 391-464.
26. Parks, W.P., Ransom, J.C., Young, H.A. and Scolnick, E.M. (1975). J. Biol. Chem. 250, 3330-3336.
27. Ringold, G.M., Lasfargues, E.Y., Bishop, J.M. and Varmus, H.E. (1975) Virology, 65, 135-147.
28. Yamamoto, K.R., Stallings, M.R., Ring, J. and Ringold, G.M. (1978) Cold Spring Harbor Symp. Quant. Biol. 42, 625-634.
29. Muhlbock, O. (1956) Acta Unio Int. Contra Cancrum 12, 665-681.
30. Nusse, R. and Varmus, H.E. (1982) Cell 31, 99-109.
31. Peters, G., Brookes, S., Smith, R. and Dickson, C. (1983) Cell 33, 369-377.
32. Sukumar, S., Notario, V., Martin-Zanca, D. and Barbacid, M. (1983) Nature 306, 658-661.
33. Dufuku, R. and Matsuzawa, A. (1983) Anticancer Res. 3, 17-34.
34. Kozbor, D. and Croce, C.M. (1984) Cancer Res. 44, 438-441.
35. Fasano, O., Birnbaum, D., Birchmeier, C., Edlund, L., Fogh, J. and Wigler, M. (1984) in Proceedings XV

Meeting of the European Tumor Virus Group, P. 152 (abst.)

36. Nusse, R., Van Ooyen, A., Cox, D., Fung, Y.K.T. and Varmus, H. (1984) Nature 307, 131-136.

37. Murray, M.J., Shilo, B-Z, Shih, C., Cowing, D., Hsu, H.W., and Weinberg, R.A. (1981) Cell 25, 355-361.

THE PROVIRAL GENOME OF RADIATION LEUKEMIA VIRUS: MOLECULAR CLONING, NUCLEOTIDE SEQUENCE OF ITS LONG TERMINAL REPEAT AND INTEGRATION IN LYMPHOMA CELL DNA

M. Janowski, J. Merregaert, J. Boniver[1] and J.R. Maisin

Department of Radiobiology, Centre d'Etude de l'Energie Nucléaire (C.E.N./S.C.K.), Boeretang 200, B-2400 Mol, Belgium, and [1]. Laboratoire d'Anatomie Pathologique, B-23, Université de Liege au Sart-Tilman, B-4000 Liège, Belgium.

The proviral genome of a thymotropic and leukemogenic C57BL/Ka mouse retrovirus, RadLV/VL_3(T+L+), was cloned as a biologically active PstI insert in the bacterial plasmid pBR322. Its restriction map was compared to those, already known, of two nonthymotropic and nonleukemogenic viruses of the same mouse strain, the ecotropic BL/Ka(B) and the xenotropic constituent of the radiation leukemia virus complex (RadLV). Differences were observed in the pol gene and in the env gene. Moreover, the nucleotide sequence of the RadLV/VL_3(T+L+) long terminal repeat revealed the existence of two copies of a 42 bp long sequence, separated by 11 nucleotides and of which BL/Ka(B) possesses only one copy.

The topography of the RadLV/VL_3(T+L+) provirus in virus-induced thymic lymphoma DNA revealed the existence of multiple integration sites.

Radiation leukemia virus (RadLV) is an in vivo passaged murine leukemia virus (MuLV) complex, isolated from thymic lymphomas of X-ray irradiated C57BL/Ka mice (1). BL/VL_3, a cell line established from a RadLV-induced thymic lymphoma, releases the $RadLV/VL_3$ viral complex (2) of which the thymotropic and leukemogenic $RadLV/VL_3$(T+L+) entity, subject of the present studies, occurs in a 1,000 fold excess over a xenotropic constituent (3). C57BL/Ka mice harbor at least three classes of nonthymotropic and nonleukemogenic (T-L-) retroviruses replicating in cultured fibroblasts of the appropriate host range. Well-characterized are a B-ecotrope, BL/Ka(B), an N-ecotrope, BL/Ka(N) and a xenotrope, BL/Ka(X) (4). The T+L+ entity is believed not to be originally present in the germ line of C57BL/Ka mice, but rather to have evolved by recombinational events between endogenous viruses (5).

We previously performed experiments (6) to determine if, as demonstrated namely in the case of the avian leukosis virus (7,8), there would be an indication that RadLV might uncover a putative cellular oncogene by adjacent provirus insertion. We observed that cell lines, established from individual $RadLV/VL_3$-induced C57BL/Ka thymic lymphomas, shared a common integration site. However, these cells represented only a minor fraction of the primary tumor cell population, since novel proviral sequences appear at different locations in the DNA of individual primary lymphomas (9). They probably were submitted to a strong selection during in vitro growth, perhaps as a consequence of provirus insertion in the vicinity of a gene involved in mitotic functions. The search for novel proviruses in mouse DNA is hampered by the presence of many cross-hybridizing endogenous provirus families. In the present work, we took advantage of the fact that the R/Cnb strain of rats is susceptible to lymphoma induction by $RadLV/VL_3$, and that rat DNA does not contain endogenous proviruses capable of hybridizing strongly to MuLV-specific probes. We will describe the absence of any obvious correlaton between the proviral integration sites and lymphomagenicity of $RadLV/VL_3$ in rats.

A variety of reports have established that the U3 portion of the retroviral long terminal repeats (LTR) and the regions coding for gp70 and p15E could all play a role in determining leukemogenicity (10–13). In order to tentatively correlate the thymotropicity and leukemogenicity of RadLV/VL_3(T+L+) with specific features of its genome, we cloned its proviral genome as a biologically active PstI insert in the bacterial plasmid pBR322. We then compared its restriction map with that of two T-L- retroviruses of the C57BL/Ka mouse, and the nucleotide sequence of its LTR with those of several leukemogenic and nonleukemogenic MuLV's.

INTEGRATION PATTERN OF THE RadLV/VL_3(T+L+) PROVIRUS IN RAT LYMPHOMA DNA

Inoculation of RadLV/VL_3 concentrates into the thymus of 15-day-old R/Cnb rats resulted in the development of thymic lymphomas after a latency period of at least 3 months. EcoRI- and Hind III-generated fragments of chromosomal DNA prepared from 2 individual tumors were first tested for their homology with a MuLV-specific ^{32}P-cDNA probe as described previously (6). Several provirus-containing fragments were detected. They yielded one single 8.3 kpb fragment (Fig. 1, lanes g and h) of which the restriction map was indistinguishable from that of RadLV/VL_3(T+L+) (see below). The absence of internal cleavage with EcoRI excluded the existence of integrated xenotropic provirus (9), and hence excluded the existence of integrate xenotropic provirus (9), and hence its role in RdhadLV/VL_3-induced tumorigenesis. A minority of EcoRII-generated subproviral fragments was however observed by examining a larger number of individual tumor DNAs (Fig. 1, lanes i to u). None of the tumors showed a common integration site. The occasional occurrence of fragments of apparently equivalent length was coincidental, as attested to by the fact that Hind III

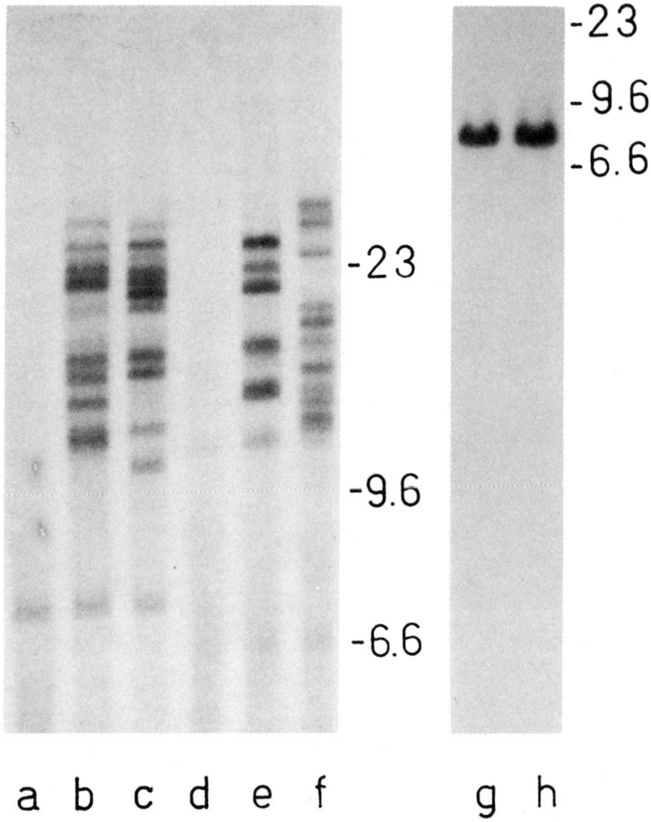

Figure 1. Provirus topography in RadLV/VL$_3$-induced rat thymic lymphomas. EcoRI analysis of control rat DNA (lane a) and of two individual tumor DNAs (lanes b and c); Hind III analysis of control rat DNA (lane d) and of the same tumor DNAs (lanes e and f); PstI analysis of the same tumor DNAs (lanes g and h, see Figure 1, next page); EcoRI analysis of control rat DNA (lanes v and w) and of 13 other individual tumor DNAs (lanes i to u). Undigested extrachromosomal DNA from a 20 h coculture of BL/RL$_{12}$-NP and BL/VL$_3$ cells (lane x), its PstI digest (lane z) and a mixture of both (lane y) are shown for molecular weight comparison. The positions of Hind III DNA fragments (in kbp) in the gels are indicated.

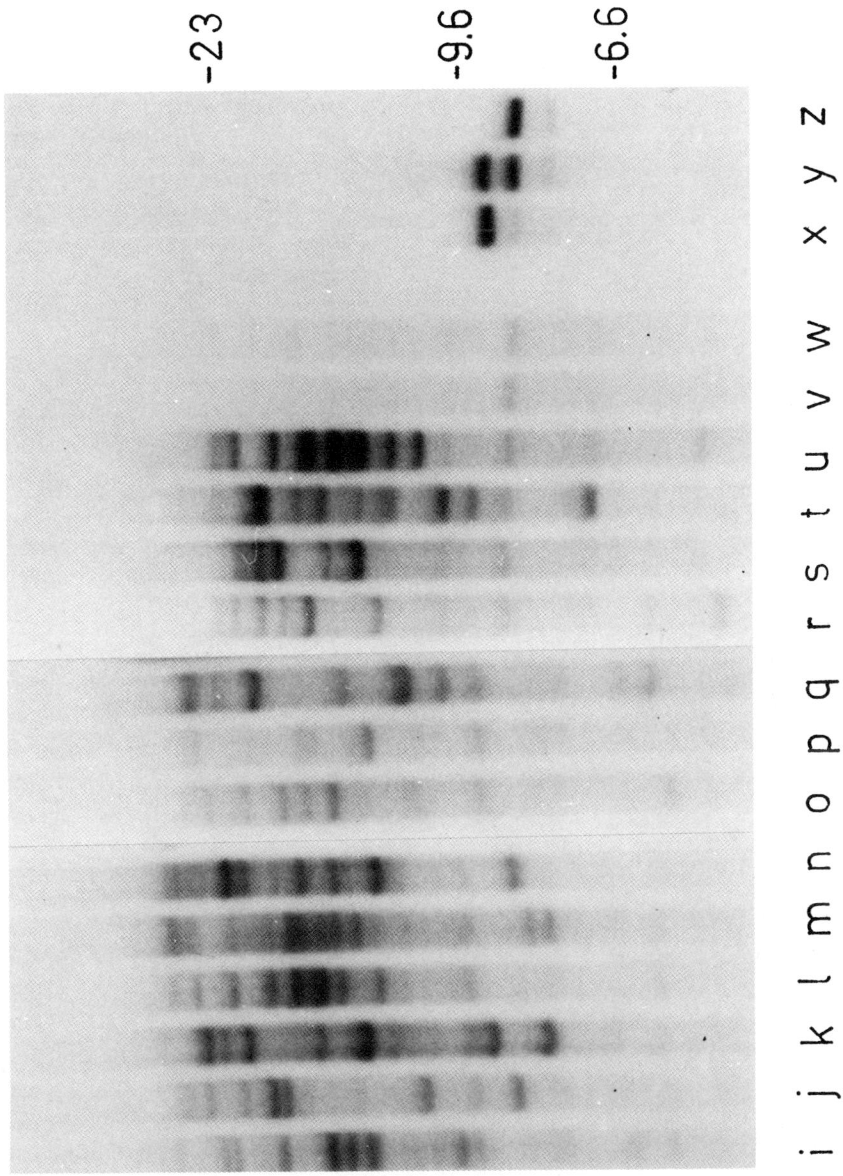

Figure 1. (Continued)

digestion of the DNAs involved in such cases did not confirm this suspicion (not shown). Our observations do not exclude the possibility that proviruses might have become integrated into specific domains of the DNA (14,15), which could be detected only by using as probes cloned cellular sequences adjacent to a tumor specific integrated provirus.

A BIOLOGICALLLY ACTIVE CLONE OF THE RadLV/VL_3(T+L+) PROVIRAL GENOME

BL/RL_{12}-NP cells were established in culture from a radiation-induced C57BL/Ka thymic lymphoma (4). They are susceptible to infection with RadLV/VL_3. During a 20h cocultivation with BL/VL_3 cells, they synthesized a 8.9 kbp long extrachromosomal proviral DNA molecule, yielding upon PstI digestion a 8.3 kpb long fragment that we cloned by insertion into the PstI site of the bacterial plasmid pBR332. The clone insert could only represent the RadLV/VL_3(T+L+) proviral genome. Indeed, transfection of SC-1 cells (16) induced the release of virus particles which were positive in tests for thymotropicity (17) and for leukemogenicity both in mice and rats. The presence of a full length LTR, reconstituted in a T4 DNA ligase-catalyzed reaction, was however necessary to obtain successful transformation.

The restriction map of the PstI insert of the recombinant plasmid (pMOL502) was established by using BamHI, BstEII, ClaI, HpaI, KpnI, PvuI, PvuII, SstII, XbaI and XhoI, used in single and in combined reactions (Fig. 2). It was indistinguishable from that of either the extrachromosomal provirus synthesized during the early stages of cocultivation of BL/RL_{12}-NP with BL/VL_3, and from that of the major proviral species which became integrated in RadLV/VL_3-induced rat thymic lymphomas. A comparison between the restriction maps of RadLV/VL_3(T+L+) and BL/Ka(B) reveals some distinct features. The first is the absence, in the former, of two restriction sites (KpnI and BstEII), located close to one another in the pol gene. The second is the absence, in BL/Ka(B), of two neighboring sites (ClaI and XbaI) in the pol gene. The third resides in the env gene, where BL/Ka(B) lacks a recognition site for SstI. Finally, a fourth dissimilarity consists in the greater length of the LTR of RadLV/VL_3(T+L+) (583 bp instead of 529), as will be seen below. At the present time, we cannot make a correlation between the T+L+ properties of the investigated retrovirus and specific features of its proviral genome. RadLV/VL_3 is devoid of mink cell focus forming (MCF) activity (3) and tentative comparisons with differences between the membrane glycoprotein structural genes of MCF and ecotropic viruses (18) should remain subject to caution. Let us note, however, that mutations in the env gene caused a loss of leukemogenicity in the case of Friend spleen focus forming virus (10). On the other hand, it has been shown that the U3 region of the LTR also may determine thymotropicity of a Balb/c MuLV (19) and leukemogenicity of SL-3 MuLV (12).

THE LTR SEQUENCE OF THE RadLV/VL_3(T+L+) PROVIRAL GENOME

We determined the nucleotide sequence (20) of the reconstituted LTR of the cloned RadLV/VL_3(T+L+) proviral genome. It was compared to those of the ecotropic BL/Ka(B) (21) and AKR MuLV's (22), the xenotropic NFS MuLV (23) and the T+L+ B-Cl-11 MuLV (19). All five LTR's contain, in the same order and approximately at the same distance from each other, the consensus CCAAT and TATAAAAA promotor sequences and the AATAAA polyadenylation signal (Fig. 2). The LTR's for which the entire nucleotide sequence is available display identical, 13 bp long inverted repeats. As in the case of B-Cl-11, RadLV/VL_3(T+L+) contains 2 copies of a relatively long direct repeat, although separated in the latter by an 11 bp sequence which interrupts the tandem arrangement. The only relevant difference between B-Cl-11 and its nonthymotropic counterpart resides in deletions and rearrangements

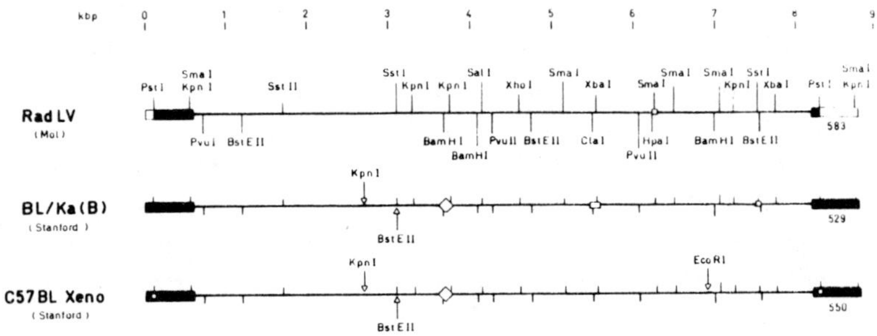


```
                10        20        30        40        50        60        70        80        90       100
RadLV     AATGAAAGACCCCACCATAAGGCTTAGCAAGCTAGCTGCAGTAACGCCATTTTGCAAGGCATGGAAAAGTACCAGAGCTGA-GTTCTCA-CAAGTT----
B-CL-11   ............TT............C.....A..............C................A...........T.......GA..AA-CAAG
AKR       ............TT............C.....A.............................G...A...........T.......GA..AA-CAAG
BL/KA(B)  ............TT............C.....A..............C.............G...A...........T.......GA..AA-CAAG
NFS                                 ............................A................-...T...-A.....----

               110       120       130       140       150       160       170       180       190       200
RadLV     -ACAAAGAAGTTTAGTTAAAG------GCTGAATAATACTGAGAAAGGGGCCGAACAGGATATCTGTGGTCAAGCACCTCGGCCCCGGCTCCGTTAGACA
B-CL-11   A....G.....AC..----..A---G....G.A.G...C.G..CTA.....A.........................TAG...----------------
AKR       A....G.....AC..----..A---G....G.A.G...C.G..CTA.....A.........................TAG.........C.A.GGCC.AG
BL/KA(B)  A....G.....AC..----..A---G....G.A.G...C.G..CTA.....A.........................TAG.........C.A.GGCC.AG
NFS       -...........G.......AATAAG.T............G..C.......A...................G.......G..........A.GGCC.AG

               210       220       230       240       250       260       270       280       290       300
RadLV     TA----------------------------------------GGCCAAACAGGATATCTGTGGCCAAGCACCT--GCCCCGGCTCAGGGCCAAAA
B-CL-11   ---------------------------GGAAAGTACCGGGACTAG.....................T.......TAGG.......C.........G.
AKR       A.CAGATGGTCCCCAGAAACAGAGAGGCTGGAAAGTACCGGGACTAG...................T.......TAGG.......C.........G.
BL/KA(B)  A.CAGATGGTCCCCAGAA----------------------------------------------------------------------------------
NFS       A.CAGATGG-------------------------------------------------------------------------------------------

               310       320       330       340       350       360       370       380       390       400
RadLV     ACAGATAGTACTCAGATAAAGTGAAACTAACAACAGTTTCTGGAAAGTCCCACCG-----CA-GTTTCA-GGTTCCCCAAACGACC-GAGAGATACCCCA
B-CL-11   ......G..C.C....A.T..CT...AC...........AA..G.--....--.AAAC---T..C...A.........G.T....G.G..TCA......
AKR       ......G..C.C....A.T..CT...AC...........AA..G.--....--.AAAC---T..C...A.........G.T....G.G..TCA......
BL/KA(B)  ----------------.T..CT...AC...........AA..G.--....--.AAAC---T..C...A.........G.T....G.G..TCA......
NFS       -------...............C.......G.......................-----T..-.......A-..........A....-.G..A......-.

               410       420       430       440       450       460       470       480       490       500
RadLV     AGCCTTATTTAAACTAACCAATCAGCTCGCTTCTCGCTTCTGTACCCGCGCTCTTTGCCCCCCCAGCCCTAGCCCTATAAAAAGGGTAAGAACTCCACAC
B-CL-11   .....C...........................-...............TA....TG...-------...T....................C......
AKR       .....C...........................-...............TA....TG...-------...T....................C......
BL/KA(B)  .....C...........................................TA....TG...-------...T...............A...C......
NFS       ..........G......................-...............T.....-....-......................................

               510       520       530       540       550       560       570       580       590       600
RadLV     --TCGGCGCGCCAGTCCTCCAACCGACTGAGTCGCCCGGGTACCCGTGTATCCAATAAAGCCTTTTGCTGTTGCATCCGAATCGTGGTCTCGCTGATCCT
B-CL-11   --..................G.TA.............................................................................
AKR       --..................G.TA.............................................................................
BL/KA(B)  AC..................G..A.............................................................................
NFS       --...-..........A...G.TA................

               610       620       630       640       650
RadLV     TGGGAGGGTCTCCTCAGAGTGATTGACTGCCCAGCTTGGGGGTCTTTCATT
B-CL-11   ...................................C..............
AKR       ...................................C............
BL/KA(B)  .................................................
```

Figure 2. Restriction map of the cloned RadLV/VL_3(T+L+) proviral genome, compared to that of BL/Ka(B) and of the xenotropic constituent of RadLV/VL_3, and the nucleotide sequence of its LTR, compared to that of B-C1-11 MuLV, AKR MuLV, BL/Ka(B) MuLV and NFS MuLV. The restriction map of the extrachromosomal DNA from a 20 h coculture of BL/RL_{12}-NP and BL/VL_3 cells, and that of the PstI fragment of the proviral species integrated in RadLV/VL_3-induced rat lymphoma DNA (see Fig. 1, lane g), were indistinguishable from that of the cloned RadLV/VL_3(T+L+) genome.

leading to the appearance of the tandem repeat (19). It is therefore tempting to draw a parallel between the compared features of RadLV/VL_3(T+L+) and Bl/Ka(B). However the LTR sequence of RadLV/VL_3 ressembles more that of the xenotropic NFS MuLV and leads us to predict that it might rather have derived from an endogenous xenotropic virus of the C57BL mouse. Furthermore, a unique 6 bp insertion upstream of the TATA box of RadLV/VL_3(T+L+) also seems to point towards a xenotropic origin (R.R. O'Neill, personal communication). Whether the T+L+ properties of RadLV/VL_3(T+L+) reside in its LTR, possibly being determined by a direct repeats acting as enhancer signals (24,25), or in other parts of its genome (possibly those which differ from the BL/Ka(B) genome) will hopefully be answered by the results of the in vitro recombination experiments which are currently under way.

ACKNOWLEDGEMENTS

This work was performed with the financial participation of the European Atomic Energy Commission (BIO-D-379-81-B), the Belgian Fonds National de la Recherche Scientifique Médicale and the European Late Effects Project Group.

REFERENCES

1. Kaplan, H.S. (1967) Cancer Res. 27, 1325-1340.
2. Lieberman M., Declève, A., Ricciardi-Castagnoli, P., Boniver, J., Finn, O.J., & Kaplan H.S. (1979). Int. J. Cancer 24, 168-177.
3. Declève A., Lieberman, M., Ihle, J.N., Rosenthal, P.N., Lung, M.L. & Kaplan, H.S. (1978) Virology 90, 23-25.
4. Lieberman, M., Declève, A., Gelman, E.P. & Kaplan, H.S. (1977) Radiation-induced leukemogenesis and Related Viruses, ed. Duplan, J.F., (North-Holland Publishing Company, Amsterdam-New York-Oxford), pp. 231-246.
5. Benade, L.E., Ihle, J.N., & Declève, A. (1978) Proc. Natl. Acad. Sci. U.S.A. 75, 4553-4557.
6. Janowski, M., Boniver, J. & Maisin, J.R. (1982) Leukemia Res. 6, 285-287.
7. Neel, B.G., Hayward, W.S., Robinson, H.L., Fang, J. & Astrin, S.M. (1981) Cell 23, 323-334.
8. Payne, G.S., Courtneidge, S.A., Crittenden, L.B., Fadly, A.M., Bishop, J.M., & Varmus, H.E. (1981). Cell 23, 311-322.
9. Grymes, R.A., Scott, M.L., Kin, J.P., Fry, K.E., & Kaplan, H.S. (1983) Prog. Nucl. Ac. Res. Mol. Biol. 29, 53-73.
10. Lung, M.L., Hartley, J.W., Rowe, W.P. & Hopkins, N.H. (1983). J. Virol. 45, 275-290.
11. Ruta, M., Bestwick, R., Machida, C. & Kabat, D. (1983) Proc. Natl. Acad. Sci. U.S.A. 80, 4704-4708.
12. Lenz, J., Celander, D., Growther, R.L., Patarea, R., Perkins, D.W. & Haseltine, W.A. (1984). Nature 308, 1467-1472.
13. Robinson, H., Blais, B.M., Tsichlis, P.N. & Coffin, J.M. (1982) Proc. Natl. Acad. Sci. U.S.A. 79, 1225-1229.
14. Nusse, R. & Varmus, H.E. (1982) Cell 31, 99-109.
15. Tsichlis, P.N., Strauss, P.G. & Hu, L.F. (1983) Nature 302, 445-449.

16. Hus, I.C., & Yang, W.K. (1977) Cancer Res. 37, 1709-1714.
17. Declève, A., Lieberman, M., Niwa, O. & Kaplan, H.S. (1974) Nature 252, 79-81.
18. Elder, J.F., Gautsch, J.W., Jensen, F.C., Lerner, R.A., Harley, J.W., & Rowe, W.P. (1977) Proc. Natl. Acad. Sci. U.S.A. 74, 4676-4680.
19. Des Groseillers, L., Rassart, E. & Jolicoeur, P. (1983) Proc. Natl. Acad. Sci. U.S.A. 80, 4203-4207.
20. Maxam, A.M., & Gilbert, W. (1980) Methods in Enzymology 65, 499-560.
21. Kim, J.P., Kaplan, H.S. & Fry, K.E. (1982) J. Virol. 44, 217-225.
22. Van Beveren, C., Rands, E., Chattopaghyay, S.L., Lowy, D.R. & Verma, I.M. (1981) J. Virol. 41, 542-556.
23. Khan, A.S. & Martin, M.A. (1983) Proc. Natl. Acad. Sci. U.S.A. 80, 2699-2703.
24. Laimins, L.A., Khoury, G., Gorman, C., Howard, B. & Gruss, P. (1982) Proc. Natl. Acad. Sci. U.S.A. 79, 6453-6457.
25. Srinivasan, A., Reddy, E.P., Dunn, C.I. & Aaronson, S.A. (1984). Science 223, 286-289.

METASTATIC POTENTIAL OF FRIEND LEUKEMIA CELLS: FIBRONECTIN INDUCES SPECIFIC ARREST, SURVIVAL AND GROWTH OF FLC IN LIVER OF DBA/2 MICE

A. Benedetto[1], C. Amici[1], W. Djaczenko[2], S. Zaniratti[1] and G. Elia[1]

1. Center of Virology, Ospedale S. Camillo, Circ.ne Gianicolense 85, 00152 Roma RM and 2. Institute of Microbiology, I University of Rome, P.le Aldo Moro 5, 00100 Roma RM

Modalities of liver and spleen infiltrations by two Friend leukemia cell (FLC) clones have been studied in DBA/2 mice by i.v. injection. The two clones applied were: a) an original 745 A clone and b) a highly fibronectin (FN) sensitive FF 16-1 clone, derived from original FLC.

The death rate of DBA/2 mice depends on the size of the 745 A inoculum while the death rate with FF 16-1 is uniformly high. The 745 A cells infiltrate only the spleens of DBA/2 mice; liver infiltrations are negligible. In contrast, FF 16-1 cells most frequently infiltrate livers, spleen infiltrations in this case being negligible. Livers of DBA/2 mice, inoculated with FF 16-1 cells, are covered by numerous nodules containing almost pure populations of FF 16-1 cells. The passage in vivo of FF 16-1 cells does not abolish their FN-sensitivity. Immunofluorescence with anti-FN antibodies of normal livers shows a continuous thin zone of FN in the sinusoids. In FF 16-1 nodules intense anti-FN fluorescence was observed in the tumor capsule, while leukemic cells are not fluorescent.

Experiments with 5-^{125}I-2'-deoxyuridine show that in livers of mice inoculated with FF 16-1 cells, in contrast to the livers of 745 A injected mice, the residual radioactivity after 2 hours of inoculation assumes significant values.

FN-sensitivity of FF 16-1 cells is probably a determinant factor, responsible for specific hepatotropism of these cells. However, other factors, such as hypothetic growth factor(s) of liver and some immunological mechanisms are probably responsible for the evolution of FF 16-1 tumor nodules in the liver.

ISOLATION OF FIBRONECTIN SENSITIVE FRIEND LEUKEMIA CELL CLONES

Murine erythroleukemia cells infected with Friend virus grow in vitro and differentiate from a pro-erythoblast-like stage to a normoblast-like stage, upon induction with different agents (1). FLC normally grow in suspension, but tend to adhere to fibroblast monolayers. By co-cultivation of FLC with human embryo fibroblasts, we selected adhesive Friend cells. After the 16th subculture, we isolated clones of FLC, referred to as FF clones, that grow as monolayers on plastic substrata, precoated either with human cold insoluble globulin (CIG) or fibroblast fibronectin (FN) and maintain the ability to differentiate upon induction by DMSO (2).

The FF 16-1 clone, characterized by the highest FN-sensitivity, and the original 745 A clone were used in all subsequent experiments. 745 A cells were routinely maintained as suspension cultures in Falcon bottles in RPMI 1640, supplemented by 10% fetal calf serum (FCS). FF 16-1 cells were instead maintained in the same medium on Falcon dishes, precoated with human CIG (Collaborative Research, Waltham, Mass. USA) at a dose of 1 ug/cm^2 FF 16-1 monolayers reached maximal density at 5 + 0.5 X$\cdot$ 10^5 cells/cm^2 and were sub-passaged by mild trypsinization at a 1:4 split ratio (3).

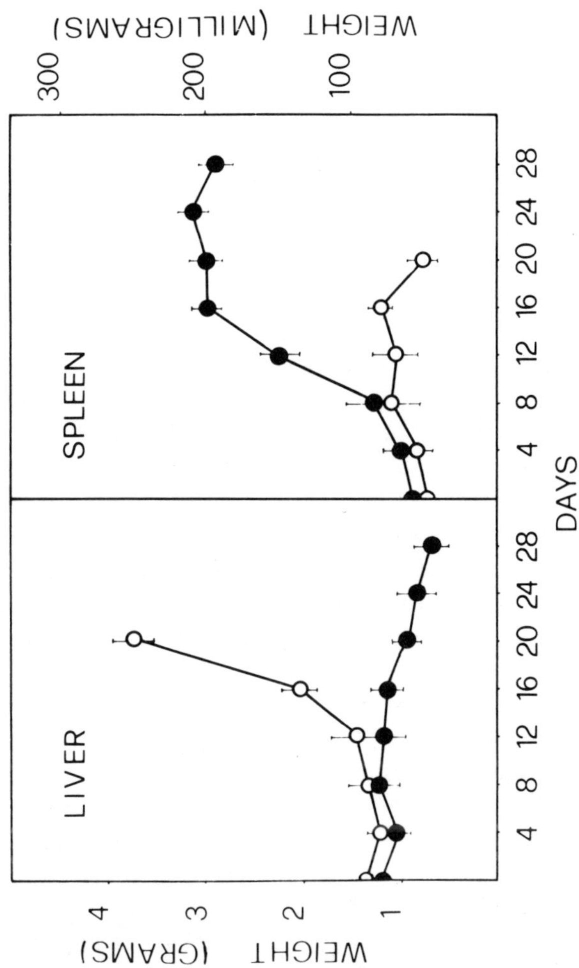

Figure 1. Variation of liver and spleen weights of mice i.v. inoculated with 745 A or FF 16-1 cells. 10^6 745 A (O--O) or FF 16-1 (●--●) cells were i.v. injected into the tail vein of DBA/2 mice. Every 4th day, 4 animals for each type of leukemic cell employed were killed and livers and spleens excised and weighed.

EFFECT OF I.V. INJECTION OF 745 A AND FF 16-1 CELLS IN DBA/2 MICE

We compared the tumorigenicity of 745 A and FF 16-1 cells after i.v. inoculation into syngeneic male two month old DBA/2 mice kept under standard conditions. Progressively increasing doses of cells, suspended in 0.3 ml of serum-free RPMI 1640, were injected into the tail vein of the mice. The observations were carried out daily. Autopsies of the dead mice were carried out immediately and weights of livers and spleens recorded. It is seen from Table 1 that the rate of mortality of mice, inoculated with FF 16-1, is higher when compared with that of animals inoculated with 745 A cells. The death rate of DBA/2 mice, inoculated with 745 A cells, depended on the size of inoculum, while the death rate of mice inoculated with FF 16-1 cells was uniformly high. The mean day of death after inoculation of 745 A was higher than that registered in mice inoculated with FF 16-1 cells. Dying mice presented posterior leg paralysis, evident 3-4 days before death, independently of the type of cells injected.

Table 1 also shows that practically only 745 A cells infiltrated spleens of DBA/2 mice, while FF 16-1 cells could be found in the spleen only occasionally. In contrast, infiltrations of livers were present only in FF 16-1 injected mice, being completely absent in 745 A injected mice at all concentrations employed. The rate of tumor infiltration in livers and spleens of injected mice was studied in the following experiment. DBA/2 mice were i.v. injected with 10^6 cells of either the FF 16-1 or 745 A clones, and, every 4th day, 4 animals for each type of injected cells were sacrificed, their livers and spleens excised and weighed.

The average weight of DBA/2 spleens on the 16th day after inoculation with 745 A cells was about three times greater than that of control mice. At the same time after inoculation with FF 16-1 cells the DBA/2 spleens were slightly reduced in weight as compared with spleens of control animals. Variations of liver weight are summarized

Table 1. Comparison of the tumorigenicity of 745 A and FF 16-1 cells injected i.v. in DBA/2 mice.

Type and number of cells injected	N° of mice dead /Total N° of mice injected	Mean day of death ± S.D.	N° of mice with metastases in spleen /Total inoculated	N° of mice with metastases in liver /Total inoculated
745 A 5x 100,000	5/30	44.2 ± 15.8	0/30	0/30
1x1,000,000	21/30	36.7 ± 14.6	5/30	0/30
2x1,000,000	30/30	21.0 ± 4.3	12/30	0/30
FF 16-1 5x 100,000	30/30	31.5 ± 10.8	0/30	26/30
1x1,000,000	30/30	22.3 ± 4.2	0/30	30/30
2x1,000,000	30/30	16.5 ± 5.0	1/30	30/30

in Fig. 1. Observations of FF 16-1 injected mice were suspended on the 20th day, when emaciation of the remaining mice occurred. The average weight of DBA/2 livers inoculated with 745 A cells was essentially constant over the whole experimental period with a slight tendency to decrease at the end of observations. In contrast, the weight of livers of DBA/2 mice inoculated with FF 16-1 cells, after a lag period of about 12 days showed a dramatic increase. On the 20th day after inoculation with FF 16-1 cells, the weight of DBA/2 livers was about 3 times that of control animals.

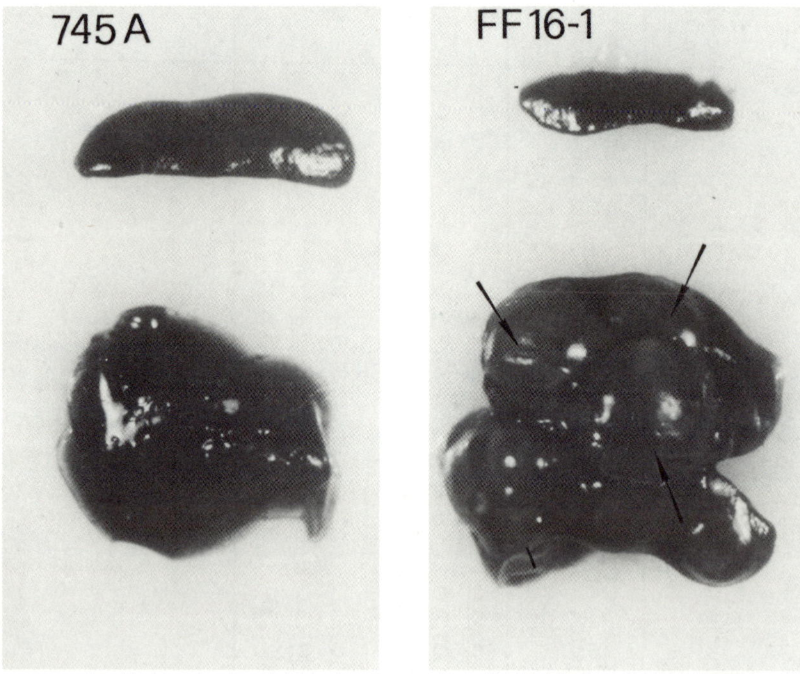

Figure 2. Gross morphology of the spleen and liver of DBA/2 mice after i.v. inoculation with leukemic cells. Spleens (upper part) and livers (lower part) were excised from mice sacrificed at 32nd day after 745 A (left) and at 19th day after FF 16-1 (right) cell inoculation. The arrows indicate tumour nodules containing FF 16-1 cells.

Differences in gross anatomy of livers of DBA/2 mice, inoculated with either 745 A or FF 16-1 cells are illustrated in Fig. 2. Livers of mice inoculated with FF 16-1 cells are greatly enlarged and contain numerous nodules of variable size covered by smooth, stretched, grayish membrane. On the 20th day after inoculation with FF 16-1 cells, livers occupied almost the whole abdominal cavity of experimental mice The nodules showed the tendency to self-enucleate and, when punctured, released large amounts of almost pure populations of FF 16-1 cells. These cells, when reseeded on FN-covered plastic surfaces, adhered firmly, indicating that the passage in vivo did not substantially modify the FN sensitivity of FF 16-1 cells.

FIBRONECTIN DISTRIBUTION IN TUMOUR INFILTRATIONS IN LIVER

Light microscopy of DBA/2 livers infiltrated with FF 16-1 cells, in Haematoxilin-Eosin preparation, shows that in the nodule area the normal hepatic tissue is greatly reduced in volume and pushed to the periphery, the central area being filled with tightly packed FF 16-1 cells (data not shown).

We paid particular attention to the distribution of FN in such nodules, which we studied by indirect immunofluorescence. Both normal and FF 16-1 cell infiltrated livers (20 days after inoculation with 10^6 cells/animal) were rapidly frozen in liquid nitrogen precooled isopenthane and cut with a cryostat set at -20°C. Frozen sections were fixed with 2.5% paraformaldeyde in phosphate buffered saline (PBS) for 30' at room temperature, washed and incubated with highly purified rabbit anti-FN antibody (Collaborative Research, Waltham, Mass., USA) and stained with FITC conjugated anti-rabbit IgG (Miles Yeda, Rehovot, Israel).

Observation was carried out using a Leitz Ortholux microscope. As seen in Figure 3a, in the normal liver the sinusoids had a continuous thin zone of anti-FN antibody

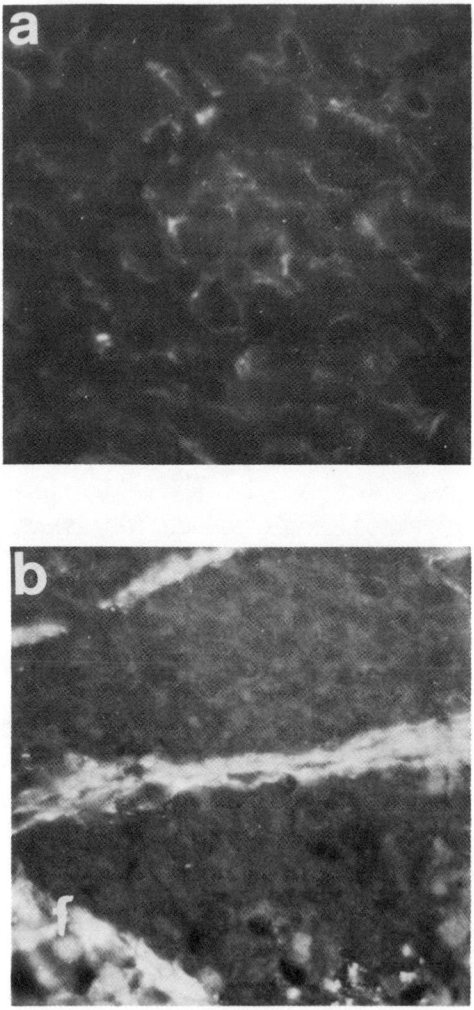

Figure 3. Indirect immunofluorescent staining of frozen liver sections with anti-FN antiserum. Pattern of anti-FN fluorescence of liver section from control, not inoculated DBA/2 mouse (a) and of a section of tumour nodules in liver of a DBA/2 mouse inoculated with FF 16-1 cells (b).

reactive material, probably located between the endothelial lining and liver epithelial cell plates. No fluorescence was observed between hepatocytes. Some anti-FN fluorescence was detected in the blood vessels. In nodules containing FF 16-1 cells, the intense anti-FN fluorescence was present in the whole area of the connective tissue capsule surrounding the nodule; leukemic cells showed hardly any anti-FN fluorescence (3b). This result indicates the stromal localization of FN, as already demonstrated in human sarcomas (4).

PREVALENT ANCHORAGE OF I.V. INJECTED FF 16-1 CELLS IN LIVER OF DBA/2 MICE

Three possibilities could be formulated to explain the ability of FF 16-1 cells, when i.v. inoculated, to produce liver tumors in DBA/2 mice: a) FF 16-1 cells are specifically anchored in some compartments of DBA/2 livers; b) FN of hepatic sinusoids stimulates the growth of FF 16-1 cells; c) some unknown mechanism protects FF 16-1 cells from cytotoxic killing.

To shed some light on the nature of the mechanism responsible for specific growth of FF 16-1 cells in the livers of DBA/2 mice, we carried out the following experiment. 745A cultures at a density of 10^6 cells/ml and FF 16-1 cell monolayers at a comparable cell density, were labelled with 1 uCie/ml of 5-^{125}I-2'-deoxyuridine (200 uCie/7.4 MBq, Amersham, UK). After 16 hours, both 745 A and FF 16-1 cultures were washed, mildly trypsinized, pelleted and resuspended in serum-free RPMI 1640 at a density of 10^7 cells/ml. Aliquots of 0.3 ml of each cell suspension were directly counted in a gamma-counter and then injected into the tail vein of DBA/2 mice. After 2 hours animals were sacrificed, their livers excised and their radioactivity determined. Blood radioctivity, measured in 0.3 ml samples taken from heart ventricles, did not differ significantly from that of the background. Results of this experiment are shown in Table 2. It is

Table 2. Recovery of radioactivity in the liver of mice inoculated by $3x10^6$ $5-^{125}I$-2'-deoxyuridine labeled 745 A and FF 16-1 cells.

Type of cell injected	Mouse	Radioactivity recovered in liver 2 hrs after cell injection / Total cell radioactivity injected x 100
745 A	1	0.8
	2	0.4
	3	0.5
FF 16-1	1	3.5
	2	4.3
	3	3.9

seen that in livers of mice inoculated with FF 16-1 cells, in contrast to the livers of 745 A injected mice, the residual radioactivity after 2 hours of inoculation assumes significant values.

Current results seem to indicate that the primary factor responsible for hepatotropism of FF 16-1 cells is their high sensitivity to exogenous FN. However, this factor alone cannot explain all the events leading to hepatic nodule formation by FF 16-1 cells as described in this report.

Experiments with $5-^{125}I$-2'-deoxyuridine demonstrate that FF 16-1 cells are preferentially and rapidly anchored in hepatic tissue. This fact does not exclude the possibility that some kind of growth factor produced by the liver is also involved in the evolution of hepatic FF 16-1 cell tumor nodules. It may be concluded that tumor infiltration of livers by FF 16-1 cells is a multifactorial phenomenon in which complex systems are involved.

REFERENCES

1. Marks, P.A. & Rifkind, R.A. (1978) in Annual Review of Biochemistry: Erythroleukemic differentiation, ed. Snell, E.E. (Annual Review Inc.), 47, 419-448.
2. Benedetto, A., Amici, C., Djaczenko, W., Zaniratti, S. & Santoro, M.G. (1981) Exp. Cell Res. 134, 219-229.
3. Benedetto, A., Amici, C., Djaczenko, W., Zaniratti, S. & Elia, G. (1982) Int. J. Cancer 30, 663-667.
4. Stenman, S. & Vaheri, A. (1981) Int. J. Cancer 27, 427-435.

THE ENVELOPE GENE OF MAMMALIAN RETROVIRUSES: ANALYSIS OF ITS STRUCTURE REVEALS SPECIFIC RECOMBINATION SIGNALS

R. Friedrich, W. Koch, B. Hackl, and W. Zimmermann

Institute of Immunobiology, University of Freiburg, Stefan-Meier-Str. 8, D-7800 Freiburg, Federal Republic of Germany

The envelope (env) gene of leukemogenic mammalian retroviruses is thought to play an important role in the induction of leukemia and in the determination of the host range of these viruses. In an effort to understand these functions in more detail we have compared the sequences of a number of env genes of leukemogenic and nonleukemogenic viruses. From these data, we have derived a general model for the structure of the env gene as well as the env gene product. Recombination of the viral DNA with cellular sequences is a prerequisite for viral replication (1) and induction of disease (13). Analysis of the viral sequences at the points of recombination has revealed a eucaryotic consensus sequence for recombination.

A MODEL FOR THE CONFORMATION OF THE ENV POLYPEPTIDE

We have compared env gene sequences of several leukemogenic and nonleukemogenic murine (2-7, and unpublished work of B.H. and R.F.) and feline (8) retroviruses. This comparison allows us to derive a general structural scheme of the env gene and the env gene coded polypeptide. It consists of two regions which seem

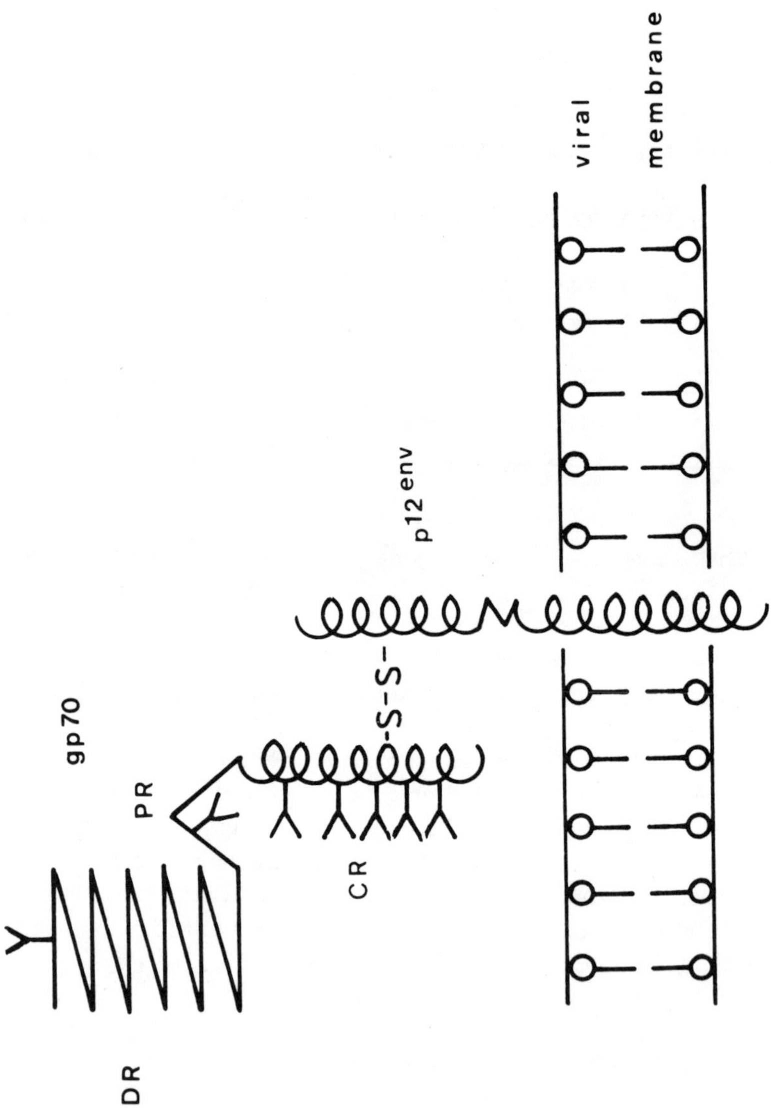

Figure 1. Model of the conformation of the env gene product. CR: constant region; DR: differential region; PR: proline rich region; Y: glycosylation sites. Zig zag lines denote possible beta sheets and beta turns and helices denote possible alpha helices.

to be different in many respects: a "constant region" (CR) comprises p15env (the nonglycosilated product of the env gene, apparent molecular weight 15,000) and about 160 amino acids of the carboxyterminal half of gp70. (the glycosilated product of the env gene, apparent molecular weight 70,000). It is very similar in all murine and feline viruses used for comparison. The N-terminal half of gp70 is essentially composed of a region which we call "differential region" (DR) since it differentiates viruses of different host tropism. Most of the sequence differences found between the env genes of the viruses are located in this region. A region rich in proline residues (16 to 36%) (PR) is located at the carboxyterminal part of the differential region at the border of the constant region. In addition to its unusual amino acid composition, this region is highly variable in ecotropic viruses.

Prediction of the secondary structure of the env polypeptide according to the rules given by Chou & Fasman (9) shows that the conformation, of the DR and CR are fairly different. While large portions of the CR consist of alpha helices, the DR is essentially free of them showing mainly beta sheets and beta turns. These data, together with the positions of hydrophobic areas, allow us to design a model for the structure of the env polypeptide (Fig. 1).

$p12^{env}$ (the mature form of $p15^{env}$) is embedded in the viral membrane with its carboxyterminal hydrophobic region. The second hydrophobic region near the N-terminus of $p12^{env}$ is linked via a disulfide bridge to a hydrophobic region in gp70. The hydrophobic character of both peptides in this region should allow intimate contact between gp70 and $p12^{env}$. Several clustered glycosylation sites suggest extensive glycosylation of the carboxyterminal part of gp70, which prevents gp70 from sinking into the membrane.

The exceptionally high proline content of the highly variable region and its hydrophilic character (3,8) suggest its location at the surface of the protein (10). This is substantiated by the existence of strong antigenic determinants in this region (11,12). We assume that this region (PR) represents a functional domain involved in receptor recognition and/or infection of the target cell. Together with the remaining part of the DR it contains most of the differences between viruses of different host tropism. We therefore believe that this part of gp70 determines the host range of the viruses.

A CONSENSUS SEQUENCE FOR DNA RECOMBINATION

The onset of leukemia in mice infected with ecotropic leukemogenic murine leukemia viruses (MuLVs)6 is invariably associated with the generation of polytropic mink cell focus forming viruses (MCFVs). Sequence comparison of ecotropic and polytropic viruses has shown that the MCFVs are recombinants between ectropic MuLVs and cellular sequences (13). These sequences are derived from endogenous, xenotropic-like viruses and replace in all MCFVs analyzed the DR of the ecotropic parent and varying amounts of neighboring sequences in pol and CR. A second substitution is located within the long terminal repeat (LTR).

One would assume that the recombinational events which lead to the exchange of defined regions of the genome are specific. To find possible signals for these exchanges we have examined the nucleotide sequences at the points of recombination. A list of sequences found near the borders of the env substitutions of several MCFVs is given in Table 1. From these sequences one can derive a general sequence of the form Y(Y)RRR(R)AC(Y), where Y stands for pyrimidine and R for purine. Characters in parentheses denote nucleotides which are not present in all cases. If this should be a more general sequence one would expect it to occur at other known recombination points also. One such position was recently found by Rechavi et al. (14) in a mouse myeloma. In this case, the LTR of an intracisternal A-particle has integrated into the cellular mos gene (14, 15). The integration point is represented

Table 1. Occurence of a possible consensus sequence for recombination. 5' and 3' denote the locations of the putative recombination signal relative to the substitution in the viral env gene.

Source	Sequence		Reference
F-MCFV pFM54B	5'	CTAGAACC	Koch et al., 1984
	3'	CAGGAACT	
pFM1/2	5'	TCAAAACC	
	3'	CGGAACC	
Deletion in pFM54B	5'	CTGAGACT	
	3'	CTGGGACG	
M-MCFV	5'	CTAGAACC	Bosselman et al.,1982
	3'	CAGGGACT	
MCF247	3'	TCAAGACG	Holland et al., 1983
Idu-MCFV	5'	CTGGAGACT	Mark and Rapp, 1983
	3'	CAGGGACT	
Deletion in IdU-MCFV		CGGGACC	
MPSV	3'	ATAGGACC	Stacey et al., 1984
c-mos insertion		CTGGGGACC	Rechavi et al., 1982
5' INS palindrome		TGGGGAC	Lebo et al., 1983
D region IgM u		CTGGGACC	Ravetch et al., 1981
D region IgM u		CAAAAACC	
J region IgM u		CTGGGGCC	
J region IgM k		CTGGGACC	Max et al., 1979
consensus sequence		**(Y)YRRR(R)AC(Y)**	

U5 and U3: unique sequences at the 5' and 3' ends, respectively, of the viral LTR; F: friend; M: Moloney; INS: insulin; IdU: iododesoxyuridine; Ig: immunoglobuline.

by the sequence CTGGGGACC which fully coincides with the consensus sequence given above. Another example of a similar sequence can be found in a region of the human insulin gene that is known for its tendency for illegitimate recombinations. This region contans repetitive sequences in which the string TGGGGAC is included. Probably the best known example for DNA recombination is the generation of the mature genes for immunoglobulins. We have found similar sequences in the D and J regions of many immunoglobulins. A few examples are given in Table 1.

In many of the cases mentioned above a complementary inverted repeat can be found downstream of the consensus sequence within about 15 to 30 nucleotides. At the 5' end of the substitution of pFM54B (Tab. 1) the inverted repeat is 24 nucleotides apart from the consensus sequence and reads GTCCTGC; at the 3' end it is 25 nucleotides apart and has the sequence GTTCCAGC. This example shows that the repeat is not strictly complementary; rather a purine is mirrored by a pyrimidine and vice versa. The presence of such a second component of the consensus sequence which is not truly complementary suggests that the mechanism which leads to the recombinational event does not involve a hairpin structure formed by a signal sequence but rather involves the interaction with an enzyme ("recombinase"). We hypothesize that this enzyme occurs in two identical or similar subunits which recognize both components of the consensus sequence on the DNA (Fig. 2). We also assume that the consensus sequence for recombination shown here represents only a subset of a more ubiquitous recombinatinal signal. The purine rich sequences TGAGC (16) which are found in switch regions of immunoglobulins seem to be related to the consensus sequence described here although they miss the characteristic dinucleotide AC. Furthermore it is possible that the proposed sequence is only part of a larger signal. Additional factors may be necessary for a successful recombinational event.

The LTRs of all murine retroviruses sequenced thus far contain the sequences TGAAAGAC and GTCTTTCA in the inverted repeats of U_3 and U_5. They are also similar to the given consensus sequence. Since U_3 and U_5 form the contact points at which a viral DNA circle is closed and integration into the cellular DNA occurs, this sequence might be the signal for the viral enzyme responsible for

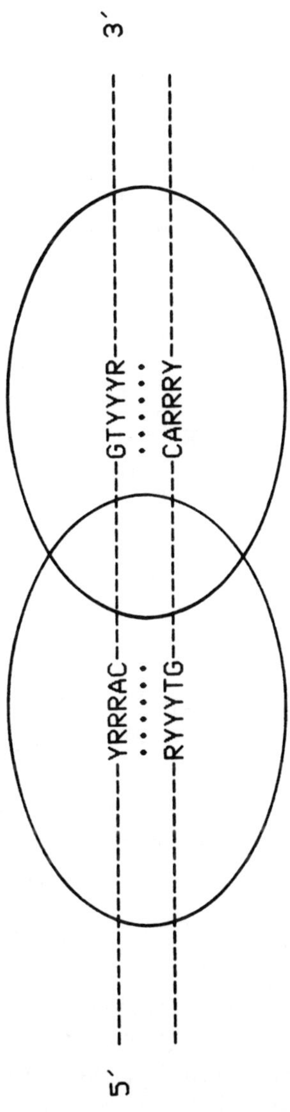

Figure 2. Model of the consensus sequence for recombination and its recognition by two subunits of a "recombinase".

integration (17), which could be related to the recombinase which recognizes the consensus sequence for recombination.

We have not found an unequivocal consensus sequence at the borders of the substitution in the LTR of MCFVs. This suggests a different mechanism for the exchange of genetic material in the LTR during the generation of MCFVs. We have shown earlier that reverse transcription from two different RNA molecules into a single DNA strand can easily occur under in vitro conditions (18). This mechanism could be responsible for the exchange of genetic material in the LTR.

The consensus sequence for recombination presented here confirms that the generation of MCFVs during the onset of leukemia is not an accidental process but rather requires specific mechanisms.

REFERENCES

1. Varmus, H. & Swanstrom, R. (1982) In: RNA Tumor Viruses, 369-512 Cold Spring Harbor, N.Y., USA.
2. Koch, W., Hunsmann, G. & Friedrich, R. (1983) J.Virol. 45, 1-9.
3. Koch, W., Zimmermann, W., Oliff, S. & Friedrich, R. (1984) J. Virol. 49, 828-840.
4. Shinnick, T.M., Lerner, R.A. & Sutcliffe, J.G. (1981) Nature 293, 543-548.
5. Lenz, J., Crowther, R., Stracesci, A. & Haseltine, W. (1982) J. Virol. 42, 519-529.
6. Bosselman R.A., van Straaten, F., van Beveren, C., Verma, I.M. & Vogt, M. (1982) J. Virol. 44, 19-31.
7. Clark, S.P. & Mak, T.W. (1983) Proc. Natl. Acad. Sci. USA 80, 5037-5041.
8. Wunsch, M., Schulz, A.S., Koch, W., Friedrich, R. & Hunsmann, G. (1983) EMBO J. 2, 2239-2246.
9. Chou, P.Y. & Fasman, G.D. (1978) Ann. Rev. Biochem. 47, 251-276.
10. Chotia, C. (1984) Ann. Rev. Biochem. 53; 537-572.

11. Nunberg, J.H., Rodgers, G. Gilbert, J.H. & Snead, R.M. (1984) Proc. Natl. Acad. Sci. USA 81, 3675-3679.
12. Bayer, H., Gruber, W., Schneider, J. & Hunsmann, G. (1984) EMBO J. 3, 1925-1930.
13. Famulari, N.G. (1983) Curr. Top. Mikrobiol. and Immunol. 103, 75-108.
14. Rechavi, G., Givol, D. & Canaani, E. (1982) Nature 300, 607-611.
15. Kuff, E.L., Feenstra, A., Lueders, K., Smith, L., Hawley, R., Hozumi, N. & Shulman, M. (1983) Proc. Natl. Acad. Sci. USA 80, 1992-1996.
16. Shimizu, A. & Honjo, T. (1984) Cell 36, 801-803.
17. Schwartzberg, P., Colicelli, J. & Goff, S.P. (1984) Cell 37, 1043-1052.
18. Novak, U., Friedrich, R. & Moelling, K. (1979) J. Virol. 30, 438-452.
19. Holland, C.A., Wozney, J. & Hopkins, N. (1983) J. Virol. 47, 413-420.
20. Mark, G.E. & Rapp, U.R. (1984) J. Virol. 50, 530-539.
21. Stacey, A., Arbuthnott, C., Kollek, R., Coggins, L. & Ostertag, W. (1984) J. Virol. 50, 725-732.
22. Lebo, R.V., Chakravarti, A., Buetow, K.H., Cheung, M.C., Cann, H. Cordell, B. & Goodman, H. (1983) Proc. Natl. Acad. Sci. USA 80, 4808-4812.
23. Ravetch, J.H., Siebenlist, U., Korsmeyer, S., Waldmann, T. & Leder, P. (1981) Cell 27, 583-591.
24. Max, E.E., Seidman, J.G. & Leder, P. (1979) Proc. Natl. Acad. Sci. USA 76, 3450-3454.

THE MAJOR HISTOCOMPATIBILITY COMPLEX (H-2) OF THE MOUSE INFLUENCES THE PHENOTYPE OF MURINE LEUKEMIA VIRUS-INDUCED LYMPHOMAS

W.L.E. Vasmel[1], M. Zijlstra[1], R.E.Y. de Goede[1], H.J. Schoenmakers[1], T. Radaszkiewics[2], and C.J.M. Melief[1]

1. Central Lab. Blood Transfusion Service and the Lab. of Exp. and Clin. Immunology of the Univ. of Amsterdam, the Netherlands, 2. Institute of Pathology, Vienna, Austria

H-2 congenic C57BL mice were inoculated neonatally with a panel of cloned ecotropic and MCF MuLV isolates. Lymphomas were characterized both for their histology and cell surface marker expression. The results indicate: 1) Synergism exists between ecotropic and MCF viruses in lymphomagenesis. 2) A single ecotropic or dualtropic MCF isolate causes a wide variety of T- and B-cell lymphomas. 3) Within a single mouse strain MuLV induced T-cell lymphomas arise earlier than B-cell lymphomas. 4) The H-2 complex influences lymphoma type. 5) The H-2 complex influences penetration of the thymus by thymotropic MCF virus. 6) These H-2 effects are correlated with H-2 linked differences in the immune responses against both MuLV particles and MuLV-infected cells. A model in which the level of the immune response is one of the main factors determining lymphoma phenotype will be discussed.

Lymphomagenesis induced by murine leukemia virus (MuLV) infection in the mouse provides an experimental model to study the immunological mechanisms involved in virus-induced tumorigenesis. Our investigations have been focused both on the role of the major histocompatibility complex (MHC) of the mouse (H-2 complex) in resistance against MuLV-induced lymphomagnesis (1-4) and on the H-2 influence on the phenotype of the MuLV-induced tumors (1,5,6). The H-2 encoded class I and class II MHC molecules regulate many immunological reactions, including anti-viral antibody responses, gamma interferon production, delayed-type hypersensitivity reactions and the strength and fine specificity of anti-viral cytotoxic T-lymphocyte responses (7).

Initial studies in our and other laboratories indicated a marked influence of the H-2 complex on both anti-MuLV immune responses (2-4, 8) and the resistance against MuLV-induced lymphomagenesis (1,9,10). Moreover, in H-2 congenic C57BL mice which received a milk-transmitted B-ecotropic MuLV a clear H-2 effect on lymphoma type was apparent (1). B10A ($H\text{-}2^a$) mice were most susceptible, had poor anti-viral immune responses and developed predominantly lymphomas of T-cell type, while the lymphomas in the more resistant B12 ($H\text{-}2^b$) strain were chiefly of B- or non-T/non-B cell type (1).

An obvious explanation for this finding would be a difference in the types of MuLV present in these H-2 congenic mice. To exclude this possibility, different host-range classes of MuLV -- ecotropic, dualtropic mink cell focus-inducing (MCF) -- were cloned from a panel of different types of lymphoma (T-, B- or non-T/non-B cell type (5)). Biochemical and immunological analysis indeed indicated extensive polymorphism in the envelope proteins in the cloned viruses, especially in the group of MCF viruses (5). This polymorphism could not be correlated to the types of tumor from which the different MuLV were cloned.

Next, it was of importance to investigate whether a virus isolated from a particular tumor type caused the same type of tumor upon neonatal inoculation. In addition, it was of interest to establish whether a cloned virus caused only one type of tumor or a spectrum of tumors. Both questions were approached by the neonatal inoculation of mice, differing for H-2, with these cloned virus isolates. The lymphomas which arose were characterized with respect to their histology as well as their cell surface markers.

In concordance with the initial observations with the milk-transmitted B-tropic ecotropic MuLV, the inoculation with cloned MuLV induced predominantly T-cell tumors in B10.A ($H-2^a$) mice, and mainly B-cell lymphomas in H+2 congenic B10 ($H-2^b$) mice (6, table 1). A single ecotropic

Table 1. Lymphoma types induced by different host-range classes of C57BL MuLV

Virus	isolated from lymphoma type	B10.A ($H-2^a$)				B10 ($H-2^b$)			
		T	nT/nB	B	mix	T	nT/nB	B	mix
MCF	T	6				3	2	2	2
E-1130	T	1	1						
Mixture		2	2			3			
MCF 1078	T	3						1	
E-1078	T							1	
Mixture		3						5	
MCF 1096	B							2	
E-1096	B								
Mixture		2		1		1		3	
E-1099	B	2	1						

or dualtropic MCF isolate caused a wide variety of T-, B- and non-T/non-B cell lymphomas (6). Furthermore, we noticed that in most cases the tumor incidence was increased by injection of a mixture of ecotropic and MCF virus (6), indicating a synergism in the tumorigenesis between these viruses. Several mechanisms can be involved in this synergism, but most likely recombination of the inoculated ecotropic and dualtropic MuLV with each other or with endogenous MuLV sequences enhances the oncogenic properties of the MuLV. This concept is supported by the finding that the DNA of T-, B- and non-T/non-B cell lymphomas often contains both reintegrated recombined MCF and ecotropic MuLV genomes (unpublished observations).

Another important observation is the fact that within a single mouse strain MuLV-induced T-cell lymphomas arose earlier than B-cell lymphomas. The most likely explanation for this finding is that mice are most susceptible to T-cell lymphomagenesis at an early stage of life, when thymic involution has not yet started. Also in man, a considerable number of acute childhood leukemias are of T-cell origin, whereas the most common adult hemopoietic neoplasia , B-CLL, is of B-cell origin (11).

Thymic penetration by MuLV proved to be inversely correlated with antiviral antibody levels (6). Thus, we suggest that mice with poor anti-viral immune responses undergo strong virus spread at an early age, leading to high level infection of the thymus and subsequently to the predominant development of T-cell lymphomas. H-2 congenic mice which mount better anti-viral immune responses are partly resistant to T-cell lymphomagenesis, but later on develop B-cell lymphomas (5,6). As an alterantive,the H-2 complex may be envisaged to dictate the nature of the immune response to the persistent infection by MuLV and therefore may dictate the pool of transformation-sensitive target cells, assuming that stimulated lymphoid cells are preferential targets for transformation.

REFERENCES

1. Melief, C.J.M., Vlug, A., de Goede, R.E.Y., de Bruyne, C., Barendsen, W. & de Greeve, P. (1980) J. Natl. Cancer Inst. 64, 1179-1189.
2. Vlug, A., Melief, C.J.M., de Bruyne, C., Schoenmakers, H. & Molenaar, J.L. (1980) J. Natl. Cancer Inst. 64, 1191-1198.
3. Vlug, A., Schoenmakers, H. & Melief, C.J.M. (1981) J. Immunol. 126, 2355-2360.
4. Vlug, A., Zijlstra, M., de Goede, R.E.Y., Hesselink, W.G., Schoenmakers, H. & Melief, C.J.M. (1983) Int. J. Cancer 31, 617-626.
5. Zijlstra, M. de Goede, R.E.Y., Schoenmakers, H., Schinkel, A.H., Hesselink, W.G., Portis, J.L., & Melief, C.J.M. (1983). Virology 125, 47-63.
6. Zijlstra, M., de Goede, R.E.Y., Schoenmakers, H., Radaszkiewicz, T. & Melief, C.J.M. (1984) Virology, in press.
7. Klein, J., Juretic, A., Baxevanis, C.W. & Nagy, Z.A. (1981). Nature (London) 291, 455-460.
8. Debré, P., Boyer, B., Gisselbrecht, S., Bismuth, A. & Levy, J.P. (1980) Eur. J. Immunol. 10, 914-918.
9. Lonai, P., Katz, E. & Haran-Ghera, N. (1982) Springer Semin. Immunopathol. 4, 373-396.
10. Meruelo, D. & Bach, R. (1983) Adv. Cancer Res. 40, 107-188.
11. Lennert, K. (1978) Malignant Lymphomas, Springer, New York.

MOUSE MAMMARY TUMOR VIRUS (MMTV) MORPHOLOGY IN THE GASTROINTESTINAL LUMEN OF SUCKLING MICE

G. Bevilacqua and A. Marchetti

Institute of Pathological Anatomy and Histology, University of Pisa, Pisa, Italy.

How the milk transmitted MMTV enters the organism is unclear. The site of entrance might be the epithelial cells of the enteric mucosa or the plaques of Peyer. The only ultrastructural study reported to date did not show viruses in the intestinal wall and hypothesized the absorption of a very small quantity of them. The electron microscopy study of the stomach and the small bowel of 8- to 10-day-old BALB/cfRIII suckling mice revealed some morphological changes of the B particles. Some of these changes were obtained in vitro by several means: swelling, breakage, bursting and the consequent release of nucleoids with angular profiles, dense cores, and the tendency to aggregate. Moreover, "head and tail" forms appear frequently as well as smaller B particles, with a diameter of about 800 A. These findings might be the expression of the denaturation of the B particles due to digestion or, at least in part, might represent a step in the absorption process of the MMTV.

The Mouse Mammary Tumor Virus (MMTV) is milk transmitted from mother to offspring in strains of mice with a high incidence of mammary tumors. The site of entrance of the MMTV is unknown; it might penetrate through the epithelial cells of the enteric mucosa or through the M cells of the plaques of Peyer, as suggested for some reoviruses (1). However, the presence of the virus has not been demonstrated in blood or tissues during the first days of life. Studies employing the noduligenic test, a technique based on the property of MMTV to induce noduligenesis after inoculation in susceptible mice, have demonstrated the presence of viral activity in the blood after about two weeks of life (2). Lymphocytes bearing high levels of MMTV antigen expression might play a role as carrier of the virus (3).

In a previous study an attempt to find viral particles by electron microscopy in the intestinal wall of suckling newborn mice was unsuccessful, and the authors suggested that a very small portion of B particles passes through the wall and is then distributed in the body in a soluble form (4). This hypothesis may be supported by the observation that there is a direct relation between incidence of mammary tumors and duration of nursing, in spite of the high viral content of the milk. The denaturation of most of the virus might explain this finding (5).

During initial electron microscopy studies on MMTV absorption in the small bowel of suckling mice our attention was drawn by some morphological changes of the MMTV particles present in the lumen of the stomach and small bowel.

Eight 8- to 10-day-old BALB/cfRIII suckling mice nursed by mothers at about the 6th pregnancy were used in order to obtain a high content of MMTV in the milk. It is known that the RIII variant of the MMTV is produced in a higher quantity than the C3H variant and that the virus release increases with the number of pregnancies (6). The stomach and the small bowel were fixed for 10 min. in glutaraldehyde or in Karnovsky's fixative immediately after removal and then sectioned. The milk found in the lumen and thin slices of the walls were fixed again for about 80 min. in glutaraldehyde or 3 hr. in Karnovsky's fixative. Fragments of about 1 mm^3 were postfixed in OsO_4

for 60 min, dehydrated, and embedded in Epon-Araldite. Thin sections were stained with lead citrate and uranile acetate and observed in a Siemens Elmiskop 1A electron microscope at 75 kV.

Based on their morphology, the B particles present in the gastrointestinal lumen usually can be assigned to one of the following groups:

1) A swollen particle with a broken envelope. Breakage occurs as a small breach, usually in an area close to the nucleoid (Fig. 1 a, b).

2) A swollen particle and burst envelope with breakage occuring at the side opposite the nucleoid. The appearance resembles a comet, with a well-defined head and a large, vaguely defined tail (Fig. 1c).

3) A swollen elongated particle with an extremely eccentric nucleoid;the envelope adheres tightly to the nucleoid. The result is an image of a "signet-ring B particle" (Fig. 2 a,b,c). The contact surface between envelope and nucleoid extends until the envelope almost entirely covers the nucleoid, giving origin to the characteristic "head and tail B particle" forms (Fig. 2 d,e,f). The neck between the head and the tail may become very thin.

4) The particle may appear as a round particle of about 850 A in which the nucleoid is tightly covered with a very adherent envelope (Fig. 2g), as though the tail had been detached following an extreme thinning of the neck. Of course, the possibility that the cutting plane passed only through the head, saving the tail, must also be considered.

5) Numerous nude nucleoids are present and frequently aggregate (Fig. 1 d,e). They show a clear angular profile and an electron dense central core (Fig. 1e, inset). They have a diameter of about 700 A, while the core measures about 400 A.

Some of these findings have been extensively obtained in vitro. "Head and tail" forms have been observed in a pH range between 5 and 8 (7) and their occurrence has been ascribed to conditions of high osmotic strength (8). B

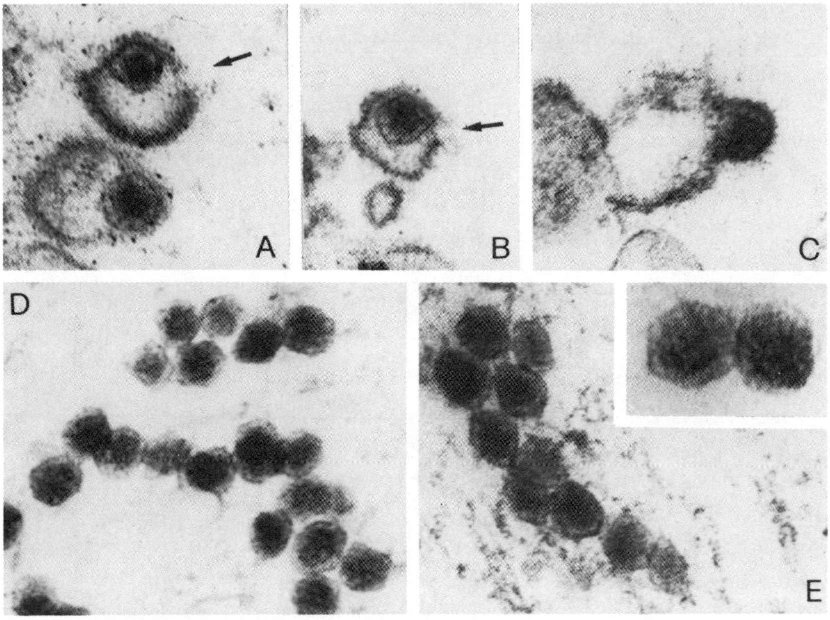

Fig. 1. a,b: arrows indicate a breach in the envelope of B particles; c: the envelope of a B particle bursts, with a comet-like image; d,e: nude nucleoids with a clear angular profile. (x 130,000; inset x 220,000)

particles have been ruptured by means of non-ionic detergents and their nucleoids isolated (9); the nude nucleoids showed a strong tendency to aggregate (10), had angular profiles, and a dense core (9).

The findings observed in the gastrointestinal lumen of suckling mice may be viewed as the result of denaturation of the B particles, a mere consequence of digestion, or as processes involved in the formation of particles that may be more easily absorbed. The MMTV has never been seen entering the intestinal cells, but the following three modes of penetration may be reasonably supposed: a) the B

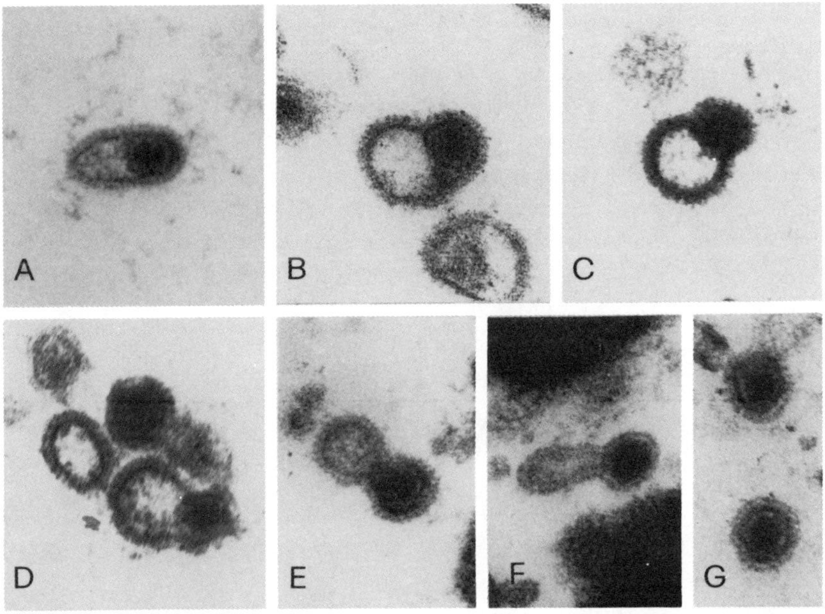

Fig. 2. a: an elongated B particle; b,c: B particles with swelling of the envelope and extreme eccentricity of the nucleoid ("signet-ring" particles); d,e,f: "head and tail" forms; g: small B particles of about 850 Å. (x 130,000)

particle may be captured whole by a cytoplasmic vacuole; b) the B particle may adhere to the cell surface, its envelope may fuse with the plasma membrane, and the nucleoid may be released into the cells; c) the nude nucleoid may be captured by a cytoplasmic vacuole. If the last hypothesis is true, the rupture of the envelopes of the B particles with the release of the nucleoids might be a crucial event. However, isolated nucleoids obtained in vitro did not prove infective when inoculated into susceptible mice (10). On the other hand, if the B particle penetrates as a whole, a reduction of its volume might be useful and this might occur with the loss of a part of the envelope, such as the "tail", and the resulting formation of smaller B particles. Moreover, the adherence of the envelope to the nucleoid might facilitate a hypothetical fusion with the plasma membrane and the subsequent release of the nucleoid.

On the basis of the findings described here, some morphological changes of the MMTV previously obtained in vitro seem to take place consistently in vivo in the gastrointestinal lumen of newborn BALB/cfRIII mice. These changes may have a role in the absorption process of MMTV. Clarification of the exact sequence of events involved in the absorption of this virus await documentation of the entrance of a MMTV particle into an intestinal cell.

REFERENCES

1. Wolf, J.L., Kauffman, R.S., Finberg, R., Dambrauskas, R., Fields, B.N., & Trier, J.S. (1983) Gastroenterology 85, 291-300.
2. Nandi, S. & McGrath, C.M. (1973) Adv. Cancer Res. 17, 353-414.
3. Dickson, C. & Peters, G. (1983) Curr. Top. Microbiol. Immunol. 106, 1-34.
4. Tanaka, H. & Tsujimura, D. (1967) Annu. Rep. Ist. Virus. Res. 10, 94-100.
5. Moore, D.H., Long, C.A., Vaidya, A.B., Sheffield, J.B., Dion, A.S., & Lasfargues, E.Y. (1979) Adv. Cancer Res. 29, 347-418.
6. Squartini, F., Pingitore, R. & Bistocchi, M. (1980) in Breast Cancer: new concepts in etiology and control, eds. Brennan M.J., McGrath C.M. & Rich M.A. (Academic Press, New York).
7. Sarkar, N.H., Moore, D.H. & Charney, J. (1973) Cancer Res. 33, 2283-2290.
8. Sarkar, N.H., Manthey, W.J. & Sheffield, J.B. (1975) Cancer Res. 35, 740-749.
9. Teramoto, Y.A., Cardiff, R.D., & Lund, J.K. (1977) Virology 77, 135-148.
10. Sarkar, N.H., Nowinsky, R.C. & Moore, D.H. (1971) Virology 46, 1-20.

MURINE RETROVIRUSES: AN ALTERNATIVE SCREENING APPROACH FOR ANTIVIRAL DRUG RESEARCH.

O. Muratore.

Institute of Microbiology, School of Medicine, Viale Benedetto XV, 10, 16132 Genova, Italy.

The development of antivirals reached "the end of the beginning" in 1980, a phrase used by Collier to summarize the intensive and cumbersome research work carried out in the previous 40 years (1). Currently there are a few antiviral agents generally accepted as efficacious. But the emergence of new problems, such as non-A and non-B hepatitis and acquired immuno-deficiency syndrome (AIDS), life-threatening infections in patients that are immunocompromised as a result of cancer therapy or organ transplantation, may require the need to increase research towards the control of viral diseases. Recently several authors have demonstrated that suramin, a drug used in the therapy of trypanosomiasis, known to inhibit the reverse transcriptase of several animal retroviruses (2), can be used to protect human T cells in vitro against infectivity and cytopathic effect of HTLV-III (3,4). Studies have begun to see if this drug and 21-tungsto-9-antimonate (HPA 23), a polyoxotungstate known for its ability to protect mice against lethal retroviral infections, can be administered to AIDS patients (5).

The observations of structural homologies between retroviruses and hepatitis B virus (6,); the recent identification of a retroviral marker in the non-A and non-B hepatitis (7); the isolation of the first human tumor virus (HTLV-I) from several hematological neoplasias of man (8) and the demonstration of a retroviral etiology in AIDS (9,10) have re-evaluated the clinical importance of retroviruses. All mammalian retroviruses require reverse transcriptase, a unique RNA-dependent DNA-polymerase, for replication (11, 12). By means of horizontal infection, the retroviral genome is integrated into the host chromosome. Reverse transcriptases of animal and human retroviruses have similar amino acid sequences (6, 13).

The epidemiological significance, the knowledge of viral replication and the presence of a unique polymerase candidate the retroviruses as an alternative screening approach for antiviral drug studies. In studying the effect of steroid hormones on various stages of the murine retrovirus replication (14), we have evaluated several parameters of the viral assays including cell plating and kinetics, media and chemical concentration, cytotoxicity, viral multiplicity of infection, antigen expression, polymerase activity and progeny production (Muratore O., in preparation).

The peculiar characteristics of the cell-virus-drug system are critical in the evaluation of the activity of antiviral synthetic compounds. Drug cytotoxicity, viral cytopathic effects and tests used are important in the assessement of antiviral activity. Drug cytotoxicity must be carefully determined for each cell line and for each compound. The cytotoxic effect of a drug may be detectable only after several days in culture. Thus short-term assays may give false indications of antiviral activity. This is the case of CA1; 3 days after infection, 10 ug/ml of CA-1 gave up to 200 fold reduction of the Friend virus titer, while cytotoxic alteration of the mouse SC-1 cell monolayer became apparent after 4 days in culture.

Several prototype strains of murine ecotropic and xenotropic retroviruses were used to determine the antiviral activity of different compounds. We have previously shown that this system can be used to evaluate

Table 1. Recovery of PFA resistant murine retrovirus strains

VIRUS STRAIN	PFA (uM)	VIRAL TITER[1]	REDUCTION (X)[2]	R.T. ACTIVITY[3]	INHIBITION (%)
AKR-4wt	-	5.47	-	221050	0
wild type	5	ND	ND	70350	68.2
	500	4.53	7.7	0	100
	1000	4.26	15.2	0	100
AKR-4mrt	-	5.99	-	245500	0
resistant	5	ND	ND	190300	22.5
	500	5.54	1.8	2600	98.9
	1000	5.50	2.1	150	99.9
MoLV-2wt	-	5.26	-	41000	0
wild type	2.5	ND	ND	24600	40
	5	ND	ND	17750	56.7
	500	4.30	8.1	0	100
	1000	2.71	354.0	0	100
MoLV-2mrt	-	5.21	-	55900	0
resistant	2.5	ND	ND	53450	4.4
	5	ND	ND	37650	32.6
	500	4.65	2.6	0	100
	1000	3.32	77.0	0	100

Virus infectivity was determined by: 1. The XC plaque assay (Log10 PFU/ml) and 3. Reverse Transcriptase (R.T.) assay (cpm/ml). Reduction values were calculated as follows : X = PFU/ml(-CA1) - PFU/ml(+CA1) / PFU/ml(+CA1). ND = Not Done.

the specific antiviral effect of trisodium phosphonoformate (PFA) (15,16), and coumermycin A1 (CA1) (17,18). CA1, at the non-cytotoxic concentration of 5 ug/ml, has a minimal but reproducible antiviral effect on murine retrovirus infectivity and replication (17). PFA is a more effective inhibitor.

Microorganisms can undergo genetic mutation, and in the process acquire specific resistance to antimicrobials, causing serious clinical problems. Resistant viruses that arise in this way modify viral products which can then influence the mode of action of a drug. Such resistant viral mutants emerge in tissue culture after only one or two passages in the presence of an inhibiting agent, apparently retaining their pathogenic properties (19).The detection of these resistant variants not only provides evidence that an inhibiting agent possesses a specific antiviral effect and does not act on host functions (17), but also suggests that clinical problems of resistance may arise in the future also for human retroviruses (16).

These facts prompted us to investigate the in vitro emergence of resistant mutants after exposure of a wild type viral population to PFA. Different strains of murine ecotropic retroviruses, which are sensitive to PFA (500-1000 uM), were inoculated into SC-1 cells as previously described (16,17). After one passage, the viral titers were diminished, in particular that of the MoLV-2 isolate (Table 1). After two passages the sensitivities of both AKR and Moloney isolates were significantly reduced. Virus propagation in the presence of 1000 uM of PFA revealed significant resistance; in particular the effect of PFA on the MoLV-2 strain decreased from a 355 to a 24 fold reduction in the viral progeny (16).

In order to give more insight into the mechanism of the antiviral activity of CA-1, we have investigated the effect of the drug on the replication of eight different ecotropic retroviruses, and we have identified one CA1 resistant strain, AKR-3, while two other virus strains tested were highly sensitive to the drug (18). These observations could suggest a specific antiviral activity of CA1; the drug may act on both cellular and viral targets (20,21).

Different antiviral compounds may act on different components of viral replication so that their contemporary use could give a synergystic antiviral effect. Our preliminary experiments indicate that the combination of CA1 and PFA results in at least an additive antiviral effect in the absence of increased toxicity (data not shown).

Further studies are needed to increase the efforts towards the understanding of the antiviral activity of the available compounds.

ACKNOWLEDGEMENTS

This work was supported by CNR grants N. 84.01841, 84.00838 and 84.02327.

REFERENCES

1. Collier, L.H. & Oxford, J. (Eds) (1980) Developments in Antiviral Therapy Academic Press, London.
2. De Clecq, E. (1979) Cancer Lett. 8,9-22.
3. Mitsuya, H., Popovic, M., Yarchoan, R., Matsushita, S., Gallo, R.C., Broder, S. (1984) Science 226:172-174.
4. Broder, S. & Gallo, R.C. (1984) New Engl. J. Med. 311:1292-1297.
5. Rozenbaum, W., Dormont, D., Spire, B., Vilmem, E., Gentilini, P., Griscelli, C., Montaigner, L., Barre-Sinoussi, F., Chermann, J.C., (1985) Lancet i:450.

6. Toh, H., Hayashida, H., Miyata, T. (1983) Nature 305:827-829.
7. Seto, B., Coleman, W.G., Jr, Iwarson, S., Gerety, R.J. (1984) Lancet: 941-943.
8 . Gallo, R.C., Reitz, M.S. Jr. (1982) J. Natl. Cancer Inst. 69:1209
9. Gallo, R.C., et al. (1983) Science 220:865-867.
10. Barre-Sinoussi, F., Chermann, J.C., Rey, F., Nugeire, M.T., Chamaret, S., Gruest, J., Dauguet, C., Axler-Blin, C., Vezinet-Brun, F., Rouzioux, C., Rozenbaum, W., Montagnier, L.. (1983) Science 220:868-871.
11. Baltimore, D. (1970) Nature 226 1209-1210.
12. Temin, H.M., Mizutani, S. (1970) Nature 226:1211-1213.
13. Patarca, R., Haseltine, W.A., (1984) Nature 30:728.
14. Varnier, O.E., and Levy, J.A. (1979) Virology 96:604-614.
15. Varnier, O.E., Repetto, C.M., Raffanti, S.P., Carloni, G. (1982) Microbiologica 5:137-141.
16. Muratore, O., Varnier, O.E., Raffanti, S.P., Schito, G.C. (1984) Eur. J. Clin. Microb. 3:447-449.
17. Varnier, O.E., Muratore, O., Raffanti, S.P., Melioli, G., Palu', G., Schito, G.C. (1984) J. Antim. Chemoth. 14:139-147.
18. Varnier, O.E., Muratore, O., Raffanti, S.P., Schito, G.C. (1984) Microbiologica in press.
19 . Hermann, E.C., Jr, Hermann, J.A. (1977) Ann. New York Acad. Sci. 284:632-637
20. Palu', G., Von Berger, J., Meloni, G.A., Masotti, L. (1984) Biochem. Pharmacol 33:147-154.
21. Francke, B., Margolin, J. (1981) J. Gen. Virol. 52:401-404.

2. Retroviruses and the Vertebrate Model System

RETROVIRUSES AND ONCOGENES IN RATS

S. Rasheed

University of Southern California School of Medicine, 1840 North Soto Street, Los Angeles, Calif., 90032.

Endogenous retroviral genes are present in all rat species including the feral rats. This virus, termed RaLV, is produced spontaneously in cultures or after treatment of cells in vitro by various chemical or physical agents. The RaLV replicates to low levels in rat cells but does not cause tumors in experimentally inoculated rats. We have isolated an acutely transforming rat sarcoma virus (RaSV) by in vitro cocultivation of RaLV productive cells with that of chemically induced tumor cultures. Unlike the previously isolated murine sarcoma viruses that are hybrids of mouse virus and cellular ras gene, the RaSV contains exclusively rat derived sequences (i.e. rat virus and ras gene). The RaSV transformed nonproducer cells produce a protein of 29,000 daltons which is distinct from all other ras oncogene encoded products in that it is synthesized as a gag-ras fusion product. Thus, the rat-cell-rat-endogenous-virus system that we have established offers a unique model to study the interaction between the endogenous virogenes and cellular genes at various stages of tumor development.

Retroviruses are ubiquitous and like other vertebrates the genomes of all rats, including the wild rats contain genetic information to produce mature C-type particles

(1-7). Although aberrant forms of C-type retroviruses have been noted in some rat tissues, no A,B or D-type of morphologic forms have yet been observed in rat cells. The rat C-type particles are called the rat leukemia viruses (RLV), although none has yet been shown to cause leukemia or other tumors in exogenously infected newborn rats or mice (1,2). However, the term RaLV is consistent with the nomenclatures of similar morphologic forms of avian and other murine retroviruses that are known to cause leukemia and lymphoma in those species.

In nature retroviruses are transmitted both vertically through the germ line (endogenous) and horizontally as exogenous infectious agents. The retroviruses of rats however, fall into only one category (i.e. those that are transmitted via the germ line). No horizontally transmitting retrovirus is known in rats. The rat endogenous virus is occasionally produced spontaneously in long term cell cultures or can be induced from the normal rat cellular DNA by treatment with halogenated pyrimidines or other chemical and physical agents (2-6). Although several RaLV strains have been isolated from the rat tumors, none has been shown to induce any pathology in experimental animals. These retroviruses therefore, have remained largely unexplored because of their low or no infectivity in vitro or in vivo. Several years ago we isolated endogenous RaLVs from rat embryo cultures that were infectious to other rat cells in vitro. These viruses provided a useful resource to study their various biologic, immunologic and biochemical properties and to study interactions between the endogenous virogenes and cellular genes in an homologous environment (i.e. rat viruses in rat cells). In this article I will summarize the major findings in rat type C virology including the genesis of the first biologically active rat sarcoma virus in vitro and a history of viral transforming genes (oncogenes) isolated from various rat strains.

THE RAT LEUKEMIA VIRUS

Although one of the most important features of retroviruses is that they occur in nature as stably integrated proviral DNA within the host cellular genome, the host-cell-tropism has played a major role in defining and classifying many avian and mammalian retroviruses. Despite the occasional isolations of the rat C-type viruses from various rat tissues including the wild rat tumors (2), it has been difficult to study the biological or biochemical properties of these viruses because they were not infectious in vitro or tumor-causing in vivo. In 1976 (1) we isolated C-type retroviruses from embryo cultures of two different rat strains, Sprague-Dawley (SD) and Fischer (Fi) (see Table 1). The endogenous RaLVs released spontaneously from these rat embryo cultures, exhibited classical properties of retroviruses, contained high levels of reverse transcriptase activity and RaLV specific major structural proteins (1). These viruses furnished material and reagents to study their virologic, biologic and biochemical properties which are discussed in the following sections.

The physical, chemical and electron microscopic data on RaLV genome are consistent with other mammalian retroviruses. The mature virion is about 90-100 nm in diameter and is released from the plasma membrane as a budding C-type particle with an electron dense central nucleoid. In a sucrose density gradient the rat viruses show a buoyant density of 1.14 - 1.15 g/ml (1). The viral genome consists of a single stranded linear 70S RNA species with a molecular weight of about 8.6×10^6 daltons. Similar to other mammalian retroviruses, the dissociated virion RNA can be seen by electron microscopy as two identical 35S molecules that are linked by a y-shaped structure involving base pairing near the 5' ends (S. Rasheed and R. Junghans, unpublished data).

The genome of a replication competent RaLV strain consists of three genes, the gag, the pol and the env, encoding the major virion structural proteins, the reverse

Table 1. Properties of Rat Leukemia Virus

1. C-Type particles budding from plasma membrane.
2. Endogenous: multiple copies of RaLV-related sequences in the genomes of both laboratory and feral rat strains.
3. Inducible by halogenated pyrimidines or other chemicals.
4. Spontaneously released in some long term embryo or tumor-derived cell cultures.
5. Viral genome ssRNA: contains reverse transcriptase and structural proteins.
6. Does not replicate in any of the known mammalian and avian cells. Poorly infectious in cells of origin i.e. ecotropic.
7. Not tumorigenic in vivo although in vitro transforming potential in long term cultures has been reported for rare strains.
8. Only one strain (SD-RaLV) known to transduce cellular transforming ras gene in vitro in the form of a stable rat sarcoma.

transcriptase and the envelope glycoproteins respectively (Fig. 1). The gag proteins are 5' -p15-pp12-p27-p10 3' and the env proteins are 5' gp70 - p15E-3'. The replication competent RaLVs also contain a reverse transcriptase enzyme which preferentially utilizes Mn++ in both the endogenous and exogenous reactions using the template primer poly (rA) oligo (dT) (1,2). However, because it is difficult to purify large quantities of RaLV reverse transcriptase, its biochemical properties have not been categorically defined although its molecular weight is expected to be in the same range as other mammalian retroviruses (i.e., 80-100,000 daltons).

The host range of rat C-type viruses is very restricted and most RaLV strains do not replicate well in vitro or in vivo. The SD- and Fi-RaLV strains that we

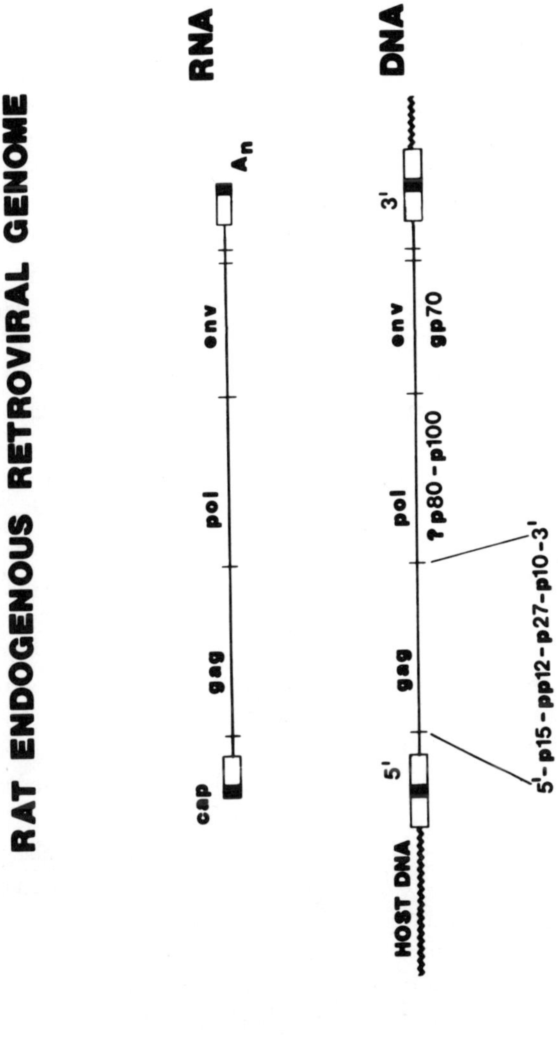

Figure 1. Rat endogenous retroviral RNA and integrated proviral DNA in the cellular genome.

isolated from SD and Fi rats respectively, are capable of replicating in exogenously infected cells from a variety of rat strains including the wild rat (1,2). However, none of the human, other primate, dog, cat, mouse, guinea pig, rabbit, or mink cells tested are susceptible to the infections with these viruses as measured by the presence of supernatant reverse transcriptase activity or the group specific (gs) antigen in the cell sonicates. Thus, the SD- and Fi-RaLV strains grow only in the rat cells and are therefore ecotropic. The wild rat leukemia virus (WR-RaLV) is also similar to other rat viruses and replicates only in the rat embryo cultures albeit to a much lower level than SD-RaLV (2).

The rat C-type viruses are neutralized by antisera made against RaLV but not by any of the antisera made against several mouse, cat or primate retroviruses. In contrast to the mouse viruses, RaLV strains isolated from rat embryo cultures, and chemically induced or spontaneous rat tumors, did not exhibit any type specific antigenic differences on the p12 or gp70 proteins (1,2). By the use of antisera made against whole disrupted virus, none of the RaLV strains tested showed any significant difference in the neutralization kinetics or interference patterns.

The cell free extracts from virus productive cells react in complement fixation tests with antiserum to the major structural core protein of RaLV (p27), but not with antisera to murine, feline, hamster and primate p30 proteins (1,2) By radioimmunoassays using highly specific antisera against isoelectric focus purfied major structural proteins of RaLV, and other murine, feline and primate viruses, some interspecies cross reactivity was detected with hamster and feline leukemia viruses but not with any other mammalian virus (1,2,8).

To define any possible structural difference in gag and env proteins of the various RaLV strains, we analyzed the major structural proteins of the RaLV isolates from Sprague-Dawley (SD), Osborne-Mendel (OM), Fischer (Fi) and feral (out-bred) rat strains. Two-dimensional trypsin-digested peptides of p27, p10 and p15 showed very similar if not identical maps for each of these respective proteins in SD-, OM-, and Fi-RaLVs (S. Rasheed and J. Lingua, unpublished observations). Analysis of a 65,000 (p65) virion protein and mixed maps of hydrolyzed radioiodinated p27 and p65 indicated peptides that were shared between the two suggesting a precursor-product relationship, similar to that described for the mouse leukemia viruses (MuLVs). Thus, in contrast to the numerous MuLV strains of both the laboratory (in-bred) and feral (out-bred) mice that can be distinguished by variations in their gag and env proteins, different strains of rat endogenous viruses cannot be separated by their major structural proteins.

Similar to other replication competent retroviruses, the RaLVs can rescue murine or feline sarcoma virus (MSV or FeSV) genomes from MSV or FeSV transformed nonproducer cell lines respectively. The pseudotype viruses produce foci in rat cells but not in mouse cells and the focus induction can be inhibited by an anti-RaLV serum (1,2).

One of the rare features of the Sprague-Dawley rat-cell-endogenous-RaLV system which distinguishes it from several other mammalian cell culture systems is the finding that the spontaneous release of endogenous SD-RALV in early passage SD-embryo cultures (passage 10-13) is associated with the transformation of the same cultures at higher passages (passages 40-50) (1,9). This was an unusual phenomenon for the rat cells because despite the frequent use of rat cultures in a number of laboratories, the release of RaLV or associated transformation was not described prior to our report (1). Infection of other rat embryo cells with SD-RaLV from high passage cultures also transformed cells but only after 40-50 passages -- i.e. after 6-7 months of virus replication (9). Moreover, exposure of SD-RaLV infected rat cells to chemical carcinogens accelerated the transformation of these cells in vitro and treatment of SD-RaLV specific antisera delayed the transformation of endogenously infected SD cultures for up to 6 months (9,10). Thus, the endogenous RaLV appears to be a critical determinant of transformation in an exogenously infected rat embryo culture.

Although most RaLV strains appear to be serologically identical, by molecular hybridization approximately 70 to 90% homology was detected among the RNAs of various RaLV strains tested. Also, about 70 to 80% of SD-RaLV RNA hybridizes to DNA from various rat strains but not with the DNAs of mouse or cat species (1). In addition to the numerous copies of RaLV-related sequences in the rat DNA, there are multiple copies of DNA sequences homologous to a unique 30S RNA, in rat cells (11,12). These sequences are defective for replication and are not related to the known retrovirus RNAs. However, the 30S RNAs resemble viruses in that they can be induced by treatment of cells with halogenated pyrimidines and packaged by a replication competent retrovirus in exogenously infected rat cells (12). The first indication that 30S RNA can be rescued and recombined with other helper retroviral or cellular genes came from the studies of two MSV strains that were isolated by serial passages of different MuLV-induced leukemia-lymphoma extracts in separate rat strains. These viruses, designated as Harvey and Kirsten strains of MSV (Ha-MSV and Ki-MSV respectively), have since been shown to be recombinants of mouse MuLV, rat 30S RNA and a rat cellular gene called ras. Although the significance of 30S RNA in sarcoma viruses is not clear, it is possible they play a role in the genetic recombination of the replicating MuLV with those of the cellular ras genes (12,13,14).

GENERATION OF THE RAT SARCOMA VIRUS

Two kinds of viruses are involved in oncogenesis: a) the acute transforming viruses that contain transforming genes, induce rapid cell transformation in vitro and cause various neoplasia including sarcoma in vivo; and b) the chronic transforming viruses that usually do not contain oncogenic sequences but cause leukemias and other lymphoproliferative diseases by various mechanisms after a long latent period. Research advances in the last decade have revealed that most of the acutely transforming viruses have arisen by recombination of the endogenous viruses of low or no pathogenicity and discrete subsets of highly conserved cellular genes called oncogenes or onc. Nucleotide sequences related to all known retroviral oncogenes have now been found in the DNAs of normal vertebrates and also some remotely unrelated species such as Drosophila and yeast (13-18). Thus, the analyses of oncogenes and their normal cellular homologues provide us with a better understanding of their roles in cancer as well as in the normal cellular development.

Although both the acutely and chronically transforming retroviruses have been isolated directly from several naturally occurring avian, murine, feline and primate host tumors, no oncogene carrying acutely transforming virus or that capable of causing leukemia after a long latent period, has yet been identified directly from a naturally occurring rat tumor. As indicated earlier only two sarcoma viruses have been isolated by long term passages of two different MuLV isolates in separate rat strains (19,20). The genomes of both of these viruses, termed Harvey and Kirsten mouse sarcoma viruses (Ha- and Ki-MSV respectively), are recombinants of mouse viral genes, rat 30S RNA and distinct rat cellular genes of the ras family (13,14). In 1978, we isolated a rapid fibroblast transforming rat sarcoma virus (RaSV) by in vitro cocultivation of an SD-RaLV productive rat culture with chemically transformed rat tumor cells (21). In contrast to Ha-MSV and Ki-MSV which are hybrids of mouse and rat genetic material, the RaSV contains exclusively rat-derived sequences, i.e., endogenous RaLV genes and the rat cellular genes. Thus, this experiment was the first example to demonstrate that the rat cellular gene ras could be recombined, packaged and transferred to another host cell in the form of an acutely transforming retrovirus (21,22).

Although a mouse and a chicken oncogene (23,24) have

been similarly rescued in vitro since our report of RaSV isolation, transduction of a cellular oncogene in vitro by a retrovirus remains an extremely rare phenomenon. Furthermore, although initially we reported the isolation of RaSV from three different chemically transformed and one polyoma virus transformed rat tumor cells (22), the rescuability from these cells was random (except for the rescue of RaSV from a culture of 4-Nitroquinoline oxide (NQ) transformed tumor cells, which was highly reproducible). Also, within a particular rat cell-rat virus system the viral and cellular sequences are more conducive to genetic recombination than in others (21,22). For example, the cellular transforming gene was not rescued when the same chemically transformed cells that had yielded RaSV were cocultivated with cultures producing other RaLV strains. Also, we were unable to rescue any oncogene when these rat tumor cells were similarly cocultivated with several other strains of replication competent murine, feline and primate retroviruses (MuLV, FeLV, RD114 and Baboon endogenous virus (BaEV)) (2). Moreover, we also tested a new RaLV strain (SG-RaLV) from a spontaneous tumor (Sarcoma Galliera-SG) that was passaged in the same rat strain (Rattus norvegicus Galliera strain) for more than 60 years (25). A transforming virus was not isolated from this tumor nor were the transforming genes rescued by SG-RaLV from various chemically or spontaneously transformed rat tumors that had yielded RaSV (22,25). However, our preliminary experiments indicate that the DNA of this spontaneous SG tumor is transfectable on NIH 3T3 mouse cells. Analysis of the DNA from SG transformed foci is now underway to identify the dominant gene/s that may be involved in the expression of this tumor but may not be rescuable by the replicating SG-RaLV. These results suggest that the ability of a retrovirus to rescue endogenous transforming genes may not depend on the passage history of the virus but perhaps accounts for the presence of unique sequences in the replicating virus that may favor the genetic recombination and generate highly oncogenic viruses.

PROPERTIES OF THE RAT SARCOMA VIRUS

The in vitro generated virus has been designated as the Rasheed strain of the rat sarcoma virus (RaSV) (16). This is an acutely transforming retrovirus that rapidly transforms rat cells in vitro and causes fibrosarcomas in rats (Table 2)(21, 22, 26). Similar to the oncogenes of all known mammalian sarcoma viruses, the RaSV oncogene (termed Ra-v-ras) is defective for replication and propagates by the use of its natural RaLV helper virus genes. Since RaLV does not replicate in any non-rat cell culture, the wild type RaSV (RaLV) also does not directly transform other mammalian cells. However, this virus readily transforms several mammalian cells including human cultures if a pseudotype virus is produced by the rescue of the defective RaSV genome by replication competent amphotropic MuLV, FeLV or BaEV (22).

Molecular cloning of RaSV provirus indicates that the transforming gene of RaSV (i.e. Ra-v-ras) is related to the cellular gene ras that is present in Ha-MSV but is distinct from that which has recombined to form Ki-MSV (27). In contrast to Ha-MSV or Ki-MSV transformed cells that express a 21,000 dalton protein (p21), the RaSV transformed cells express a protein of 29,000 daltons (p20) (22,28,29). This distinction was first recognized when an antiserum to p21 protein of Ha-MSV immunoprecipitated p29 from the RaSV transformed non-producer cells but the sera from RaSV tumor bearing rats did not immunoprecipitate p21 of Ha-MSV (28). Also, antiserum to whole disrupted RaLV also immunoprecipitated p29 from various extracts of RaSV transformed cells but did not recognize p21 protein from Ha-MSV transformed cells. Thus, there was a one-way cross-reaction of p29 with the ras induced p21 protein. To determine which RaLV-related protein was present in Ra-v-ras, we used antisera to various RaLV gag and env protens to immunoprecipitate RaSV transforming p29 protein. Antiserum to RaLV gag-p15, but not those made against other RaLV structural protein (p27, p12, p10 and gp70),

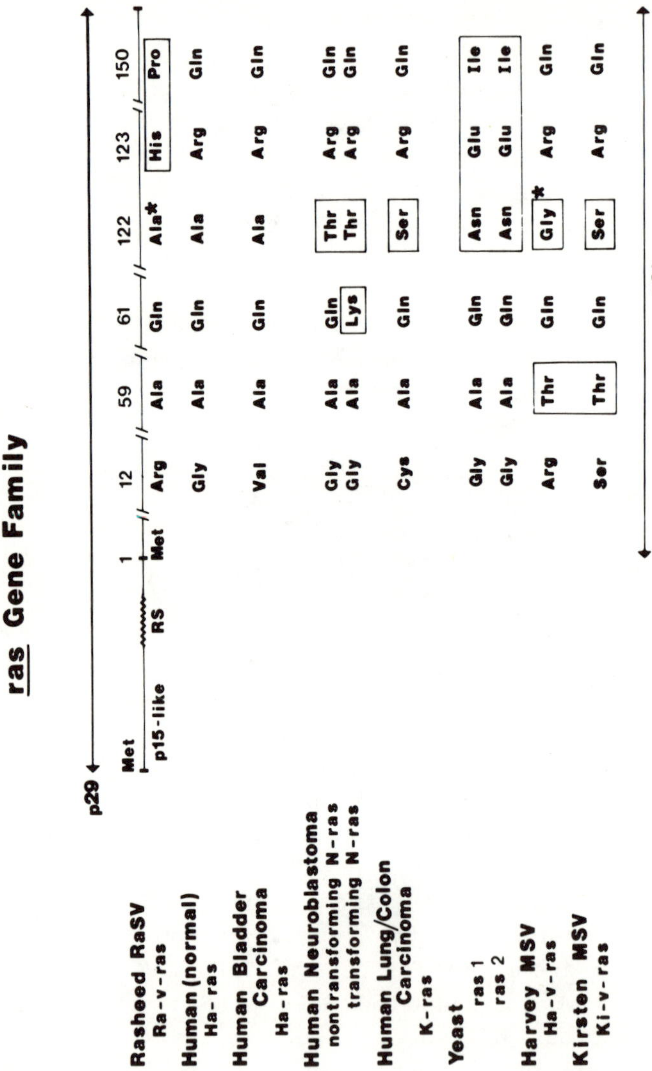

Figure 2. Comparison of the amino acid residues of the known ras genes at selected positions of interest. Shaded amino acids at position 12 indicates a change from the normal (nontransforming) glycine residue. Boxed amino acids at other positions indicate differences from concensus residue found at that position. Sequence data from (17, 18, 31, 34, 36).

immunoprecipitated p29, suggesting that the transforming protein of RaSV is expressed as a gag-ras fusion protein (28,29).

The ras-encoding transforming proteins of the viral oncogenes Ha-v-ras and Ki-v-ras have been localized on the inner surface of the plasma membrane (30). Immunofluorescence staining of the RaSV transformed non-producer cells by sera from these tumor bearing rats indicated both cytoplasmic and membrane staining on 70-80% of the cells. Some of these sera also showed "stippled" staining of the entire surface of the nucleus but not nuclear membrane. Since these sera were heat inactivated (56°C for 30') and absorbed 3-6 times with normal syngenic rat tissue extracts, it appears that this dot-like nuclear staining is specific for RaSV transformed cells. Fractionation of cellular organelle and immunoprecipitation of these antigens is now underway to characterize these proteins.

Nucleotide sequence analysis of Ra-v-ras indicated a large open reading frame of 747 nucleotides which included a 5'-gag-p15-like region, an RaSV-specific DNA termed "RS" and Ha-v-ras related c-ras gene (Fig. 2). The first ATG codon of Ra-v-ras coincides with the RaLV gag-p15 initiation codon (31). This codon is also the first translational signal for p29 which is translated from a single transcript. Comparison of the nucleotide sequence and the encoded amino acid residues of Ra-v-ras with those of other oncogenes and retroviral genes indicated significant homology of the first 32 amino acid residues of RaSV with several retroviral gag p15 regions. Thus, the p15-related amino acids that are present in RaSV appear to have been conserved in most mammalian retroviral gag-p15 regions but are not related to any of the avian retroviral structural proteins. It is noteworthy that these 32 amino acids are also retained in almost the exact same sequence in the Abelson (Ab) transforming MuLV (32,33). Although the significance of this sequence in the transforming retroviruses is not well understood, their presence was thought to be essential for Ab-MuLV induced transformation

Table 2. Sarcoma viruses that have incorporated ras oncogenes of rats.

	KIRSTEN-MSV	HARVEY-MSV	RASHEED-RaSV
PATHOGENESIS IN RATS	Sarcoma erythroleukemia	Fibrosarcoma erythroleukemia	Fibrosarcoma
ONCOGENE	Ki-v-ras	Ha-v-ras	Ra-v-ras
METHOD OF ISOLATION	In vivo passage of MuLV (C3H strain) in Wistar rats.	In vivo passage of Moloney MuLV in Chester-Beaty rats	In vitro cocultivation of RaLV productive cells with chemically induced tumor cells
RECOMBINANT OF	MuLV+30S RNA+Ki-ras	MuLV+30S RNA+Ha-ras	RaLV and c-ras
ONCOGENIC PROTEIN	Ki-ras encoded p21	Ha-ras encoded p21	gag-ras encoded fusion protein p29
PHOSPHOAMINOACID	Threonine	Threonine	Serine
GTP-BINDING	yes	yes	yes
CELLULAR LOCATION OF ONCOGENIC PROTEIN	Plasma membrane	Plasma membrane/ cytoplasm	Cytoplasm and nucleus (?)

(33). Our preliminary transfection experiments with deletion mutants of the molecularly cloned RaSV did not show classical foci of transformed cells, indicating that the 32 amino acids of the gag p15 portion of Ra-v-ras may also be important for the induction and/or maintenance of transformation. Thus although the Ra-v-ras contains cellular ras (c-ras) sequence related to Ha-v-ras, the gene product as shown by biologic, immunologic and nucleic acid sequence analysis is distinct from those of Ha-v-ras, Ki-v-ras or human c-ras oncogenes.

A cluster of 6 residues ("RS" in Figure 2) in the amino terminus of the p29 do not show homology with any of the known viral proteins or with the nucleotide sequences of other oncogenes including those of Ha-v-ras or Ki-v-ras. This RaSV specific DNA (RS) that links the RaLV gag-p15 with the ras sequence consists of a perfect palindrome flanked on both sides with an inverted repeat. It is possible that this sequence plays an important role in the genetic recombination of RaLV and cellular ras gene.

Although the p21-like portion of Ra-v-ras is similar to Ha-v-ras in the nucleotide and amino acid sequences, a non-gag-fused protein (i.e., exclusively ras-induced p21) is not expressed in RaSV transformed cells and a gag fusion protein is not seen in any of the Ha-MSV and Ki-MSV transformed cells. This difference in the transcriptional activities of Ra-v-ras and Ha-v-ras is mainly due to differences in the genetic make-up of the two oncogenes. The mechanisms by which these oncogenes have been transduced in the form of sarcoma viruses is not well understood but the specificity of genetic recombination appears to depend largely on the replicating viral sequences. Thus, whereas the interaction of an endogenous, weakly infectious, RaLV with rat cellular genes (i.e., within a homologous system of rat virus and rat cells) may potentiate fusion of gag p15-like sequence or the RS-DNA with c-ras to generate RaSV, the gag or the RS-DNA may not be necessary when a highly infectious oncogenic mouse virus (MuLV) rescues a rat oncogene in the form of Ha-MSV

Moloney MuLV has now been shown to carry strong promoter sequences whose integration into a foreign rat DNA may have been sufficient to activate, transcribe and package a dominant c-ras gene in the form of a sarcoma virus.

A major portion of the Ra-v-ras is homologous to the Ha-v-ras sequence including the mutation of glycine to arginine at the 12th amino acid codon of the ras-encoded protein. A mutation of glycine at this position in the normal gene to any other amino acid has now been shown to be a crucial determinant for oncogenic activity in both human and viral oncogenes (34,35).

Alignment of the nucleotide sequences of the p21-like region of Ra-v-ras with those of all other known ras genes including the human oncogenes indicated several differences in the Ra-v-ras gene encoding sequence. One major difference that distinguishes Ra-v-ras from all the ras containing viral oncogenes is the presence of alanine at position 59 of the p21-like protein encoding region (Figure 2). This is important because unlike the protein products of several mammalian and avian oncogenes that have tyrosine specific protein kinase activities, the ras gene products of Ki-MSV and Ha-MSV catalyze their own phosphorylation (i.e. autophosphorylate themselves). Thus, the phosphoamino acid of both Ha-MSV and Ki-MSV encoded p21 is phosphothreonine. Although the Ha-v-ras and Ki-v-ras were derived from distinct cellular ras genes, they are autophosphorylated at the same amino acid residue threonine at position 59. Although the threonine substitution in this position has been reported to be important in the oncogenic activation of Ha-v-ras and Ki-v-ras oncogenes, this mutation is not present in Ra-v-ras which contains alanine at position 59. In this respect the Ra-v-ras gene is similar to the other ras genes including those isolated from yeast or the normal and activated human oncogenes from bladder carcinoma (17,18,33-45).

One of the most interesting properties of the ras gene product p21 is that the autophosphorylating activity at the threonine residue uses a guanine nucleotide triphosphate (GTP) as the phosphate donor rather than the adenosine triphosphate (ATP) which is used by other tyrosine specific phosphokinases (46,47). The strong affinity with GTP implies that the transforming function of ras induced p21 may involve the metabolism of guanine nucleotides (46,47). The Ra-v-ras is also GTP binding, although the p29 appears to be phosphorylated at the serine residue (46,47) and the phosphoamino acid in the transforming protein is a phosphoserine. Since a small amount of serine form was also detected in the normal cellular ras gene related to Ha-v-ras, it indicates that the Ra-v-ras transduced by RaLV is more closely related to the normal genes of rats and humans than those present in Ha-MSV.

A change from glutamine to lysine at amino acid residue 61 of the N-ras encoded transforming protein is regarded as a critical determinant of the oncogene. This residue is unchanged in all other ras encoded proteins including the p29 protein of Ra-v-ras (Table 2).

The amino acid residue 122 of the p21-like region of Ra-v-ras is alanine. This residue is variable in all known viral and cellular ras genes but it is similar to that of human normal and activated bladder carcinoma ras oncogenes (Figure 2). Thus, in this region the p21-like region of Ra-v-ras encoded p29 is different from Ha-MSV and Ki-MSV viral oncogenes. Two additional changes at amino acid residues 123 and 150 of the p21-like protein are seen in Ra-v-ras encoding p29 that are not seen in any of the known ras oncogene encoding proteins including those of yeast and Drosophila (15-18). Although we do not yet know whether any of these changes in Ra-v-ras are critical for transformation, it is possible that they may have been caused by the chemical carcinogens that were used to originally transform the rat cells prior to or since its transduction in the form of a sarcoma virus.

CELLULAR HOMOLOGUES OR ras GENES

Although it was proposed in 1969 that the oncogenes of retroviruses are present in normal cells (48), their cellular origin was demonstrated in 1973/74 by nucleic acid hybridization of cDNA probes of Ha-MSV and Ki-MSV with cellular and retroviral RNAs (49,50). This finding was subsequently confirmed and extended by Stehelin et al. (51) and Spector et al. (52) who showed for the first time that cellular homologues or proto-oncogenes of the avian viral oncogene src were highly conserved during the evolution of species (15). The proto-oncogenes of almost all the known viral oncogenes have now been identified in all vertebrates such as Drosophila and yeast (15-18).

The cellular homologues of all the viral ras genes have now been isolated directly from several human tumors (15-45). Studies with human ras oncogenes demonstrated that single point mutations can convert normal cells to neoplastic growth (35-45). Thus, the activated c-ras genes homologous to both Ha-v-ras and Ki-v-ras genes appear to be mutated at the 12th codon in the human T24 bladder carcinoma and lung/colon carcinoma respectively and at the amino acid residue 61 position in another ras gene, the N-ras of the human neuroblastoma (43). Activation of cellular homologues of Ha-v-ras, Ki-v-ras and N-ras genes by single point mutations have also been shown in some chemically induced tumors of mice and at least one tumor each of rat and the guinea pig (53-55). In Ra-v-ras, although the 12th and 61st codons of the p21-like sequence are similar to those present in Ha-v-ras p21, four additional amino acid residues at 59, 122, 123 and 150 are distinct from Ha-MSV or Ki-MSV viral oncogenes. Moreover, the 59th and 122nd residues of Ra-ras are identical to the normal and human bladder cancer oncogenes (31,34). These genetic changes apparently produce conformational changes in the protein that allows for the expression of the transformed state in these tumors (35-45). In addition to the conformational changes due to several genetic mutations in the viral oncogene of RaSV, the unique property that distinguishes it from all other ras encoded proteins is the synthesis of a single gag-ras fusion product. Since all the RaSV strains that were isolated in our laboratory or elsewhere, regardless of the origin of the rat tumors (21,22,28,29), showed the same gag-fuson protein, it is tempting to speculate that the endogenous gag-p15 related region first recombined with the normal ras gene to form a hybrid cellular gene with the help of the RS sequence (similar to the movable genetic elements (56)), and then the hybrid gene was transduced by the replicating RaLV. Molecular cloning of ras genes with the use of probes containing RS and other specific regions is now underway to resolve this question.

Although we have isolated an activated ras gene in the form of a sarcoma virus, the phenomenon may represent one of a number of possible late steps in carcinogenesis. Moreover, since cancer is a multi-step process, several molecular interactions other than point mutations may also produce both qualitative and quantitative changes in a proto-oncogene. These include DNA rearrangements, translocations, gene amplification, promoter activation, or synergistic or cooperate effects of two or more proto-oncogenes. The rat cell-endogenous virus system that we have studied allows us to use new approaches to analyzing molecular events at various stages of cancer development in a controlled cell culture system. A sequential analysis of the genetic changes from the normal to pretransformed to fully transformed cells may aid in a better understanding of the molecular pathways necessary for subsequent clonal evolution and progression of tumor cells.

ACKNOWLEDGEMENTS

This investigation was supported by grant CA 27246 from the National Cancer Institute. I thank Dr. G.L. Norman for his help in making charts and reading the manuscript and M. Benitez for its preparation.

REFERENCES

1. Rasheed, S., Bruszewski, J., Rongey, R.W., Roy-Burman, P., Charman, H.P., & Gardner, M.B. (1976) J. Virol. 18, 799-803.
2. Rasheed, S., Charman, H., & Gardner, M.B. (1978) Virology 89, 605-609.
3. Bergs, V.V., Pearson, G., Harish, C., & Turner, W. (1972) Int. J. Cancer 10, 165-173.
4. Chopra, H.C., Bogden, A.E., Zellijadt, I., & Jansen, E.M. (1970) Eur. J. Cancer 6, 287-290.
5. Freeman, A.E., Gilden, R.V., Vernon, M.L., Wolford, R.G., Hugunin, P.E., & Huebner, R.J. (1973) Proc. Natl. Acad. Sci. U.S.A. 70, 2415-2419.
6. Gazzolo, L., Simkovic, D., & Martin-Berthelon, M.C. (1971) J. Gen. Virol. 12, 303-311.
7. Klement, V., Nicolson, M.O., Nelson-Rees, W., Gilden, R.V., Oroszlan, S., Rongey, R.W. & Gardner, M.B. (1973) Int. J. Cancer 12, 654-666.
8. Charman, H.P., White, M.H., Rahman, R., & Gilden, R.V. (1976) J. Virol. 17, 51-59.
9. Rasheed, S., Freeman, A.E., Gardner, M.B. & Huebner, R.J. (1976) J. Virol. 18, 776-782.
10. Rasheed, S., Young, H. & Gardner, M. (1979) J. Natl. Canc. Inst. 63, 745-750.
11. Tsuchida, N., Gilden, R.V. & Hatanaka, M. (1974) Proc. Natl. Acad. Sci. U.S.A. 71, 4503-4507.
12. Scolnick, E.M., Vass, W.C., Howk, R.S. & Duesberg, P.H. (1979) J. Virol. 29, 964-972.
13. DeFeo, D., Gonda, M.A., Young, H.A., Chang, E.H., Lowy, D.R., Scolnick, E.M. & Ellis, R.W. (1981) Proc. Natl. Acad. Sci. U.S.A. 78, 3328-3332.
14. Ellis, W.R., DeFeo, D., Shih, T.Y., Gonda, M.A., Young, H.A., Tsuchida, N., Lowy, D.R. & Scolnick, E.M. (1981) Nature 292, 506-510.
15. Bishop, M.J. (1983) Ann. Rev. Biochem. 52, 301-354.
16. Coffin, J.M., Varmus, H.E., Bishop, J.M., Essex, M., Hardy, W.D., Martin, G., S., Rosenberg, N.E., Scolnick, E.M., Weinberg, R.A. & Vogt, P.K. (1981) J.

Virol. 40:943-957.
17. Shira Neuman-Silberberg, F., Schejter, E., Hoffmann, F.M. & Shilo, B. (1984) Cell 37, 1027-1033.
18. Powers, S., Kataoka, T., Fasano, O., Goldfarb, M., Strathern, J., Borach, J., & Wigler, M. (1984) Cell 36, 607-612.
19. Harvey, J.J. (1964) Nature 204, 1104-1105.
20. Kirsten W.H. & Mayer, L.A. (1967) J. Natl. Cancer Inst. 39, 311-335.
21. Rasheed, S., Gardner, M.B. & Huebner, R.J. (1978b) Proc. Natl. Acad. Sci. U.S.A. 75, 2972-2976.
22. Rasheed, S. (1980) Cold Spring Harbor Symp. Quant. Biol., XLIV, 779-786.
23. Rapp, U.R., Todaro, G.J. (1978) Science 201, 821-823.
24. Stavnezer, E.D., Gerhard, S., Binari, R.C. & Balazs, I. (1981) J. Virol. 39, 920-934.
25. Varnier, O.E., Raffanti, S.P., Muratore, O., Repetto, C.M., Pippia, P., Tilloca, G., Melone, M.A., Ivaldi, G. & Rasheed, S. (1985) Europ. J. Cancer & Clinic. Onc.21, 97107. .
26. Rasheed, S. & Young, H.A. (1982) Virology 118, 219-224.
27. Gonda, M.A., Young,H.A., Elser, J.E., Rasheed, S., Talmadge, C.B., Nagashima, K., Li, C., Gilden, R.V. (1982) J. Virol. 44, 520-529.
28. Young, H.A., Shih, T.Y., Scolnick, E.M., Rasheed, S. & Gardner, M.B. (1979) Proc. Natl. Acad. Sci. U.S.A. 76, 3523-3527.
29. Young, H.A., Rasheed, S., Sowder, R., Benton, C.V. & Henderson, L.E. (1981) J. Virol. 38, 286-293.
30. Willingham, M.C., Pastan, I., Shih, T.Y., & Scolnick, E.M. (1980) Cell, 19, 1005-1014.
31. Rasheed, S., Norman, G.L. & Heidecker, G. (1983) Science 221, 155-157.
32. Witte, O.N., Rosenberg, N.E. & Baltimore, D. (1979) Nature 281, 396-398.
33. Prywes, R., Foulkes, J.G., Rosenberg, N. & Baltimore, D. (1983) Cell 34, 569-579.
34. Capon, D.J., Chen, E., Levinson, A., Seeburg, P. &

Goeddel, D. (1983) Nature 302,33-36.
35. Tabin, C.J., Bradley, S.M., Bargmann, C.I., Weinberg, R.A., Papageorge, A.G., Scolnick, E.M., Dhar, R., Lowy, D.R. & Chang, E.H. (1982) Nature 300, 143-149.
36. Premkumar Reddy, E., Reynolds, R.K., Santos, E. & Barbacid, M. (1982) Nature 300, 149-152.
37. Murray, M.J., Shilo, B., Shih, C., Cowing, D., Hsu, H. & Weinberg, R.A. (1981) Cell 25, 355-361.
38. Shih, C. & Weinberg, R.A. (1982) Cell 29, 161-169.
39. Shilo, B. & Weinberg, R.A. (1981) Proc. Natl. Acad. Sci. U.S.A. 78, 6789-6792.
40. Shimizu, K., Goldfarb, M., Suard, Y., Perucho, M., Li, Y., Kamata, T., Feramisco, J., Stavnezer, E., Fogh, J. & Wigler, M.H. (1983) Proc. Natl. Acad. Sci. U.S.A. 80, 2112-2116.
41. Taparowsky, E., Suard, Y., Fasano, O., Shimizu, K., Goldfarb, M. & Wigler, M. (1982) Nature 300, 762-765.
42. Parada, L.F., Tabin, C.J., Shih, C. & Weinberg, R.A. (1982) Nature 297, 474-478.
43. Shimizu, K., Goldfarb, M., Perucho, M. & Wigler, M. (1983) Proc. Natl. Acad. Sci. U.S.A. 80, 383-387.
44. Pulciani, S., Santos, E., Lauver, A.V., Long, L.K., Robbins, K.C. & Barbacid, M. (1982) Proc. Natl. Acad. Sci. U.S.A. 79, 2845-2849.
45. Chang, E.H., Furth, M.E., Scolnick, E.M. & Lowy, D.R. (1982). Nature 297, 479-483.
46. Shih, T.Y., Papageorge, A.G., Stokes, P.E., Weeks, M.O. & Scolnick, E.M. (1980) Nature 287, 686-690.
47. Papageorge, A., Lowy, D. & Scolnick, E.M. (1982) J. Virol., 509-519.
48. Huebner, R.J. & Todaro, G.J. (1969) Proc. Natl. Acad. Sci. U.S.A. 64, 1087-1094.
49. Scolnick, E.M. & Parks, W.P. (1974) J. Virol. 13, 1211-1219.
50. Scolnick, E.M., Rands, E., Williams, D. & Parks, W.P. (1973) J. Virol. 12, 458-463.
51. Stehelin, D., Varmus, H.E., Bishop, J.M. & Vogt, P.K. (1976) Nature 260, 170.
52. Spector, D.H., Smith, K., Padgett, T., McCombe, P.,

Roulland Dussoix, D., Moscovici, C., Varmus, H.E. & Bishop, J.M. (1978) Cell 13, 371.

53. Balmin, A. & Pragnell, I.B. (1983) Nature 303, 72-74.
54. Sukumar, S., Notario, V., Martin-Zarca, D. & Barbacid, M. (1983) Nature 306, 659-661.
55. Sukumar, S. Science 223, 1197-1199.
56. Temin, H.M. (1974) Virology 6, 669-688.

TARGET CELLS FOR AVIAN LEUKEMIA VIRUSES REVISITED

C. Moscovici

Tumor Virology Laboratory, Research Service, VAMC, and Department of Pathology, College of Medicine, University of Florida, Gainesville, Fla., 32602, U.S.A.

The pathogenesis and molecular functions of the avian retroviruses have been comprehensively reviewed in recent years (1-3). This presentation will focus on three replication-defective avian tumor viruses that are responsible for causing, in a relatively short period of time, acute leukemias in chickens. The involvement of these viruses with the hemopoietic system of the chicken stimulated investigators to search for and to characterize the corresponding in vitro target cells present in hemopoietic organs. In vitro assays for growing target cells for all known acute leukemia viruses are now available and have been described in the literature (4,5).

The three leukemic viruses to be considered are: avian myeloblastosis virus (AMV), which infects and transforms cells of the myeloid series; avian erythroblastosis virus (AEV), which transforms cells of erythroid nature, and E26 virus, which has the interesting property of causing two different types of leukemia in both the chicken and the quail (6).

AMV-TARGET CELLS, THE PHENOTYPE OF TRANSFORMED CELLS, AND DIFFERENTIATION MARKERS

AMV is an oncogenic retrovirus that causes a rapid leukemia in chickens and transforms specific hemopoietic cells in culture. The oncogene of AMV, v-myb, is a truncated version of c-myb (7). v-myb encodes the transforming protein, $p45^{v\text{-}myb}$, located in the nucleus (8,9).

Experiments that are aimed at the characterization of AMV target cells in chicken bone marrow, by density, velocity sedimentation, adherence, and phagocytic activity, indicate that the target cells for AMV are recruited among cells located just beyond the stage of the myeloid progenitors -- i.e., CFC (colony-forming cell) (10) -- and are already committed toward the macrophage lineage (11).

In addition, in vitro studies from my laboratory did establish that functionally differentiated macrophages obtained from bone marrows or secondary yolk sac cultures can also serve as target cells for transformation (3). Our findings were challenged by a group of investigators who suggested that the cultures we used for the focus assay were contaminated with myeloblasts, which are considered to be the immediate precursors of granulocytes (12). This problem was later carefully reexamined by Durban and Boettiger (13), who were able to demonstrate that the number of contaminating immature cells in macrophage cultures is less than 1 in 5,000 and therefore does not account for the high level of transformation obtained in the focus assay. No correlation was found between the granulocyte-lineage cells and the number of AMV transformed cells observed in yolk sac cultures infected with AMV. Furthermore, they reconfirmed that the target cells for this virus are recruited among the mononuclear-phagocytic lineage; therefore, the leukemia induced by this virus should be classified as a monocytic leukemia.

The AMV-transformed cells can be maintained in culture

for long periods of time (14). They were obtained either from colonies of transformed bone marrow or yolk sac cells, from foci of macrophage cultures, or from the peripheral blood of moribund leukemic chickens. Regardless of their origin, they are morphologicaly the same and have the same functional and surface properties (Table 1).

These cells are mostly nonadherent and round, and are about 10 um in diameter. Their large and eccentric nucleus is surrounded by a rim of cytoplasm containing small granules. The presence of surface markers, characteristic of macrophages, on the membrane of AMV-transformed cells has been investigated (10,15,16). It was found that receptors for the Fc part of immunoglobulins are expressed on the surface of these cells, whereas receptors for the C3 component of complement are not expressed. Both receptors were present on normal avian macrophages. Moreover, AMV-transformed cells could engulf latex particles (phagocytosis mediated by nonspecific receptors). However, phagocytosis mediated by Fc receptors did not occur, which indicated that these receptors are not functional. The search for enzymatic and antigenic surface markers has shown the presence of ATPase, the expression of a macrophage-related antigen. Finally, when treated with phorbol myristate acetate, AMV-transformed cells adhere to the surface of the culture flask and differentiate into macrophages (17).

Transformation of hemopoietic target cells by avian retroviruses leads to the proliferation of cells that display distinct phenotypes of differentiation. The markers that are present on the normal hemopoietic cells are missing from the transformed cells. AMV-transforming activity is well documented and shows that all stages of macrophage differentiation, from the committed progenitor to the mature macrophage, may serve as targets for transformed progeny cells (11). A model showing how AMV interacts with the myelomonocytic lineage is therefore proposed (Figure 1). The model may be valid for other related myeloid viruses (MC29*, MH2, OK10, CMII), and is consistent with all the data obtained to date. It

Table 1. Expression of myeloid differentiation parameters by hemopoietic cells transformed by AMV.

		Surface receptors*		Phagocytosis*		Enzyme activities§		Cell surface antigens§		
Cell type	Adhesiveness	Fc	C3	Nonspecific	Immune	Acid P'tase	ATPase	Myeloblast	Macrophage	Erythrocyte
normal macrophages	+ + +	95–98	75	97	95	+ + +	+ + +	+	+ + +	–
AMV-transformed	–	9–73	1	35–85	0	+	+ + +	+ + +	+	–

* = Percentage of positive cells.

§+ = slightly positive, + + + = strongly positive, – = not detectable.

Data from Moscovici and Gazzolo (3) modified.

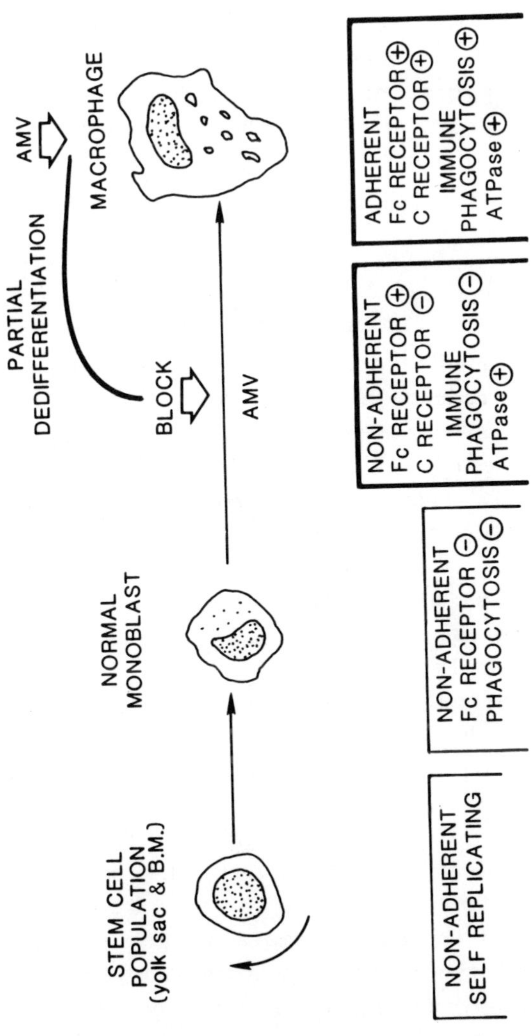

AMV INTERFERENCE WITH MYELOID DIFFERENTIATION IN VITRO: A PROPOSED MODEL

proposes that these viruses transform cells at late stages of the myeloid lineage. Target cells to be transformed must express some or all of the differentiation parameters of mature macrophages (partial dedifferentiation). Nevertheless, infection can occur in immature cells, but transformation will be triggered when these immature cells acquire some of the differentiation markers. According to this model we can postulate that when precursor cells for the lineage are infected, transformation or leukemia arises only after some cellular maturation has occurred (9).

---

*Although MC29-induced transformation and leukemia have not been fully considered in this review, I should clarify the controversial findings revolving around MC29-induced effects on hemopoietic cells both in vivo and in vitro (18). In vitro MC29 transforms macrophages as AMV does. The phenotype of the transformed cells however is quite different for each virus used (i.e., myelomonoblastic nongranulated cells with AMV, versus poorly defined macrophage-like cells with MC29), which suggests that different target cells are specifically involved within the same cell lineage. On the other hand the leukemia obtained with MC29 has been classified as myelomonocytic leukemia (18). In our experience (unpublished), a myelomonocytic leukemia is induced only when embryonated eggs are injected with MC29 through the chorioallantoic vein. Hatched chickens injected with the same virus by different routes developed only a stem cell leukemia accompanied by solid tumors. Attempts to grow tumors cells of the granulocytic type have always failed. These results suggest that MC29-transforming events cover a broader range of differentiating cell compartments, which remain to be defined.

E26 VIRUS-ERYTHROID AND MYELOID LEUKEMIA AND IDENTIFICATION OF TARGET CELLS

The avian leukemia virus E26 is a replication-defective oncogenic retrovirus whose genome shares nucleotide sequences with v-myb and c-myb (19,20). The E26 genome contains an additional nucleotide sequence, termed v-ets, which is derived from a cellular gene, c-ets (20-22). The oncogenic properties of E26 differ considerably from AMV. E26 transforms cells of the myeloid and erythoid lineage and can induce myeloid and erythoid leukemia in the chicken (6,23). The question is still not answered whether the differences in oncogenicity between AMV and E26 are caused by different modes of expression of myb-related nucleotide sequences of the two viruses, or by the presence of v-ets sequences in the E26 genome. The response of hemopoietic cells to E26 virus infection and the identification of the target cells present in the chick embryo and in the bone marrow of young chickens have been reported (24). The data indicate that E26 virus is capable of interfering with both the erythoid- and myeloid-committed cells. In addition, a larger number of target cells was found to be within the precursor and the uncommitted-progenitor cell pool when embryonic hemopoietic tissues were compared with adult bone marrows. Cells at both the primitive streak and the 12-somite stages contain a higher percentage of immature progenitors than do adult bone marrows cells. Upon infection, three different types of colonies were obtained, namely pure erythroid, pure myeloid, and a mixed colony containing cells of both lineages. Even after several passages, cultures derived from colonies of mixed lineage contain a self-replicating bipotent target cell.

In conclusion, E26 virus may be the first avian retrovirus that can infect and transform a bipotent (uncommitted erythroid-myeloid) hemopoietic cell as well as a myeloid and erythroid-committed progenitor cell. Our data also showed that E26-transformed erythroid cells, when derived from embryonic tissues, tend to escape the block in differentiation, hence hemoglobinization of more mature erythroid cells occurs. This is in contrast with E26-transformed erythroblasts derived from adult bone marrows, which remain immature and therefore do not exhibit any further change in their transformed phenotype. Further work is in progress to examine this question.

A model describing the possible pathway of E26 virus infection with both cell lineages is presented in Figure 2.

AEV-TARGET CELLS AND DIFFERENTIATION

AEV is a retrovirus that can cause erythroblastic leukemia and sarcomas in susceptible birds in a short period of time. The virus transforms cultures of chicken fibroblasts and hemopoietic precursor cells of erythroid lineage (2). The AEV genome is defective, in that it does not produce reverse transcriptase. In addition, many of the env and gag genes have been deleted (25); therefore, AEV progeny is produced only in the presence of a helper virus that supplies replicative functions. It has been found that the oncogenic potentials of AEV pertain to sequences derived by recombination with the genome of avian vertebrates (26). Oddly enough, the recombinational event produced a virus containing two oncogenes, namely v-erbA and v-erbB encoding two proteins $p74^{gag\text{-}erbA}$ and $p61\text{-}68^{erbB}$, respectively (27). The existence of these two gene products prompted the question of whether one or both proteins are necessary for the full oncogenic expression of AEV both in vitro and in vivo. Frykberg et al. (28) and Sealy et al. (29,30) independently constructed deletion mutants in both the v-erbA and v-erbB genes, and the results of the two groups are essentially the same. The data show that the ability of AEV to induce erytholeukemia in chickens and transform fibroblast cells in culture depends on the expression of $p61\text{-}68^{erbB}$ (mutant v-erbA^{-}B^{+}). In contrast, the mutant, which is incapable of synthesizing $p61\text{-}68^{erbB}$ (mutant v-erbA^{+}B^{-}), lacks

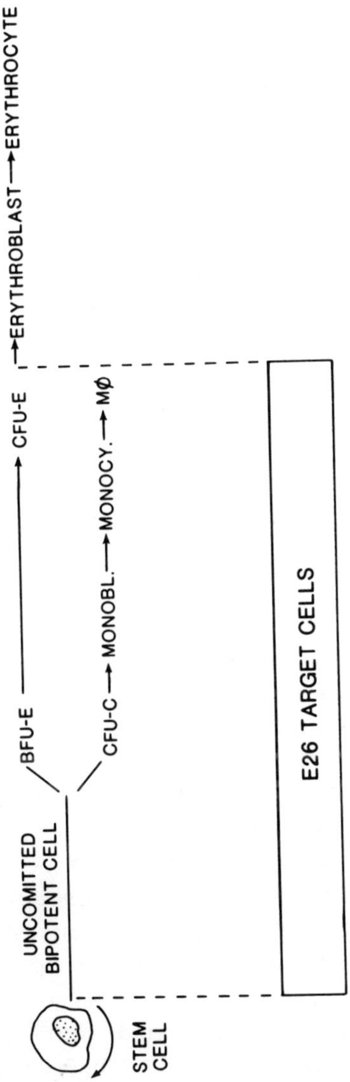

E26 INTERFERENCE WITH TWO HEMOPOIETIC PROGENITOR CELL-POPULATIONS

transforming activity in vitro. Its role in leukemogenesis remains to be assessed more rigorously.

The characterization of AEV target cells for in vitro transformation of bone marrow cells has been reported (31,32). Briefly, AEV target cells are recruited within the BFU-E compartment. After infection the maturation of the CFU-E proceeds, but it is blocked at the CFU-E stage, as described by Gazzolo et al. (33). The CFU-E cells express late erythroid markers but have acquired a self-renewal potential that will impair terminal differentiation.

Several observations in the literature reported that virus-transformed cells may at times escape the block, resulting in partial or total spontaneous differentiation (34-37).

In examining the response of embryonic tissues of various ages after infection with E26 virus, we observed that erythroblast-like cells produced from virus-transformed blastoderms showed a definite level of spontaneous differentiation up to the terminal stage of erythrocytes (24) (see earlier in this review). These studies prompted us to reexamine the transforming activity of AEV in early and late embryonic tissues, and the data obtained may be summarized as follows:

a) In the embryonic tissues examined (primitive streak, 12 somites, yolk sac at different ages) the target cell for AEV is not in the BFU-E compartment as it is in the adult bone marrow. The embryonic target cell probably resides in an earlier compartment either just preceding the CFU-E or within the CFU-M stage, or both.

b) All embryonic transformed colonies obtained after infection with wild type AEV show a high percentage of hemoglobinization.

c) Colony-derived transformed cells display CFU-E markers (Im^{+}), but unlike normal CFU-E they have acquired self-renewal potential. Recloning of these transformed CFU-E results once again in partially hemoglobinized colonies (38). A schematic model for AEV interaction with target cells is presented (slightly modified from the one

AEV INTERFERENCE WITH ERYTHROID DIFFERENTIATION PATHWAY

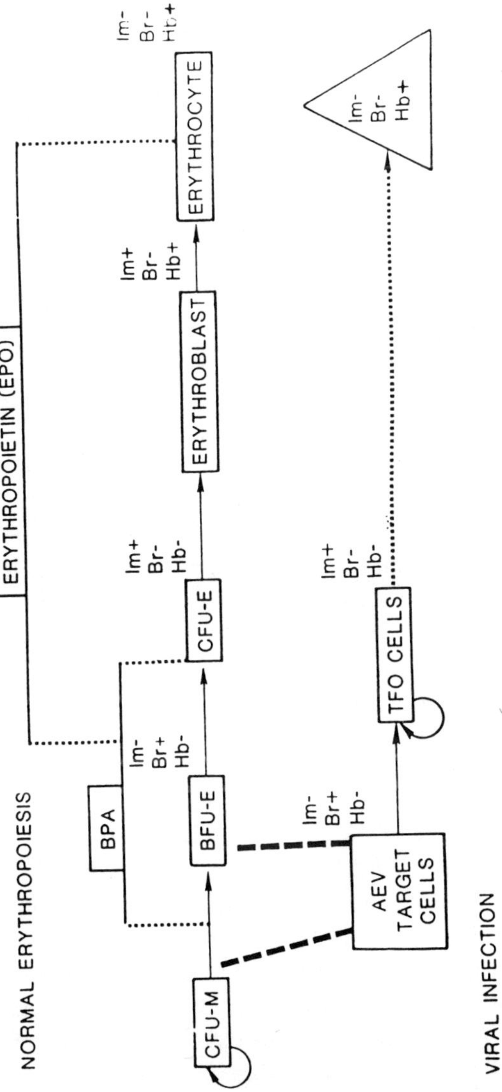

proposed by Gazzolo and Samarut, 31) (Figure 3). The upper section of the scheme illustrates the erythrocytic differentiation pathway characterized by specific antigens expressed during maturation: Immature antigen (Im), brain antigen (Br), and Hemoglobin (Hb). "Plus" and "minus" signs refer to expression of markers. The lower part of the scheme represents the identification of target cells belonging to two different compartments: a) the BFU-E in the bone marrow, and b) the CFU-M and/or pre-BFU-E in the embryo. Target cells from both compartments differentiate to CFU-E-transformed cells after infection. In the case of bone marrow, the CFU-E are blocked at this stage, undergoing self-renewal. By contrast, embryo-derived CFU-E partially escape the block (horizontal dotted line) to terminal differentiation (triangle).

Spontaneous differentiation has been observed by Graf and Beug (39) when transformation was induced by infection with a v-erbA deletion mutant (v-erb$A^{-}B^{+}$). They suggested that terminal differentiation is probably due to the absence of the B-erbA gene. Our results, however, indicate that self-renewal, together with differentiation occurs with wild type AEV. It remains to be proved whether the use of embryonic hemopoietic cells provides a different environment, which may influence the full oncogenic expression of the virus.

Although we seemingly have a better knowledge of the target cell for each virus and have improved our methods for detecting differential markers in transformed cells, we are still far from fully understanding how viral gene products interact with cell differentiation. It has become apparent that all retroviruses do not follow similar patterns when they interact with the hemopoietic system. In the case of AEV and AMV, for instance, it seems that the virus can express its transforming potential only when the infected cell has reached a certain stage along its differentiation pathway. Conversely, in the case of E26, cells at all stages of differentiation are competent for transformation.

Many questions remain unanswered, two of which are

particularly pertinent: Is the presence of as-yet-unidentified differentiating factors interfering with full viral expression in the embryo? Or is there a regulator lacking in the embryonic tissue, but present in the adult tissue, which prevents full transforming activity of the virus?

Therefore, the spontaneous differentiation observed in embryonic transformed cells adds a new dimension to the understanding of virus-cell interaction. Whether these findings have a broader implication remains to be seen. Answers to these questions will help clarify the complex problem of how disruption of the hemopoietic program occurs.

ACKNOWLEDGMENTS

This work was supported by National Cancer Institute Grant CA-10697 and by the Medical Research Service of the Veterans Administration.

REFERENCES

1. Bishop, J.M. (1982) Sci. Am. 246, 68-78.
2. Graf, T. & Stehelin D. (1982) Biochim. Biophys. Acta 651, 245-271.
3. Moscovici, C. & Gazzolo, L. (1982) Adv. Viral Oncol. 1, 83-106.
4. Dodge, W.H., & Moscovici, C. (1973) J. Cell. Physiol. 81, 371-386.
5. Graf, T., von Kirchbach, A. & Beug H. (1981) Exp. Cell Res. 131, 331-343.
6. Moscovici, C., Samarut, J., Gazzolo, L. & Moscovici, M.G. (1981) Virology 113, 765-768.
7. Klempnauer, K.H., Ramsay, G., Bishop, J.M., Moscovici, M.G., Moscovici, C., McGrath, J.P. & Levinson, A.D. (1983) Cell 33, 345-355.
8. Klempnauer, K.H., Symonds, G., Evan, G.I. & Bishop,

J.M. (1984) Cell 37, 537-547.
9. Bishop, J.M. (1983) in: Normal and Neoplastic Hematopoiesis (A.R. Liss, New York) 9, 1-30.
10. Gazzolo, L., Moscovici, C., Moscovici, M.G. & Samarut J. (1979) Cell 16, 627-638.
11. Boettiger, D. & Durban, E.M. (1984) J. Virol. 49, 841-847.
12. Graf, T. & Beug, H. (1978) Biochim. Biophys. Acta 516, 269-299.
13. Durban, E. & Boettiger, D. (1981) J. Virol. 37, 488-492.
14. Moscovici, M.G. & Moscovici, C. (1980) in: In Vivo and In Vitro Erythropoiesis: The Friend System, ed. Rossi G.B., (Elsevier/North Holland Amsterdam), 503-514.
15. Beug, H., von Kirchbach, A., Doederlein, G., Conscience, J.F. & Graf, T. (1979) Cell 18, 375-390.
16. Durban, E.M. & Boettiger, D. (1981) Proc. Natl. Acad. Sci USA 78, 3600-3604.
17. Pessano, S., Gazzolo, L. & Moscovici, C. (1979) Microbiologica 2, 379-392.
18. Langlois, A.J., Fritz, R.B., Heine, U., Beard, D., Bolognesi, D.P. & Beard, J.W. (1969) Cancer Res. 29, 2056-2074.
19. Roussel, M., Saule, S., Lagrou, C., Rommens, C., Beug, H., Graf, T. & Stehelin D. (1979) Nature 281, 452-455.
20. Bister, K., Nunn, M., Moscovici, C., Perbal, B., Baluda, M.A. & Duesberg, P.H. (1982) Proc. Natl. Acad. Sci. USA 79, 3677-3681.
21. Leprince, D., Gegonne, A., Coll, J., de Taisne, C., Schneeberger, A., Lagrou, C. & Stehelin, D. (1983) Nature 306, 395-397.
22. Nunn, M., Seeburg, P.H., Moscovici, C. & Duesberg, P.H. (1983) Nature 306, 391-395.
23. Radke, K., Beug, H., Kornfeld, S. & Graf, T. (1982) Cell 31, 643-653.
24. Moscovici, M.G., Jurdic, P., Samarut, J., Gazzolo, L., Mura, C.V. & Moscovici, C. (1983) Virology, 129, 65-78.
25. Bister, K. & Duesberg, P.H. (1979) Proc. Natl. Acad.

Sci. USA 76, 5023-5027.

26. Bishop, J.M. (1982) Adv. Cancer Res. 37, 1-32.
27. Sheiness, D., Vennstrom, B. & Bishop, J.M. (1981) Cell 23, 291-300.
28. Frykberg, L., Palmieri, S., Beug, H., Graf, T., Hayman, H.J. & Vennstrom, B. (1983) Cell 32, 227-228.
29. Sealy, L., Privalsky, M.L., Moscovici, G., Moscovici, C. & Bishop, J.M. (1983) Virology, 130, 155-178.
30. Sealy, L., Moscovici, G., Moscovici, C. & Bishop, J.M. (1983) Virology 130, 179-194.
31. Beug, H., Palmieri, S., Freudenstein, C., Zentgraf, H. & Graf, T. (1982) Cell 28, 907-919.
32. Samarut, J. & Gazzolo,L. (1982) Cell 28, 921-929.
33. Gazzolo, L., Samarut, J., Bouabdelli, M. & Blanchet, J.P. (1980) Cell 22, 683-691.
34. Marks, P.A. & Rifkind, R.A. (1978) Annu. Rev. Biochem. 47, 419-448.
35. Fibach, E., Treves, A. & Rachmilewitz, E.A. (1983) Cancer Res. 43, 4136-4141.
36. Hankins, D.W. (1983) J.Natl.Canc.Inst. 70, 725-734.
37. Waneck, G.L. & Rosenberg, N. (1981) Cell 26, 79-89.
38. Jurdic, P., Bouabdelli, M. & Moscovici, M.G. (in press) Cell Differ.
39. Graf, T. and Beug, H. (1983) Cell 34, 7-9.

FELINE RETROVIRUSES

O. Jarrett

University of Glasgow Veterinary School, Bearsden, Glasgow, Scotland

Feline leukemia virus (FeLV) is the exogenous retrovirus of cats. In addition, three types of endogenous retroviral DNA are found in cat cells but are not usually expressed as infectious virus. These are represented by multiple copies of the RD114 provirus, FeLV-related proviruses and FeLV-related long terminal repeats (LTRs). FeLV is the only one of these known to cause disease. Most cats which are exposed naturally to FeLV recover and are immune. However, some become permanently infected and are then at high risk of developing a FeLV-related disease. Many of these diseases are neoplastic, such as leukemias and fibrosarcomas but the majority are non-malignant conditions like anaemia and immunosuppression. Interactions between FeLV and cellular genes appear to be important in the pathogenesis of at least some of these diseases. Acutely pathogenic, defective viruses which are recombinants between FeLV and the myc gene have been isolated from T-cell leukaemias and recombinants between FeLV and seven other proto-oncogenes have been isolated, as feline sarcoma viruses, from fibrosarcomas. Hence, transduction of proto-oncogenes by FeLV appears to be an essential process in many cases of FeLV-induced neoplasia.

The most important feline retrovirus is feline leukaemia virus (FeLV) which is transmitted by contact among cats and causes several serious diseases mainly in those cats which develop a persistent infection. When DNA of cells from a cat with a permanent FeLV infection is examined, however, four types of retroviral DNA are found in chromosomal DNA. The complete exogenously-acquired FeLV genome is present, of course, and is expressed leading to the production of large quantities of infectious virus. In addition there are three other types of retroviral DNA which are endogenous to cells of the domestic cat.

ENDOGENOUS RETROVIRUS DNA

The first endogenous retrovirus to be discovered in cat cells was RD114 (1). This designation was given to a virus which was isolated from human cells transplanted into feline embryos and, when subsequent isolations were made, was used to describe this group of endogenous retroviruses. RD114 viruses are very closely related to baboon endogenous viruses but are only distantly related to FeLV and other mammalian retroviruses (2). In the DNA of cells of domestic cats there are multiple copies of the viral genome which may be activated spontaneously, as occurred with RD114 in vivo and further isolates in vitro, or following exposure of normal cat cell cultures to inducing agents (3). RD114 viruses are xenotropic, infecting, for example, human cells but not cat cells. It is generally considered that these viruses do not play a part in the pathogenesis of any feline disease.

The second type of endogenous retroviral DNA, unlike RD114, is closely related to FeLV. This DNA occurs in multiple, genome-sized copies flanked by long terminal repeats (LTR) but has yet to be identified as an infectious virus indicating that the genome is either defective or is very strongly repressed, or that the virus may have a host range which does not include the cells normally used for FeLV isolation (4,5). While each cat has 8-10 copies of the endogenous provirus the distribution of these copies within cellular DNA varies between cats (6).

The restriction enzyme pattern of endogenous DNA is very similar to FeLV in the centre of the genome but is less related towards the ends. In fact the U3 regions of the LTRs of FeLV and endogenous provirus have no homology with the result that cloned FeLV U3 DNA is extremely useful as a probe to identify the exogenous virus in cellular DNA (6). The significance of endogenous FeLV DNA in the pathogenesis of feline disease is not clear but a possible interaction between this DNA and exogenous FeLV DNA in the generation of novel recombinant viruses involved in erythroid hypoplasia is discussed below.

An intriguing finding is that in addition to the genome-sized copies of FeLV-related DNA there are approximately 150 copies of the endogenous LTR in cellular DNA (6). These elements appear to be mobile but their origin and function, if any, is unknown.

FELINE LEUKAEMIA VIRUS

FeLV has the same particle and genomic structure as other mammalian retroviruses. Of particular importance in the biology of FeLV is the oganization of the spikes on the viral envelope which are composed of the env gene products, gp70 and p15(E). Structures on the spikes determine, first, the specificity of the virus-cell interactions by mediating the binding of virus to cell receptors, and secondly the induction of virus neutralising antibody.

Three subgroups of FeLV (A,B or C) are recognised by their capacity to attach to different cellular receptors (7). All virus isolates contain FeLV-A. Viruses of subgroups B and C are never found alone but always in combination with FeLV-A so that the possible content of isolates is FeLV-A, FeLV-AB, FeLV-AC or FeLV-ABC. About half of isolates contain FeLV alone and half are mixtures of FeLV-A and B (8). It appears that FeLV-B is dependent on FeLV-A for natural transmission within phenotypic mixtures (9). While FeLV-C is rare, occurring in only about 2% of all isolates, it is isolated from one-third of cats with severe anaemia (10). Antigenic analysis by neutralisation indicates that all FeLV-A viruses are very closely related but that there is considerable heterogeneity within subgroups B and C (11).

THE OUTCOME OF EXOGENOUS FeLV INFECTION OF CATS

The major transmission cycle of FeLV is by free, infectious virus transferred from persistently infected carrier cats to susceptibles either in saliva or prenatally across the placenta (12,13). Following contact infection the virus grows in the oropharynx and spreads in macrophages and lymphocytes to local lymphoid tissue and then to the central haemopoietic tissue in the bone marrow (14). There is extensive viral growth in the marrow with the result that virus is released into the blood and is thereby disseminated to many other tissues.

There are several possible consequences of FeLV infection. The major division is between the establishment of a permanent, productive carrier state, or recovery. The outcome depends largely on the age of the cat and the dose of virus to which it is exposed. Thus, young kittens are more susceptible to infection than older cats and a higher proportion become carriers (15). Also, cats infected with high doses of virus, as in multiple cat households, are more likely to become carriers than those animals infected with small doses as in the free-range cat population (12).

In the development of the carrier state there appears to be virus-specific immunodepression. With the growth of FeLV in lympho-haemopoietic cells and in epithelial tissue there is a persistent viraemia and infectious virus is excreted from the mouth and transmitted via saliva and placenta to complete the productive trasmission cycle. Carrier cats have a very high risk of developing disease (16).

In the abortive infection which procedes recovery the extent of spread of virus throughout lympho-haemopoietic tissue is variable and there may or may not be transient viraemia (14,17). The apparent elimination of virus is due to an immune response associated with clearance of virus and virus-infected cells. Neutralising antibodies are found in recovered cats and play an important part in recovery (18,19). A cell mediated immune response is also considered to be involved. Recovered cats appear to be equivalent to non-infected cats in terms of survival (16).

In many cats which apparently recover from infection the virus takes a considerable period to be eliminated and during that time non-productive but provirus-containing cells are present in the bone marrow and other lymphoid organs. This virus may be activated in vivo by administration of corticosteroids (20) or in vitro by culture of aspirated bone marrow cells (21). The proportion of these latently infected cells declines with time (22,23). It is likely that the latent stage is mediated by an immune response but the mechanism by which latency is maintained is not yet known. Virus does not appear to be transmitted by contact from these animals (22). Whether or not they have a greater risk of developing FeLV-related diseases than uninfected cats, or cats which quickly eliminate FeLV following infection, remains to be seen. There may be a special category of cats, however, which transmits virus. In these animals the repression of the provirus is not completely controlled as indicated by the release of viral p27 into the blood and there is some evidence that they can transmit infectious virus to their young kittens although the route of infection is not yet established. (A. Pacitti and O. Jarrett - unpublished).

FeLV-RELATED DISEASES

The mechanisms involved in the development of several of these diseases have begun to be understood. In particular, lymphosarcoma, fibrosarcoma and anaemia have been studied in detail.

Thymic lymphosarcoma is a type of leukaemia which appears to originate in the bone marrow where transformed T-cells arise and then home in to the site of the thymus (24). The tumour cells are clonal as indicated by common integration sites of FeLV provirus in tumour cell DNA (6). The structure of FeLV proviruses and their association with cellular oncogenes in tumour DNA has been studied recently. The frequent rearrangement of the myc gene by FeLV in T-cell lymphosarcoma suggests that interactions between the virus and this proto-oncogene are important in the selection of leukaemic cells (25). Two types of interaction have been observed. In the first, integration of FeLV occurs close to the c-myc gene in an analogous fashion to findings in B-cell lymphomas induced by avian leukosis virus (26). As in the chicken, insertion of the exogenous provirus adjacent to myc has been found in experimentally-induced feline leukaemia. The question of whether FeLV promoters or enhancers of transcription act on the myc gene in this situation in the cat is unresolved. While in the FeLV-associated tumours which have been studied the level of myc transcription was considerably higher than an FeLV-negative lymphosarcoma, in contrast to the situation with avian leukosis virus myc transcripts were not linked to viral LTRs.

A second, and more frequent, type of FeLV-myc interaction was observed in naturally occurring T-cell leukaemias in cats (25,27,28). In these transduction of myc sequences by the virus occurred resulting in a recombinant FeLV-myc genome in which some viral sequences were replaced with myc DNA. Transcription of the myc gene was raised markedly in these tumours. Not only was this structure present in tumour cell DNA, but the recombinant virus was transmissible to fibroblasts in culture. Further, an inoculum containing the recombinant virus produced T-cell tumours in kittens in the remarkably short incubation period of 12 weeks (D.E. Onions, unpublished). These results indicate that the appearance of a recombinant FeLV-myc virus in a cat has dramatic consequences resulting in leukaemia.

Another malignant FeLV-related condition which has been studied in detail is fibrosarcomas. Fibrosarcomas have been observed in cats viraemic with FeLV. From cells of several of these tumours acute transforming viruses have been isolated in association with FeLV. All of these tumours, which represent 6-12% of cat tumours, have been of the multicentric type and most have occurred in cats under 5 years of age (29). These feline sarcoma viruses (FeSV) cause fibrosarcomas when inoculated into kittens and transform fibroblasts in vitro. The structure of the genome of several FeSV isolated has been examined (30). Each virus is a recombinant between FeLV and a cellular oncogene with deletion of FeLV sequences analogous to the FeLV-myc viruses described above. Thus far, seven separate proto-oncogenes have been transduced by FeLV in addition to myc.

The most studied non-malignant condition associated with FeLV is erythroid hypoplasia (10,31,32). From about one-third of cases of severe anaemia which were examined, FeLV of subgroup C was isolated (10). Inoculation of four separate isolates of FelV-C into kittens produced an identical syndrome of erythroid hypoplasia. This condition is the consequence of a failure of differentiation of an erythroid precursor cell, the BFU-E, brought about by infection with FeLV-C (10,33). The molecular mechanism by which the block in differentiation occurs is unclear but would appear to involve a very specific, rapid and direct effect of the virus on this particular cell type. The failure to isolate FeLV-C from healthy cats has led to the suggestion that each FeLV-C virus arose de novo in an individual cat as a result of recombination between exogenous FeLV and endogenous FeLV-like DNA sequences in cat cells (19). However, direct evidence of this origin of FeLV-C is not yet available.

This brief review of feline retroviruses and FeLV-related diseases highlights the fact that the pathogenesis of a variety of these conditions involves interactions between FeLV and cellular genes. In particular, it appears, that the generation of recombinants of FeLV and proto-oncogenes by transduction is a relatively common occurrence which is often associated with neoplasia. It will be interesting to determine if this mechanism is involved in the pathogenesis of naturally occurring tumours by retroviruses in other species.

REFERENCES

1. McAllister, R.M., Nicolson, M., Gardner, M.B., Rongey, R.W., Rasheed, S., Sarma, P.S., Huebner, R.J., Hatanaka, M., Oroszlan, S., Gilden, R.V., Kabigting, A., & Vernon, L. (1972) Nature New Biol. 235, 3-6.
2. Barbacid, M., Stephenson, J.R., & Aaronson, S.A. (1977) Cell 10, 641-648.
3. Livingston, D.M. & Todaro, G.J. (1973) Virology 53, 142-151.
4. Okabe, H., Twiddy, E., Gilden, R.V., Hatanaka, M., Hoover, E.A. & Olsen, R.G. (1976) Virology 69, 798-801.
5. Koshy, R., Gallo, R.C. & Wong-Stahl, F. (1980) Virology, 103,434-445.
6. Casey, J.W., Roach, A., Mullins, J.I., Burck, K.B., Nicolson, M.O., Gardener, M.B. & Davidson, N. (1981) Proc. Natl. Acad. Sci. USA 78, 7778-7782.
7. Sarma, P.S. & Log, T. (1973) Virol. 54, 160-169.
8. Jarrett, O., Hardy, W.D.Jr., Golder, M.C. & Hay, D. (1978) Int. J. Cancer. 21, 334-337.
9. Jarrett, O. & Russell, P.H. (1978) Int. J. Cancer 21, 466-472
10. Onions, D., Jarrett, O., Testa, N., Frassoni, F., & Toth, S. (1982) Nature 296, 156-158.
11. Russell, P.H. & Jarrett, O. (1978) Int. J. Cancer 21, 768-778.
12. Hardy, W.D.Jr., Old, L.J., Hess, P.W., Essex, M. & Cotter, S.M. (1973) Nature 244, 266-269.
13. Jarrett, W., Jarrett, O., Mackay, L., Laird, H., Hardy, W.D.Jr. & Essex, M. (1973b) J. Natl. Cancer

Inst. 51, 833-841.

14. Rojko, J.L., Hoover, E.A., Mathes, L.E;, & Olsen, R.G. (1979) J. Natl. Cancer. Inst 63, 759-768.
15. Hoover, E.A., Olsen, R.G., Hardy, W.D.Jr., Schaller, J.P. & Mathes, L.E. (1976) J. Natl. Cancer Inst.. 57, 365-369.
16. McClelland, A.J., Hardy, W.D. Jr., Zucherman, E.E. (1980) In: Feline Leukemia Virus, pp. 121-131. Eds. W.D. Hardy, Jr., M. Essex and A.J. McClelland. Elsevier, New York.
17. Jarrett, O., Golder, M.C., & Stewart, M.F. (1982) Vet. Rec. 110, 225-228.
18. Hardy, W.D.Jr., Hess, P.W., MacEwen, E.G., McClelland, A.J., Zuckerman, E.E., Essex, M., Cotter, S.M. & Jarrett, O. (1976) Cancer Res. 36, 582-588.
19. Russell, P.H. & Jarrett, O. (1978) Int. J. Cancer 22, 351-357.
20. Post, J.E. & Warren, L. (1980) In:Feline Leukaemia Virus pp 151-155. ed. W.D. Hardy,Jr. M. Essex & A.J. McClelland. Elsevier, New York.
21. Rojko, J.L., Hoover, E.A., Quackenbush, S.L. & Olsen, R.G. (1982) Nature 298, 385-388.
22. Madewell, B.R. & Jarrett, O. (1983) Vet.Rec. 112,339-342.
23. Pedersen, N.C., Meric, S.M., Ho, E., Johnson, L., Plucker, S., & Theilen, G.H. (1984) Feline Pract. 14, 32-48.
24. Hoover, E.A., Perryman, L.E. & Kociba, G.J. (1973) Cancer Res. 33, 145-152.
25. Neil, J.C., Hughes, D., McFarlane, R., Wilkie, N.M., Onions, D.E., Lees, G. & Jarrett, O. (1984) Nature 308, 814-820.
26. Hayward, W.G., Neel, B.G. & Astrin, S.M. (1981) Nature 290, 475-480.
27. Levy, L.S., Gardner, M.B. & Casey, J.W. Nature 308, 853-856.
28. Mullins, J.I., Brody, D.S., Binari, R.C. Jr. & Cotter, S.M., (1984) Nature 308, 856-858.
29. Hardy, W.D. Jr., (1980) In:Feline Leukemia Virus, pp.

79-118. Eds. W.D. Hardy, Jr., M. Essex and A.J. McClelland. Elsevier, New York.

30. Besmer, P. (1983) Curr. Top. Microbiol. Immunol. 107, 1-27.
31. Hoover, E.A., Kociba, G.J., Hardy, W.D.Jr. & Yohn, D.S. (1974) J. Natl. Cancer. Inst. 53, 1271-1276.
32. Mackey, L., Jarrett, W., Jarrett, O. & Laird, H. (1975) J. Natl. Cancer Inst; 54, 209-217.
33. Boyce, J.T., Hoover, E.A., Kociba, G.J. 1981) Exptl. Haematol. 9, 990-1001.

BOVINE LEUKEMIA VIRUS, A DISTINGUISHED MEMBER OF THE HUMAN T LYMPHOTROPIC VIRUSES FAMILY

A. Burny[1,3], C. Bruck[2], Y. Cleuter[1], D. Couez[1], J. Deschamps[1], J. Ghysdael[1], D. Gregroire[1], R. Kettmann[1,3], M. Mammerickx[2,3], G. Marbaix[1], D. Portetelle[1,3] and L. Willems[1,3].

1. Department of Molecular Biology, University of Brussels, 67, Rue des Chevaux, 1640 Rhode-St-Genèse, 2. National Institute for Veterinary Research, 99 Groeselenberg, 1180 Uccle, and 3. Faculty of Agronomy, 5800 Gembloux, Belgium

The Bovine Leukemia Virus (BLV) has many structural and functional characteristics in common with Human T lymphotropic Viruses (HTLVs). The most striking feature of these retroviruses is the existence of a Long Open Reading frame (LOR) located at the 3' side of the provirus between the right end of the 3' side of env gene and the left end of the Long Terminal Repeat (LTR). It is believed that the LOR protein product is of critical importance in the induction process of the tumor phase of bovine leukemia.

Prevention of BLV infection will be attempted through vaccination. To that aim, careful study of BLV envelope glycoprotein epitopes has shown that epitopes F, G and H play a major role in biological activities of the virus. Their native structure depends upon glycosylation of the peptide backbone.

Enzootic bovine leukemia has been known as an infectious disease for the last century (1-8). The agent, a retrovirus with morphological properties reminiscent of -- but not identical to -- those of the type C group, was discovered in 1969, in short-term in vitro cultures of lymphocytes from animals with persistent lymphocytosis (PL) (9). This condition, characterized by long lasting lymphocytosis, had been associated with bovine leukemia for a number of years and was considered a preleukemic state. (reviewed, 1 and 2). Circulating virus, however, had not been encountered and this was soon explained by the heavy load of circulating anti BLV antibodies found in PL animals (10,11). During this period, it was commonly thought that all leukemia viruses were related. BLV, however, did not seem to obey this widely accepted rule (12).Thus from the start, bovine leukemia seemed peculiar in the sense that viremia could not be shown and that PL animals carried heavy loads of anti-BLV antibody.

The oncogenic potential of BLV was demonstrated in sheep (13-15) and later in goats (16,17). Successful propagation of BLV in fetal lamb kidney cells (18) opened the road to characterization and analysis of BLV provirus structure, BLV cloning and sequencing, and the establishment of very sensitive methods of detection of BLV infection. The virus was shown to be able to infect animal species foreign to the subclass of ruminants, such as capybaras, pigs, rabbits, primates, etc. Computer-assisted analyses of sequencing data have clearly demonstrated that BLV and HTLVs are related members of the same large family (19-22), a new family of retroviruses acting in trans via a protein product encoded by the proviral genome. Some members of this new family induce chronic leukemias in sensitive animals; some are the causative agents of immunodeficiencies; and a number of them can act as killing or transforming agents depending upon parameters that are currently not understood.

The first interesting finding derived from annealing experiments between ^{3}H-BLV-cDNA and tumor DNA from BLV(+) animals was the observation that the labeled probe was hybridizing to tumor DNA and not to normal bovine DNA. The immediate and clearcut conclusion of these experiments was that BLV was an exogenus virus, unrelated to the bovine genome (23,24). All together, these experiments confirmed that enzootic bovine leukemia was an infectious disease and justified the sanitary policy aimed at eradication of the disease by elimination of infected recipients. The exogenous character of BLV was stressed again later on when clones and subclones of BLV proviral DNA became available (25).

To our surprise after examination of about 45 tumors from BLV infected animals, it appeared that all tumors carried at least the 3' portion of one BLV provirus. No tumor was found that was not the outcome of the clonal expansion of a BLV containing cell. On the contrary, PL lymphocytes appeared as a polyclonal population of cells, some containing a provirus, others being reactive cells with no trace of provirus integration (26,27). When several tumors of the same animal were examined, they all generally harbored the provirus(es) at the same location(s) indicating that a unique tumor clone was propagating in the animal,giving rise to a number of tumors in the various organs. Only once did we observe the simultaneous presence of two tumor clones in one animal. Long latency, clonality of tumors and constant presence of BLV footprints, were solid arguments pointing to BLV as a necessary participant in the onset of the neoplastic process.

For the virus to play a role in neoplasia, it was thought that it implied expression of the provirus. Poly A(+) RNA was extracted by various methods from tumor material selected for absence of necrotic lesions, and was immediately frozen in liquid nitrogen. Liquid or dot-blot hybridizations led to the same conclusion, namely that no expression of any part of BLV provirus and/or immediately flanking sequences was detectable in cells of fully developed tumors (28).

From these data, it could be inferred that either BLV expression was never required for the tumor cell to take off or was no longer required in the tumor cells once the switch from the normal to the neoplastic state had been turned on. Approach to the solution of the above alternatives led us to investigate the site of integration of BLV provirus in various tumors, considering that the provirus, although silent, could evoke expression of neighboring genes through a downstream promotion effect (29) or through a more distant enhancer effect (30). To that end, the 3' proximate flanking DNA sequencs from 3 tumors were cloned and used as probes with DNA extracted from some 45 tumors. The conclusions reached were the same for the 3 probes: the restriction profile obtained was the same for calf thymus DNA and all the tumor DNAs examined. In the tumor of origin, the flanking DNA probe recognized 2 bands, due to the fact that the provirus integrated solely in one chromosome of a given pair.

Statistical calculations made from the above data showed that if a preferential domain for BLV integration existed, it had to be extremely large (31). These assumptions were indeed verified in experiments with hamster-bovine cell hybrids. A number of these were available from which bovine chromosomes had segregated. This material was ideal to answer the question whether provirus integration could occur in the same chromosome in all cases, even if the integration domain was large (32). The data depicted in Figure 1., clearly demonstrated that the DNA of a given clone hybridized to one (or two) probe(s) and not to the third one, thus excluding the possibility that the provirus had to integrate in a given chromosome in order to lead to transformation.

Given the fact that the 3' end of a provirus was systematically present in the tumor cell, it was argued that this proviral region was bearing the necessary information required to transform the target cell. We also hypothesized that after transformation, extinction of provirus expression is mandatory in order to allow the neoplastic cells to escape immune surveillance while proliferating. BLV provirus sequencing (21,22) has given credit to the above assumptions. As in HTLV-I and HTLV-II

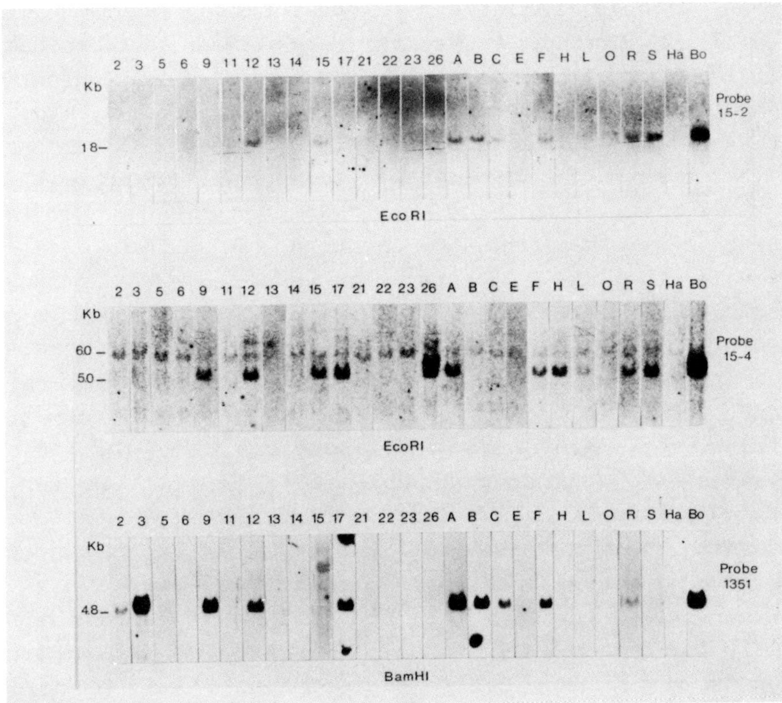

Figure 1. Restriction analysis of hamster x bovine hybrid DNAs. (A) ten micrograms each of normal parental hamster cell DNA (lane Ha), normal parental bovine DNA (lane Bo), and 25 hamster x bovine hybrid DNAs (lanes 2 through S) were digested to completion by EcoRI. The DNA was depurinated and transferred to nitrocellulose. The filters were hybridized for 48 h with 0.007 ug (10^9 cpm/ug) of ^{32}P-labeled probe 15-2 per ml. Autoradiography was carried out after a 5 day exposure. B. Same as in (A), but with ^{32}P-labeled probe 1351 (0.010 ug/ml, $3x10^8$ cpm/ug). Exposure time was 3 days. (The molecular weights of all native DNAs was 50 kb, as estimated by electrophoresis in 0.8% agarose gels with lamda phage DNA as the molecular weight marker).

genomes (33–35), the BLV proviral genome contains a long open reading frame (LOR) located in the so-called px region (21) and transcribed in BLV-infected cells as a 2,1 kb mRNA (R. Mamoun, T. Astier, R. Kettmann, J. Deschamps, N. Rebeyrotte, and B. Guillemain, personal communicaton). The protein coded for by the LOR sequence acts as a potent activator of BLV transcription (C.A. Rosen, J.G. Sodroski, R. Kettmann, A. Burny, and W.A. Haseltine, submitted) just as previously discovered for HTLV (34,35). It is worth noting here that the LOR protein of HLTV-I does not activate the BLV LTR and vice-versa. Rather stringent specificity has developed here. It is also remarkable that even if expression of BLV provirus is most probably important in initiation of cell transformation, it is no longer required (and is indeed suppressed!) in tumor cells, even maintained in tissue culture for several passages (R. Kettmann, unpublished). Experiments carried out with normal circulating lymphocytes and tumor cells also indicated that none of the presently known oncogenes was grossly overexpressed in BLV-induced tumors. On the contrary, it was recently found that B-lym expression was easily detected in normal lymphocytes but totally suppressed in tumor cells. Even if B-lym plays a role in the tumorization process, it is extinct in the fully developed tumor (L. Willens, unpublished).

Intensive research has been carried out to characterize the biologically active epitopes located on BLV envelope glycoprotein gp51 (36,37). Production of a battery of monoclonal antibodies directed against gp51 has allowed the identification of 3 closely located epitopes, named F, G and H, responsible for the biological properties of the virus, namely infectivity and syncytia induction. That these 3 epitopes are well exposed at the outside of the virus or at the surface of the infected cell was demonstrated by the fact that recently infected cattle only react against these 3 epitopes (38). With time however the immune reaction broadens to encompass all epitopes of the surface glycoprotein.

Table 1. Evolution of antibody levels of sheep born from an enzootic bovine leukosis infected mother (BLV-).

Date	M. 374			M. 375			M. 378			M.379		
	AGID gp	AGID p 24	RIA gp	AGIG gp	AGID p 24	RIA gp	AGID gp	AGID p 24	RIA gp	AGID gp	AGID p 24	RIA gp
17-04-73	+++++	–	76880	+++++	+	89040	ND	ND	ND	ND	ND	ND
12-07-73	+++	–	5250	+++	–	6020	+++++	–	–	+++++	+	56730
23-10-73	–	–	320	–	–	500	++	–	1540	+	–	2510
05-11-74	–	–	0	–	–	0	–	–	0	–	–	< 100
12-11-75	–	–	0	–	–	0	–	–	0	–	–	0
14-10-76	–	–	0	–	–	0	–	–	0	–	–	0
26-09-77	–	–	0	–	–	0	–	–	0	–	–	0
10-10-77	–	–	0	–	–	0	–	–	0	–	–	0
24-10-77	–	–	0	–	–	0	++	–	310	++	–	560
07-11-77	–	–	0	–	–	0	++	–	590	++++	–	1570
22-11-77	–	–	0	–	–	0	+++	–	1690	++++	–	3170
05-12-77	–	–	0	–	–	< 100	+++	–	3210	++++	–	4350
20-12-77	–	–	0	++++	–	2350	++++	–	4390	++++	–	7280
03-01-78	–	–	< 100	++++	–	5590	++++	–	6690	++++	–	7660
23-01-78	–	–	0	+++++	–	9960	++++	–	12830	++++	–	10290
29-08-78	–	–	0	+++++	++	130200	+++++	–	27160	++++	–	35460
01-03-79	–	–	< 100	+++++	++	239660	+++++	–	49710	+++++	–	31180

Table 1. Evolution of antibody levels of sheep born from an enzootic bovine leukosis infected mother (BLV-). Animals were given two series of oral inoculations with blood from an enzootic bovine leukosis infected cow (BLV+); the first at birth and the second at 4 years. Infection trials at birth failed; infections at 4 years were successful except in animal M. 374.

M. 374 -- female, born 05-03-73, mother M. 319 (BLV+) -- and M. 375 -- female, born 05-03-73, mother M. 319 (BLV+) -- were inoculated orally with blood B. 907 (BLV+) from birth to 13-04-73 and with blood B. 82 (BLV+) from 26-09-77 to 28-10-77.

M. 378 -- female, born 08-05-73, mother M. 330 (BLV+) -- and M. 379 -- female, born 08-05-73, mother M. 321 (BLV+) -- were inoculated orally with blood B.907 (BLV+) from birth to 25-06-73 and with blood B. 82 (BLV+) from 26-09-77 to 28-10-77.

Monoclonals directed against F, G or H are unreactive toward p46, the non-glycosylated precursor of gp51 or toward gp51 heat-denatured at 100°C in the presence of sodium dodecylsulfate and blotted on nitrocellulose. This indicates that the three monoclonals recognize a conformation and not a sequence (39) . Such an observation is of basic importance, establishing that the native configuration of F,G,H is dependent upon glycosylation. Design and tailoring of efficient anti BLV vaccines have obviously to cope with the difficulties of reproducing a three dimensional structure imposed on the glycoprotein by the sugar residues. Most probably, expression of gp51 will have to be carried out in host vector systems that provide adequate glycosylation.

The basic question that arises deals with the possibility of mounting an efficient protective barrier against BLV infection, considering that most virus propagation occurs via the cellular route. Experiments carried out by Mammerickx et al. (49) (Table 1) propose a positive answer to that question. Data detailed in Table 1, show that lambs harboring passive antibodies are fully protected against challenges with massive amounts of infected cells. As soon, however, as passive antibody titers have fallen to very low values, animals become fully sensitive to the challenging infectious material. Provided that the vaccination procedure used offers a protection of comparable efficacy to that of passive immunity, it seems quite reasonable to assume that vaccintion will be a method of choice to block spread of BLV infection.

If we assume -- and this seems to be a reasonable assumption -- that an efficient immune protection will have to be dircted against F, G and H, it remains to be seen if F, G and H are well conserved determinants present in all possible BLV variants. To that end we carried out a survery of the reactivity of a number of BLV isolates with our panel of monoclonal antibodies.

Somewhat to our surprise, it appeared that animal vdM 7628 carried a BLV strain almost devoid of epitope F whilst all animals of the MM herd had a BLV strain lacking epitope G and from which epitope H was almost missing (40). Thus far, however, we have not found a BLV isolate devoid of all three F, G, H epitopes. We thus tentatively conclude that vaccines against BLV must contain in the right configuration the three epitopes F, G and H.

The feasibility of a vaccine preventing BLV infection calls for in-depth analysis of the possibilities of using the same approach to achieve protection against HTLV-I and HTLV-II, etiologic agents of human T cell leukemias, and LAV/HTLV-III, a novel subgroup of viruses, strongly suspected to be the agents responsible for AIDS (Acquired Immune Deficiency Syndrome). That BLV and the HTLVs belong to the same family was suggested by the homology of amino acid sequences found in BLV and HTLV-I p24s (19-20). A remote but significant relatedness between BLV and LAV/HTLV-III was recently illustrated by immunogold reactions performed on lymphoid tissues of prodromic AIDS patients (41). The antibodies used in these studies were directed against BLV and HTLV-I structural proteins. These last data were confirmed and extended recently by Thiry et al. (L. Thiry, S. Sprecher-Goldberger, J. Cogniaux, P. Jacquemain, A. Burny, D. Portetelle, N. Clumeck, N. and S. Cran, unpublished) who showed significant reactivities of BLV anti p24 and gp51 antibodies and cell extracts of LAV/HTLV-III infected human lymphocytes. Extracts of the same cells but non infected were devoid of any reactivity. It is of interest to note here that rabbits infected by BLV die, with high frequency, of a wasting disease reminiscent of immune deficiency. We often observed that anti BLV antibody titer fluctuates up and down, until a sharp drop to about zero precedes death by just a few hours. It is at the same time remarkable that the plasma immunoglobulin concentration of these animals remained absolutely normal.

The data accumulated thus far indicate that BLV and the HTLVs (LAV) belong to a new family of retroviruses, derived most probably from a common ancestor. The relevant virus systems will provide answers to a few puzzling questions such as:

1. What are the mechanisms of leukemogenesis that involve expression of a virus gene and lead to chronic leukemia ?
2. What are the parameters that condition cell killing or its neoplastic transformation. Answers to these questions will bring deeper insight into the intricacies of cell proliferation and differentiation.

ACKNOWLEDGEMENTS

The work performed in the authors' laboratory was helped financially by the Belgian Ministry of Agriculture and the Funds cancerologique de la Caisse Generale d'Epargne et de Retraite - DC, RK, GM and LW are fellows of the Fonds National e la Recherche Scientifique. DG is a fellow of Institut pour la Recherche Scientifique dans l'Industrie et l'Agriculture.

REFERENCES

1. Burny, A., Bex, F., Chantrenne, H., Cleuter, Y., Dekgel, D., Ghysdael, J., Kettmann, R., Leclercq, M., Leunen, J., Mammercikx, M. & Portetelle, D. (1978). Adv. Cancer Res. 28, 251-311.
2. Burny, A., Bruck, C., Chantrenne, H., Cleuter, Y., Dekegel, D., Ghysdael, J., Kettmann, R., Leclercq, M., Leunen, J., Mammercikx, M. & Portetelle, D. (1980). Bovine Leukemia Virus: Molecular Biology and Epidemiology. In "Viral Oncology" (G. Klein, ed.) pp. 231-289, Raven Press, New York.
3. Burny, A., Bruck, C., CLeuter, Y., Couez, D., Dekegel, D., Deschamps, J., Ghysdael, J., Gilden, R.V., Kettmann, R., Mammerickx, M., Marbaix, G. & Portetelle, D. (1984). Leukaemogenesis by Bovine Leukaemia Virus. In: "Mechanisms of Viral Leukaemogenesis" (J.M. Goldmann and O. Jarrett, eds) pp. 229-260. Churchill Livingstone, Edinburgh.
4. Burny, A., Bruck, C., Couez, D., Deschamps, J., Ghysdael, J., Kettmann, R., Mammerickx, M., Marbaix, G. & Portetelle, D. (1984). Enzootic Bovine Leukemia: its Relevance as a Model System for Human T cell Leukemia. In: "Human T-cell Leukemia/Lymphoma Viruses" (R.C. Gallo, M. Essex, L. Gross, eds) pp. 17-24. Cold Spring Harbor Laboratory, Cold Spring Harbor, New York.
5. Ghysdael, J., Bruck, C., Kettmann, R. & Burny, A. (1984). Bovine Leukemia Virus, Curr. Top. Microb. Immunol. 112, 1-19.
6. Portetele, D., Bruck, C., Mammerickx, M. & Burny, A. (1984). Bovine Leukosis: Recent Developemnts with use of Monoclonal antibodies and ELISA Tests. In "Recent Advances in Virus Diagnosis" (M.S. McNulty, J.B. Ferran, eds.) pp. 157-170., Martinus Nyhoff, Boston.
7. Burny, A., Bruck, C., Cleuter, Y., Couez, D., Ceschamps, J., Ghysdael, J., Kettmann, R., Mammerickx, M., Marbaix, G. & Portetelle, D. (1985) Bovine Leukemia Virus: A New Mode of Leukemogenesis.

In"Advance in Viral Oncology". (G. Klein, ed.) in press.
8. Mussgay, M. & Kaaden O.R. (1978) Progress in Studies on the Etiology and Serologic Diagnosis of Enzootic Bovine Leukosis. Curr. Top. Microb. Immunol. 79, 43-72.
9. Miller, J.M., Miller, L.D., Olson, C., & Gillette, K.G. (1969) J. Natl. Cancer Insti., 43, 1297-1305.
10. Miller, J.M. & Olson, C. (1972) J. Natl. Cancer Inst., 49, 1459-1462.
11. Ferrer, J.F., Avila, L. & Stock, N.D. (1972) Cancer Res., 32, 1864-1870.
12. Ferrer, J.F., (1972). Cancer Res., 32, 1872-1877.
13. Wittmann, W. & Urbaneck, D. (1969) Arch. Exp. Vererinaery Med, 23, 709-713.
14. Mammercikx, M. (1970) Exper. Anim., 3, 285-293.
15. Olson, C., Miller, L.D., Miller J.M. & Hoss, H.E. (1972) J. Natl. Cancer Inst., 49, 1463-1467.
16. Olson, C., Kettmann, R., Burny, A. & Kaja, R. (1981) J. Natl. Cancer Inst. 67, 671-675.
17. Kettmann, R., Mammerickx, M., Portetelle, D., Gregoire, D. & Burny, A. (1984) Leukemia Res., in press.
18. Van der Maatern, M.J. & Miller, J.M. (1976). Bibl. Haematol. 43, 360-362.
19. Oroszlan, S., Copeland, T.D., Kalyanaraman, V.S., Sarngadharan, M.G., Schultz, A.M. & Gallo, R.C. (1984) Chemical Analysis of Human T-cell Leukemia Virus Structural Proteins. In: "Human T-cell Leukemia/Lymphoma Viruses". (R.C. Gallo, M. Essex, L. Gross, eds.) pp 101-110. Cold. Spring Harbor Laboratory, Cold Spring Harbor, New York.
20. Orszlan, S., Sarngadharan, M.G., Copeland, T.D., Kalyanaraman, N.S., Gilden, R.V., & Gallo, R.C. (1982) Proc. Natl. Acad. Sci. USA, 79, 1291-1295.
21. Rice, N.R., Stephens, R.M., Couez, S., Deschamps, J., Kettmann, R., Burny, A. & Gilden, R.V. (1984) Virology, in press.
22. Sagata, N., Yasunaga, T., Tsuzuku-Kawamura, J.,

Ohishi, K., Ogawa, Y. & Ikawa, Y. (1984) Proc. Natl. Acad. Sci. USA, in press.

23. Kettmann, R., Portetelle, D., Mammerichx, M., Cleuter, Y., Dekegel, D., Galoux, M., Ghysdael, J., Burny, A. & Chantrenne, H. (1976) Proc. Natl. Acad. Sci. USA 73, 1014-1018.
24. Callahan R., Leiber, M.M., Todaro, G.J., Graves, D.C., & Ferrer, J.F. (1976) Science 192, 1005-1007.
25. Deschamps, J., Kettmann, R. & Burny, A. (1981) J. Virol., 40, 605-609.
26. Kettmann, R., Cleuter, Y., Mammerickx, M., Meunier-Rotival, M., Bernardi, G., Burny, A. & Chantrenne, H. (1980) Proc. Natl. Acad. Sci. USA 77, 2577-2581.
27. Kenyon, S.J., & Piper, C.E. (1977). Infect. Immun., 16, 898-903.
28. Kettmann, R., Deschhamps, J., Cleuter, Y., Couez, D., Burny, A. & Marbaix, G. (1982). Proc. Natl. Sci. USA 79, 2465-2469.
29. Hayward, W.S., Neel, B.G., & Astrin, S.M. (1981) Nature 290, 475-480.
30. Payne, G.S., Bishop, J.M. & Varmus, H.E. (1981) Nature 295, 209-213.
31. Kettmann, R., Deschamps, J., Couez, D., Claustriaux, J.J., Palm, R. & Burny, A. (1983) J. Virol. 47, 146-150.
32. Gregoire, D., Couez, D., Deschamps, J., Heuertz, S., Hors-Cayla, M.C., Szpirer, J., Szpirer, C., Burny, A., Huez, G. & Kettmann, R. (1984) J. Virol. 50, 275-279.
33. Seiki, M., Hattori, S., Hirayama, Y., & Yoshida, M. (1983) Proc. Natl. Acad. Sci. USA 80, 3618-3622.
34. Sadroski, J.G., Rosen, C.A. & Haseltine, W.A. (1984) Science 225, 281-285.
35. Haseltine, W.A., Sodroski, J.G., Patarca, R., Briggs, D., Perkins, D. & Wong-Staal, F. (1984) Science 225, 419-421.
36. Bruck, C., Mathot, S., Portetelle, D., Berte, C., Granssen, J.D., Herin, P. & Burny, A. (1982). Virology 122, 342-352.

37. Bruck, C., Portetelle, D., Burny, A. & Zavada, J. (1982) Virology 122, 353-362.
38. Bruck, C., Portetelle, D., Mammerickx, M., Mathot, S. & Burny, A. (1984). Leukemia Res. 8, 315-321.
39. Bruck, C., Rensonnet, N., Portetelle, D., Cleuter, Y., Mammerickx, M., Burny, A., Mamoun, R., Guillemain, B., Van der Maaten, M.J., & Ghysdael, J. (1984) Virology, 136, 20-31.
40. Mammerickx, M., Portetelle, D., Burny, A. & Leunen, J. (1980) Zentrabl. Veterinaermed B., 27, 291-303.
41. Feremans, W.W., Menu, R., Goldman, M., Schandene, L., Portetelle, D., Cleuter, Y., J., Dustin, P., Wybran,

ASSOCIATION OF ULTRAVIOLET-INDUCED RETROVIRUS EXPRESSION WITH ANCHORAGE-INDEPENDENT SURVIVAL IN RAT EMBRYO CELLS

W.A. Suk

Laboratory of Cellular and Molecular Oncology, In Vitro Toxicology Program, Northrop Services, Inc., P.O. Box 12313, Research Triangle Park, N.C. 27709

Our previous studies have shown that carcinogens (chemical or physical) induce an enhancement of anchorage-independent (AI) survival in aggregate form, a premalignant phenotype in retrovirus-infected Fischer rat embryo (RIFRE) cells. A specific role for the nontransforming retrovirus genome has been shown in the expression of AI survival: uninfected Fischer rat embryo (FRE) cells are relatively unresponsive to treatment with chemical carcinogens, whereas RIFRE cells are highly responsive. However, exposure of FRE cells to increasing doses (500-2000 uJ/cm^2) of ultraviolet (UV) irradiation induced AI survival dose dependently. Cells isolated in aggregate form were allowed to reattach and, upon reaching confluency, were subcultured. The replated UV-exposed cells subsequently showed changes in their cellular morphology as well as growth in semisolid agar, indicating their neoplastic potential. In an attempt to explain the enhanced cell survival in FRE cells following their exposure to UV, the cells were assayed for the presence of endogenous retrovirus by immunofluorescence. The FRE cells were exposed to UV, refed on supplemented media, and the presence of virus was antigenically determined with goat anti-Moloney virus. Endogenous retrovirus expression was detected dose-dependently at similar UV exposure levels used in the expression of increased cellular AI survival. The results show that UV-induced activation of endogenous retrovirus expression in rat embryo cells is associated with the induction of AI survival, a phenotype that precedes the acquisition of morphological or neoplastic transformation.

Previous studies have shown that nontransforming retroviruses play a significant and specific role in promoting the expression of transformation (1-6). Fischer rat embryo cells infected with Rauscher leukemia virus (RLV) were reported to be susceptible to chemically induced neoplastic transformation (1,3,6). Low passage FRE cell cultures were resistant to spontaneous transformation, chemically induced transformation, or transformation by murine retroviruses; however, cultures chronically infected with retrovirus had an increased sensitivity to transformation by chemical carcinogens (3,6). Chemical transformation was also seen when low-passage FRE cells were infected with a xenotropic retrovirus (5), or when the endogenous rat leukemia virus was induced by treatment with a halogenated pyrimidine (2). It was further shown that active viral synthesis is a prerequisite for chemically induced transformation (3), and if this synthesis is inhibited by virus specific antisera, chemically induced cell transformation is also inhibited (4,5).

Proliferation of cells in an AI state in semisolid medium has been considered a confirmation of neoplastic transformation (7). The ability of transformed cells to aggregate and/or survive in liquid media above a base layer of solid agar is considered an extension of their anchorage independence and has been used to confirm transformation of a variety of cells exposed to either viruses or chemicals (8,9). Anchorage-independent survival as an indicator of neoplastic transformation has been measured and applied to RLV-infected FRE cells (10). Recently, a number of modifications have been made in the assay that have increased its sensitivity and reproducibility (11,12) and have enabled the RIFRE cells to respond to chemical carcinogen treatment dose dependently. The data also showed that cells exhibiting carcinogen-mediated enhancement of AI survival subsequently progressed to a transformed phenotype (12).

We have also shown in the AI assay that the nontransforming retrovirus increases the differential in enhanced survival response in infected cultures (12). To more fully understand this aspect of the system, we examined the effect of UV irradiation on infected and uninfected FRE cells. In this communication we report that UV irradiation induces AI survival in infected and uninfected cells; in uninfected cells there is a concomitant induction of endogenous retrovirus expression.

The AI survival of both cell lines was determined using a previously described procedure (15). Anchorage-dependent media control and solvent control cells, when suspended in medium above an agar base layer, showed a rapid decline in cell survival; however, cells that had been treated with carcinogen did not undergo the destructive process that took place in control cells, indicating specificity.

The comparative effects of chemical and physical carcinogens on RIFRE and FRE cells are shown in Table 1. Two chemical carcinogens, 7,12-dimethylbenzanthracene (DMBA) and benzo(a)pyrene (B(a)P), were used to compare the responsiveness of the two cell lines in the AI survival assay; these agents, as well as others, have also been shown in RIFRE cells to respond dose-dependently (12). The passage level of the two cell lines was similar. The chemical carcinogens enhanced the expression of AI survival when RLV was present, but did not do so when the retrovirus was absent. DMBA at 0.1 and 1.0 ug/ml enhanced the expression of AI survival 247 and 605%, respectively , in RIFRE cells, but only 16 and 20% respectively, in FRE cells; B(a)P at 0.5 and 5.0 ug/ml increased AI survival 144 and 161%, respectively, in RIFRE cells, whereas no response was detected in FRE cells. The cytotoxicity of both carcinogens in these cells lines was comparable Thus, this enhanced survival response in chemically treated cells appears related to the presence of the retrovirus.

Several reports on cellular transformation induced by UV irradiation have recently appeared (13,14). We have also recently shown the transforming potential of UV irradiation in RIFRE cells using AI survival as an endpoint (15). The cells were seeded at 6.66 x 10^3 cells/cm^2 in 100 mm petridishes, and incubated for 24 h, at which time the medium was removed from the experimental dishes and the cultures were exposed to UV light (254 nm) at an intensity of 100 uJ/cm^2. Cultures were refed with EMEM and incubated for 72 h. The procedure then followed the replication/recovery and agar phases of the AI survival assay (12). Exposure of RIFRE and FRE cells to increasing doses of UV irradiation caused an enhancement of AI survival in both cell lines; the reponses were dose-dependent (Table I). UV irradiation at 500, 1000, and 2000 uJ/cm^2 induced AI survival 110, 138, and 385% respectively, in RIFRE cells, and 77, 106, and 215%, respectively, in FRE cells. Although the enhanced survival response was somewhat higher in the RIFRE cells, it was comparable to the FRE cells. The cytotoxicity observed in both cell lines was comparable. It appears, therefore, that UV irradiation is capable of inducing AI survival in rat cells, whether they are retrovirus-infected or not.

Cells taken directly from the assay after the four day agar phase were plated into 25 cm^2 flasks to establish cell cultures. Upon reaching confluence, these cultures were passaged biweekly and examined macroscopically and microscopically for changes in their cellular morphology (1,6,12). The control cells remained normal in appearance while the chemically treated and UV-treated cells showed loss of contact inhibition (data not shown). In correlative studies, these same cells were seeded into semisold agar at 5x10^5 cells per 60 mm dish according to the procedure of MacPherson (16). This anchorage independent phenotype was selected because of the relationship between malignant potential and the ability

Table 1. Association of retrovirus with anchorage-independent survival and growth phenotypes in Fisher rat embryo cells

Treatment[b]	% Cyto-toxicity[c]	Mean No Cells + SD[d] ($x10^3$)	% Enhanced Survival[e]	Growth in Semisolid Agar[f]
		RIFRE Cells[a]		
Medium	0	40.0±2.1	0	-
500 uj/cm^2	73	84.0±3.6	110	+
1,000 uj/cm^2	82	95.0±4.7	138	NT[g]
2,000 uj/cm^2	84	194.0±3.6	385	+
DMSO,0.1 %	0	40.0±3.2	0	-
DMBA,0.1 ug/ml	74	138.8±5.4	247	NT
DMBA,1.0 ug/ml	88	282.4±6.7	605	+
B(a)P,0.5 ug/ml	50	104.4±3.1	144	+
B(a)P,5.0 ug/ml	62	97.6±4.4	161	NT
		FRE Cells (a)		
Medium	0	31.3±3.1	0	-
500 uj/cm^2	79	55.3±2.9	77	-
1,000 uj/cm^2	79	64.7±3.0	106	+
2.000 uj/cm^2	88	98.7±3.7	215	+
DMSO, 0.1 %	0	36.7±2.1	0	-
DMBA,0.1 ug/ml	75	42.7±5.6	16	-
DMBA,1.0 ug/ml	85	44.1±5.0	20	-
B(a)P,0.5 ug/ml	70	38.5±5.9	5	-
B(a)P,5.0 ug/ml	62	36.0±5.9	-2	NT

(a) The RIFRE cells used in this assay have been described previously (10,12). The FRE cells were received from Dr. J. Poiley and were also previously described (12). The cells were cultivated in Eagle's minimum essential medium with 10% fetal bovine serum and grown in 37° C incubators with a water-saturated atmosphere of 5% CO_2 in air; no antibiotics were used.

(b) The cultures were treated with varying concentrations of DMBA or B(a)P for three days or exposed to UV light (254 nm) at an incidence of 100 uJ/cm^2/sec; UV-exposed cells were immediately refed with medium. Seventy-two h later; the cultures (chemical- and UV-treated) were refed for an additional three-day incubation period. They were subsequently trypsinized, adjusted for cytotoxicity, and overlaid at 6 x 10^5 cells per 60 mm dishes containing 1% agar Noble medium. Viable cell counts using trypan blue exclusion were made following four days in suspension in medium above agar.

(c) Cytotoxicity was determined at the end of the additional three-day incubation period (replicative recovery phase) prior to suspending the cells above agar; cells dissociated at this time were counted for subsequent assay procedures. The cellular toxicity is expressed as a percentage of the solvent control and media control for chemical- and UV-treated cultures, respectively.

(d) The mean and standard deviation of the number of viable cells counted (X 10^3) determined on three dishes at the end of the four day agar phase.

(e) The enhanced survival response is expressed as the number of anchorage-independent surviving viable cells induced by carcinogen treatment relative to the solvent of medium control cells: % Enhanced Survival is defined as the Treated VCN less the Control VCN, divided by the Control VCN, and then multiplied by 100. The VCN equals viable cell number.

(f) Cells were maintained in culture for up to eight passages; periodically 5 x 10^5 cells per 60 mm dish were tested for growth in semisolid agar (16).

of cells to grow in semisolid agar (7). The results of these studies are also shown in Table 1. The frequency of expression of growth in semisolid agar correlated with enhanced cell survival that had been shown in the assay performed some weeks prior, indicating progression to this malignant phenotype.

Induction of endogenous retrovirus from cells primarily of mouse origin, has been reported with UV irradiation (17,18). Therefore, retrovirus expression was antigenically examined with goat anti-Moloney virus (19) on FRE cells in an attempt to explain the enhanced cell survival following UV exposure. Exposure to increasing doses of UV induced endogenous retrovirus expression is shown in Figure 1. In all immunofluorescence experiments, the peak induction occurred between 48 and 72 h. The UV dose-response curve shows that the virus induction frequency increased with UV exposure reaching an optimum at 2000 uJ/cm^2. The assay detects cells producing infectious retrovirus but may also detect cells producing only viral protein resulting from partial expression or induction of defective viral foci. Retrovirus expression was detected at UV exposure similar to those that caused the enhancement of AI survival and subsequently morphological and malignant phenotypes.

The enhancement of AI survival by carcinogens appears to be a preneoplastic event associated with progression to neoplastic transformation and is relevant to the carcinogenic process. The system presented in these studies appears to require retrovirus. The molecular mechanisms underlying the retrovirus-dependent transformation of rat embryo cells are not yet determined. Recent work by Land et al. (20), Newbold and Overell (21), and Ruley (22), gives a molecular clue to the multihit character of carcinogenesis. The process of carcinogen-induced immortality/establishment that predisposes cells to further progression to malignancy, yields cellular functions beyond those achieved by transforming oncogenes alone. The present study provides a

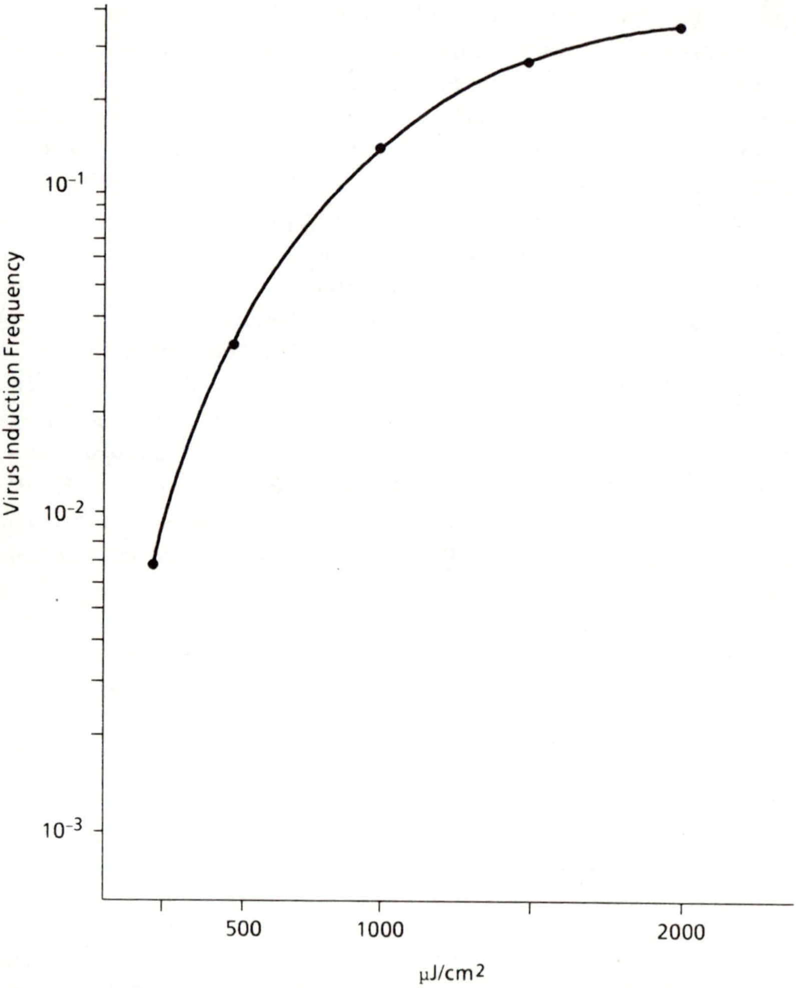

Figure 1. Dose-response relationship for UV induction of endogenous retrovirus from FRE cells. Monolayer cultures were exposed to increasing doses of UV irradiation (254 nm) and subsequently refed on medium supplemented with 10^{-6} M hydrocortisone, 0.2 ug/ml polybrene. At the end of 48 h, cell counts were done and coverslips were harvested for immunofluorescence assay (19). The data are expressed as:

$$\text{virus induction frequency} = \frac{\text{Fraction cells induced}}{\text{Fraction cells viable}}$$

valuable system for investigation of the molecular nature of these events associated with the progression to neoplastic transformation, as well as the role of the retrovirus in the expression of this process.

ACKNOWLEDGEMENTS

The author thanks Joan Humphreys, Perry Hays, and John Arnold for their technical assistance; and Dr. Raymond W. Tennant for his continued interest and support. This research was sponsored by NIEHS/NTP Contract N01-ES-15798.

REFERENCES

1. Freeman, A.E., Price, P.J., Zimmerman, E.M., Kelloff, G.J. & Huebner, R.J. (1973) in Unifying Concepts of Leukemia, eds. Dutcher, R.M. & Chieco-Bianchi, L. (Bibliotheca Haematologica), No. 39, pp. 617-634.
2. Freeman, A.E., Gilden, R.V., Vernon, M.L., Wolford, R.G., Hugunin, P.E. & Huebner, R.J. (1973) Proc. Natl. Acad. Sci USA 70, 2415-2419.
3. Price, P.J., Suk, W.A. & Freeman, A.E. (1972) Science 177, 1003-1004.
4. Price, P.J., Bellew T.M., King, M.P., Freeman, A.E., Gilden, R.V. & Huebner, R.J., (1976) Proc. Natl. Acad. Sci. USA 73, 152-155.
5. Price, P.J., Suk, W.A., Peters, R.L., Gilden, R.V., & Huebner, R.J. (1977) Proc. Natl. Acad. Sci. USA 74, 579-581.
6. Price, P.J. & Mishra, N.K. (1980) in Advances in Modern Environmental Toxicology eds Mishra, N., Dunkel, V. & Mehlman, M. (Senate Press, Inc. New Jersey), Vol. 1, Mammalian cell transformation by chemical carcinogens, pp. 213-239.
7. Shin, S., Freedman, V.N., Risser, R. & Pollack, R. (1975) Proc. Natl. Acad. Sci. USA 11, 4435-4439.
8. Cho, H., Cutchins, E., Rhim, J. & Huebner, R. (1976) Science 194, 951-953.

9. Steuer, A.F., Hentosh, P., Diamond, L. & Ting, R.C. (1977) Cancer Res. 37, 1864-1867.
10. Traul, K.A., Takayama, K., Kachevsky, V., Hink, R.J. & Wolff, J.S. (1981). J. Appl. Toxicology 1, 190-195.
11. Suk, W.A., Humphreys, J.E., Arnold, J.D. & Hays, E.P. (1983). Proc. Am. Assoc. Cancer Res. 24, 401.
12. Suk, W.A., Poiley, J.A., Raineri, R., Steuer, A.F. & Tennant, R.W. (in press) Environmental Mutagenesis.
13. Chan, G.L. & Little, J.B. (1979) Br. J. Cancer 39, 590-593.
14. Ananthaswamy, H.N. & Kripke, M.L. (1981) Cancer Res. 41, 2882-2890.
15. Suk, W.A. & Arnold, J.D. (1984) Proc. Am. Assoc. Cancer Res; 25, 528.
16. MacPherson, I. (1969) In Fundamental Techniques in Virology, eds. Abel, K. & Salzman, N.P. (Academic Press, New York), pp 274.
17. Hellman, K.B., & Brewer, P.P. (1979) Mutation Res. 62, 205-212.
18. Niwa, O. & Sugahara, T. (1979) J. Natl. Cancer Inst. 62, 329-335.
19. Tennant, R.W., Farrelly, J.G., Ihle, J.M., Kenney, B.C. & Brown, A. (1973). J. Virol. 12, 1216-1225.
20. Land, H., Parada, L.F. & Weinberg, R.A. (1983). Nature 304, 596-602.
21. Newbold, R.F. & Overell, R.W. (1983) Nature 304, 648-651;
22. Ruley, H.E., (1983) Nature 304, 602-606.

PARTICIPATION OF 7S L RNA IN REVERSE TRANSCRIPTION BY AN AVIAN RETROVIRUS

P. J. Chen, A. Cywinski & J. M. Taylor

The Institute for Cancer Research, Fox Chase Cancer Center, Philadelphia, PA, USA.

In the endogenous reaction of a melittin-disrupted avian retrovirus, SE21Q1b, there is significant reverse transcription of a cellular RNA, the 7S L RNA. Many of the characteristics of this synthesis are analogous to the process by which a retrovirus genome is reverse transcribed and subsequently integrated into the host genome. These findings of reverse transcription of a cellular RNA are thus of potential relevance to an understanding of processed genes and certain pseudogenes.

Nucleotide sequencing studies of DNA from higher eucaryotes has revealed that many genes exist as sets of related but non-identical copies. In many of these sets there are copies that have features consistent with the interpretation that they arose from a master gene by a process involving reverse transcription and subsequent integration in germ line cells (1). Such putative gene copies include species that are called processed genes, pseudogenes and Alu-like elements (1,2). Examples of processed genes include tubulins (3) and ribosomal proteins (4). However the genes involved in such reverse transcription events may be the small nuclear RNA's such as U1, U2, and U3 (5). Also, the RNA templates may not necessarily be RNA polymerase II transcripts. Conceptually it is also possible that RNA polymerase III transcripts, such as 7S L RNA, may be converted to pseudogenes by reverse transcriptase.

Although the observations with processed genes and certain other pseudogenes are highly suggestive of reverse transcriptase involvement, there has been little success in even partially reconstructing such events (5). We need to know the details of the postulated reverse transcription and integration events: such as the source of the reverse transcriptase in germline cells, the possible role of copackaging the reverse transcriptase and cellular RNA in a retroviral particle, the mechanism of priming of the reverse transcription and strategy for the subsequent completion and integration of the reverse transcript.

Our studies open an avenue of attack to some of these questions. We have studied DNA synthesis in the endogenous reaction of melittin-disrupted avian retrovirus particles. With wild type virus such endogenous reactions begin with the tRNA-primed copying of the viral RNA genome (6). We have concentrated on the reverse transcription that occurs in the virions that are released from a virus-transformed quail cell clone, SE21Q1b, that was first isolated and characterized by Linial and coworkers (7). These cells contain a single provirus with a defect such that the virus particles released contain cellular rather than viral RNA. Our initial studies showed that in the endogenous reaction of SE21 particles some cellular RNA species were reverse transcribed using tRNA-sized species as primers (8). The DNA produced included a major discrete-sized species that we have now found by hybridization procedures to be related to the cell 7S L RNA. This DNA species was isolated, end-labeled and sequenced. It was predominantly 134 b long although there were additional species that are one, two or three nucleotides shorter at the 3'-end. The sequence, as shown in Fig. 1, is complementary to the 5'-terminus of the 303 b human 7S L RNA (9). We have shown that the tRNA-sized

```
SE21 cDNA     3'    NNNNAGC GCGCCACCGC GTGCGGACAT CAGGGTCGAT GAGCCCTCCG
              5'    NNNNTCG CGCGGTGGCG CACGCCTGTA GTCCCAGCTA CTCGGGAGGC

Human 7S L    5' AGGCGCCGGG CGCGGTGGCG CGTGCCTGTA GTCCCAGCTA CTCGGGAGGC
                         10         20         30         40         50

SE21 cDNA        ACTCGGGCGG CCTAGCGAAC TCGGGTCCTC AAGACCCGAC GTCACGCGAT
                 TGAGCCCGCC GGATCGCTTG AGCCCAGGAG TTCTGGGCTG CAGTGCGCTA

Human 7S L       TGAGGCTGGA GGATCGCTTG AGTCCAGGAG TTCTGGGCTG TAGTGCGCTA
                         60         70         80         90        100

SE21 cDNA        ACGGCTCGCC NGCAGGCGCG ATTCGGGCCG TAG-TAT
                 TGCCGAGCGG NCGTCCGCGC TAAGCCCGGC ATC-ATA

Human 7S L       TGCCGATCGG GTGTCCGCAC TAAGTTCGGC ATCAATATGG TGACCTCCCG
                        110        120        130        140        150
```

Figure 1. A comparison between the sequence of the 134 b DNA species synthesized by the SE21 virus and the 5' terminal 150 b of human 7S L RNA (9). The 134 b species was purified by hybrid selection to a clone of human 7S L DNA, labeled at the 5'-end with polynucleotide kinase and sequenced by the procedure of Maxam and Gilbert. Uncertain nucleotide determinations are indicated by N.

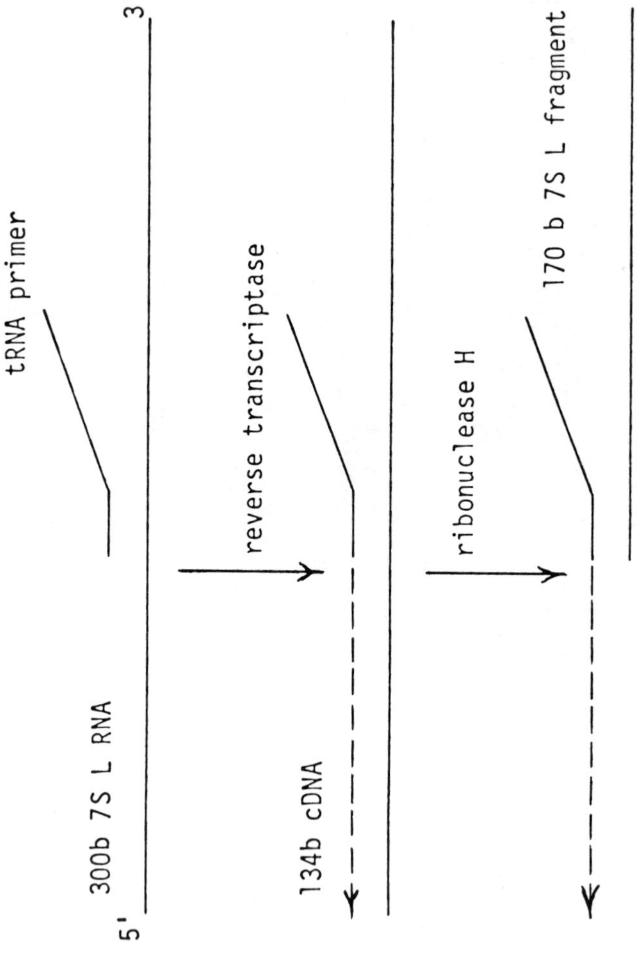

Figure 2. The reverse transcription of 7S L RNA as it occurs in the endogenous reaction of melittin-disrupted SE21 virus.

primer is unique both in size and sequence. It contains modified nucleotides as expected for a tRNA, and it is not tRNA.trp, the primer that is used in the endogenous reaction of wild type virus in the reverse transcription of the viral genome (6). Our interpretation of the data of the reverse transcription of the 7S L RNA is shown in Fig. 2. Also, as indicated in Fig. 2, we have obtained results suggesting that subsequent to the synthesis of the 134 b species, the corresponding region of the 7S L RNA is removed, presumably by the ribonuclease H activity of reverse transcriptase. Our evidence for this conclusion is that reverse transcription is followed by the appearance of a novel 170 b RNA species that is related to the 3'-end of the 7S L RNA.

The 7S L RNA is an abundant cellular RNA (about 250,000 copies per cell (9)) and recently has been shown to be the nucleic acid component of the signal recognition particle which functions in the transfer of specific nascent proteins through membranes (10). Other workers have shown that cellular 7S L RNA is normally present within wild type retrovirus particles and on a molar basis is as abundant as the viral genome itself (11). In fact, 7S L RNA was first found as a species present in Rous sarcoma virus (12). Thus in our studies with the mutant virus SE21 it is not unexpected that the 7S L RNA would be present or even that it could be reverse transcribed. However, as summarized in table 1, the most interesting aspect is that many features of this reverse transcription are analogous to the reverse transcription of a retroviral genome. As far as the first four items in the table, this analogy is very strong. To understand item 5 it should be explained that the 95 nucleotides at the 5'-end of human 7S L are homologous to Alu-like sequences (9). Such sequences are highly abundant at the DNA level for higher eucaryotes and can be present in stable cellular RNA species (2). Thus the reverse transcripts of 7S L RNA may proceed, by analogy to the R sequence at the 5'-end of the retrovirus genome (6), by a transcriptional jump to another RNA species. Item 6 is included in the table to

Table 1. A speculative comparison of strategies for the reverse transcription of avian retrovirus RNA and of cellular 7S L RNA.

	avian retrovirus RNA	cellular 7S L RNA
1. Reverse transcription in an endogenous reaction of disrupted virions	+	+
2. Minus strand DNA synthesis primed by a unique tRNA	+ (=trp)	+ (identity not yet known)
3. Synthesis of a minus strand strong stop DNA	+ (=101 b)	+ (=134 b)
4. Removal of transcribed RNA by RNase H	+	+
5. Transcriptional jump for further minus strand synthesis	+ (via R sequence)	? (possibly via Alu-like sequences)
6. Subsequent synthesis of plus strand DNA	+ (leading to LTR)	?
7. Integration of reverse transcript	+	? (certain Alu-like elements are good candidates)
8. Generation of a direct repeat of cellular DNA at integration site	+	? (certain Alu-like elements are good candidates)

indicate that as yet we have no information regarding plus strand DNA synthesis from the 7S L. Item 7 is to point out that the 134 b species, if integrated, would be similar in size and sequence to the 129 b Alu-like elements of the mouse and the 134 b elements of the Chinese hamster (2). Furthermore, as indicated in item 8, Alu-like elements are frequently found flanked by small direct repeats (2), just as occurs for integrated retrovirus DNA (6).

In conclusion, much more information is yet needed to understand the role of reverse transcriptase in the synthesis and generation of processed genes. However, the present studies on the reverse transcription of cellular 7S L RNA may provide an accessible system and our results suggest that the process may by much more analogous to retrovirus genome replication than previously considered.

ACKNOWLEDGMENTS

This work was supported by Public Health Service grants CC-22651, CA-06927-20, and RR-05539 from the National Institutes of Health, grant MV-7 from the American Cancer Society, and by an appropriation from the Commonwealth of Pennsylvania. We are grateful to Drs. Elizabetta Ullu and Robert Krumlauf for helpful discussions and the 7S L clones essential to this work. Also we thanks Drs. Bill Mason and Julie Smith for critical comments and Ms. Helene McGinley for preparation of the manuscript.

REFERENCES

1. Sharp, P.A. (1983) Nature 301, 471-472.
2. Jelinek, W.R. & Schmidt, C.W. (1982) Ann. Rev. Biochem. 51, 813-844.
3. Raff, E.C., Fulle, M.T., Kaufman, T.C., Kemphues, R.J., Rudolf, J.E., & Raff, R.A. (1982) Cell 28, 33-40.
4. Dudov, K.L., & Perry, R.P. (1984). Cell 37, 457-468.

5. Bernstein, L.B., Mount, S.M. & Weiner, A.M. (1983) Cell 32, 461-472.
6. Varmus, H.E. (1983) In Mobile Genetic Elements, Shapiro, J. ed., pp. 411-503.
7. Linial, M., Medieros, E. & Hayward, W.S. (1978) Cell 15, 1371-1381.
8. Taylor, J.M. & Cywinski, A. (1984) J. Virol. 51, 267-271.
9. Ullu, E., Murphy, S. & Melli, M. (1982) Cell 29, 195-201.
10. Walter, P. & Blobel, G. (1983)Cell 34, 525-533.
11. Erikson, E., Erikson, R.L., Henry, B. & Pace, N.R. (1973) Virology 53, 40-46.
12. Bishop, J.M., Levinson, W.E., Sullivan, D., Fanshier, L., Quintrell, N. & Jackkson, J. (1970) Virology 42, 927-937.

DIFFERENT RETROVIRUSES SHOW DIFFERENT SUSCEPTIBILITIES TO 2-DEOXY-D-GLUCOSE

L. Thiry, S. Sprecher-Goldberger, J. Cogniaux-LeClerc, A. Burny, D. Portetelle and H.A. Blough

Institut Pasteur du Brabant, Faculty of Science of Université Libre de Bruxelles, Faculty of Agronomy, Gembloux, Belgium and University of Pennsylvania School of Medicine, Philadelphia, Pa., USA

Three cell lines chronically producing different retroviruses were treated with 5 and 10 mM 2-deoxy-D-glucose and assayed for viral protein synthesis with a solid phase radioimmunoassay. In A204 cells producing M7 strain of Baboon Endogenous Virus (BaEV), the drug decreased the amount of cell receptors to this virus, with a parallel inhibition of virus release, as tested with a syncytium forming units assay. Viral p24 and gp first accumulated in parallel within the cells and then decreased. BILN virus, another BaEV strain, was found to differ from the M7 strain by at least one epitope of the gp and was much more susceptible to inhibition by 2-deoxy-D-glucose. Cells infected with this strain were killed by the drug, in contrast to virus-free cells. In ovine FLK cells producing Bovine Leukemia Virus (BLV), the drug specifically inhibited synthesis of the viral gp-51, with no effect on the viral p24, and no evidence of intracellular accumulation of viral components.

Inhibitors of glycosylation may allow the formation

of polypeptide chains which are the normal counterpart of the protein moieties of glycoproteins, but these polypeptides may be unable to participate in cleavage processes of polyprotein precursors or in maturation of virions. We have here studied the possible consequential effects of cell treatment with 2-deoxy-D-glucose on the synthesis of retrovirus proteins. We chose to study the retroviruses for which well documented antibodies were available. Also, titration of BaEV can be performed by taking advantage of the fact that these viruses are able to fuse RSa cells. Each biological unit forms discrete syncytium on monolayers of these cells. The human A204(M7) cell line chronically producing M7 strain of BaEV was treated with 5 and 10 mM 2-deoxy-D-glucose for 1 day, or with repeated daily doses for 5 days (Table 1). Release of BaEV syncytium forming units was decreased to 38% and 51% after a 10 mMdose of drug for 1 day, and a 5 mM dose for 5 days, respectively. Virus release was completely abolished after a 10 mM dose for 5 days. Even the latter treatment did not decrease cell growth, as tested by counting the

Table 1. Action of 2-deoxy-D-glucose on the release of BaEV(M7) from A204(M7) cells; as detected by production of syncytium forming units (SFU)

	Period of drug treatment (days)	
2-deoxy-D-glucose	1	5
10mM	97 ± 18*	5 ± 2
5mM	231 ± 28	98 ± 26
None	252 39	194 + 36

* 200 ul of supernatant medium of A204(M7) cells producing BaEV were seeded in 4 wells containing semi-confluent RSa cells. Syncytia were counted after 24 hours at 37° C. Results show the mean of syncytia plus or minus S.D.

number of viable cells with the use of trypan blue. Synthesis of viral and cellular antigens within the cells was then studied by testing the ability of total crude cell extracts to bind mouse monoclonal antibodies prepared in our laboratory (1). Synthesis of viral glycoprotein was not selectively modified by drug treatment but rather there was a parallel effect on the amount of antigenic determinants of the viral core protein and of the envelope glycoproteins (Table 2). It must be stressed that this assay does not measure glycosylation of the later proteins but only the presence of the polypeptide moieties. In extracts of A204(M7) cells treated for 1 day with 5mM 2-deoxy-D-glucose, threshhold was a twofold increase of viral polypeptides, indicating that virus maturation or release was inhibited. However, this treatment did not significantly reduce the amount of syncytium forming units in the supernatant of the culture, as shown in table 1. This parodox may indicate that virions which were already mature at the moment of drug treatment could normally be released into the medium. Prolonged treatment with 5mM 2-deoxy-D-glucose for 5 days decreased polypeptides of viral gp and coreprotein to 66 and 79%, respectively. Increasing drug concentration to 10 mM did not enhance the inhibiting effect on the synthesis of viral polypeptides, although inhibition of syncytium forming units release was augmented. This also favors the hypothesis that the drug does not affect early events of the virus infectious cycle, but rather processes related to maturation. In this respect, it was interesting to find that synthesis of cell receptors to the virus, as detected by monoclonal antibody D12, was partly inhibited by 2-deoxy-D-glucose. Degree of inhibition parallelled that of syncytium forming units found in culture medium. We have previously provided evidence that mature BaEV virions contain determinants of the cell receptors (2). Thus, it is possible that the main effect of 2-deoxy-D-glucose is to inhibit virus maturation via action on a determinant of the cell membrane. This determinant does not seem necessary for cell viability, since the number of viable cells was not affected.

Table 2. Solid phase radioimmunoassay using monoclonal antibodies to detect BaEV and cellular antigens in A204(M7) cells treated with 2-deoxy-D-glucose [a]

Monoclonal antibodies	Drug concentration (mM)	Period of Treatment (days)	
		1	5
A6, anti BaEV gp	10	2640[b]	1896
	5	3319	1819
	0	1407	2772
B9, anti BaEv gp	10	670	701
	5	847	610
	0	467	904
F12, anti BaEV core protein	10	3471	1654
	5	3825	1629
	0	1983	2075
D12, anti BaEV cell receptor	10	4550	2730
	5	5413	3855
	0	6025	4409

[a] A204(M7) cells; with or without drug treatment, were suspended at a concentration of 10^6 cells per ml in phosphate buffered saline with protease inhibitors (2mM Tosyl lysine chloromethylketone and phenyl methyl sulfonyl fluoride); they were frozen at -80°C for at least 2 hours and then thawed and sonicated. Fifty ul of cell extracts were distributed in the wells of Microtest III flexible assay plates (Falcon 3911) and left to dry overnight. Fifty ul of a 5% bovine serum albumin solution were then added for 1 hour at 37°C followed by 50 ul of antibodies diluted 1:50. After 2 hours at 37°C wells were washed 3 times and then filled with 50 ul containing 25,000 counts/min of Protein A; iodinated each month in this laboratory. After 1 hour at room temperature; wells were washed 3 times; dried for 20 min. at 70°C, and then distributed into tubes for counting in a gamma counter.

TABLE 2, continued

---

[b] Mean of cpm of ^{125}I Protein A bound; for tests run in quadruplicate. Standard Deviations (not shown) were plus or minus 10 percent. Background of ^{125}I protein A bound to cells without antibody was 100 to 150 cpm.

We were surprised to find that the BILN strain of BaEV produced by the Fcf2th canine cell line was much more susceptible to the action of 2 deoxy-D-glucose than the M7 strain was (Fig. 1). A 2mM concentration nearly completely abolished viral protein synthesis within 24 hours and higher drug concentrations significantly decreased the number of viable cells. Control virus-free FCf2th canine cells were completely resistant to drug toxicity (not shown). This indicates that Fcf2th (BILN) cells were killed by the drug because of the presence of the virus, another interesting way of limiting viral infection. Up to now, no differences had been described between various isolates of BaEV. However, we found that FCf2th (BILN) cells do not bind antibody B9 while A204(M7) cells do (Fig. 1). We have shown that antibody B9 addresses to an epitope of BaEV(M7) gp which is distinct from the epitope recognized by antibody A6 (1). The latter epitope must play a part in virus fixation since antibody A6 neutralizes the virion, in contrast to antibody B9. It will be interesting to investigate why lack of epitope recognized by antibody B9 renders the infected cells so highly susceptible to the action of 2-deoxy-D-glucose.

Results shown above indicate that exquisite differences between two retrovirus strains have great impact on their susceptibility to 2-deoxy-D-glucose. Thus, it would be hazardous to extrapolate drug sensitivity to other retrovirus groups. Members of the human HTLV-AIDS retrovirus group are the most interesting targets for drug action. We have not yet studied the action of 2-deoxy-D-glucose on HTLV-III or LAV, due to lack of appropriate anti-gp antibodies. Such antibodies are

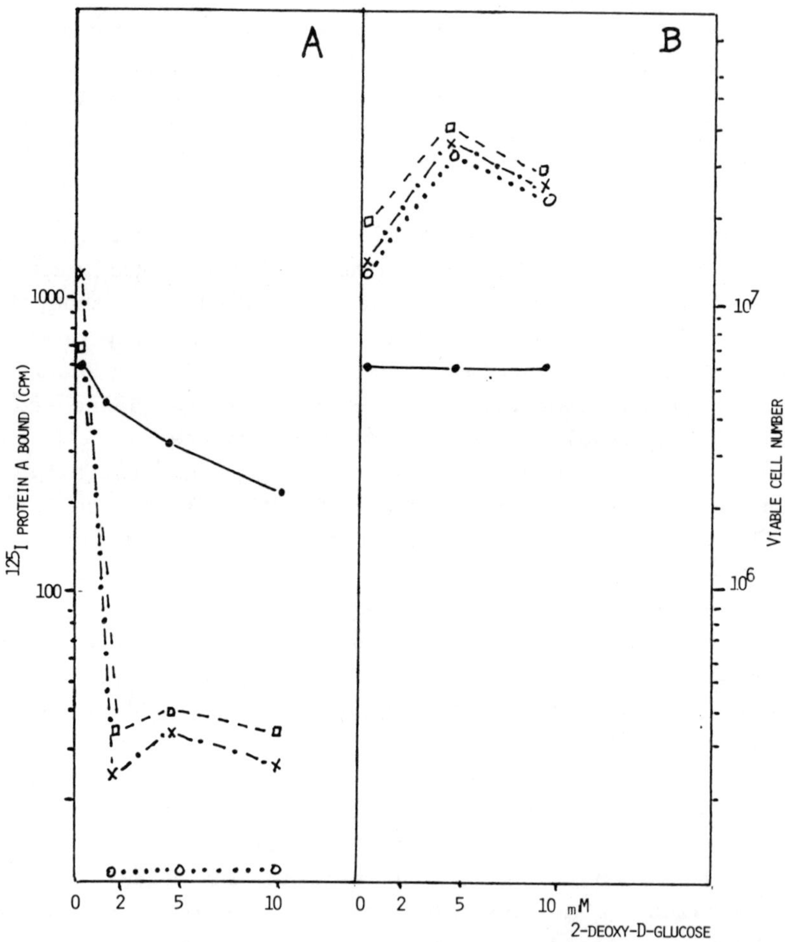

Figure 1. Compared susceptibility of BILN and M7 strains of BaEV to 2-deoxy-D-glucose. FCf2th cells producing BILN virus (A) and 204 cells producing M7 virus (B) were grown for 24 h with various concentrations of 2-deoxy-D-glucose and cells extracts were tested for binding of monoclonal antibodies A6 (x), F12 (□) and B9 (O). Ordinate indicates the amount of cpm of ^{125}I protein A bound, as indicated in Table 2. Solid line (●) shows the number of cells counted with trypan blue.

Table 3. Bovine Leukemia Virus (BLV) antigens in FLK cells treated for 5 days with 5 mM 2-deoxy-D-glucose

	Binding of ^{125}I labeled Protein A 2 (cpm) to cells grown with drug	no drug
Rabbit immune sera	cpm*	cpm
anti BLV p24	13750	13337
anti BLV gp-51	4205	6928
Mouse monoclonal 16D4		
anti BLV gp-51	3283	4601

*The assay was performed as described in Table 2.

available for Bovine Leukemia Virus (BLV) (3), a virus which shares morphological and reverse transcriptase features with the HTLV-LAV group, as well as amino acid sequences of p24 (4), and antigenic cross reactivity (5). FLK cells from an ovine cell line chronically producing BLV were treated for 1 day, and repeatedly for 5 days, with 5mM 2-deoxy-D-glucose, and cell extracts were tested for the presence of viral p24 and gp-51, using monospecific rabbit hyperimmunesera raised against these purified proteins, and a mouse monoclonal antibody prepared against BLV gp-51. Viral protein synthesis was not modified after a 1 day treatment (not shown) but 5 daily doses specifically decreased gp-51 synthesis to 61%, with no effect on p24 synthesis (Table 3). The number of viable cells was not decreased.

Our results stress the point that a given inhibitor of glycosylation can disrupt retrovirus synthesis machinery in various ways. However, since the three retroviruses studied here grow in different types of cells, it is not clear whether host or virus determined drug susceptibility. Attempts to grow the three viruses in the same cell line are in progress.

ACKNOWLEDGMENTS

We thank Léopold Tack and Jacques Stienon for their technical assistance, and Janine Herinckx for preparing the manuscript. This work was supported by grants from the Caisse Générale d'Epargne et de Retraite and from Fonds de la Recherche Scientifique Médicale.

REFERENCES

1. Cogniaux, J., Olislager, R., Sprecher-Goldberger, S. & Thiry, L. (1982) J. Virol. 43, 664-672.
2. Thiry, L., Cogniaux-LeClerc, J., Olislager, R., Sprecher-Goldberger, S. & Buekens, P. (1983) J. Virol. 48,697-708.
3. Portetelle, D., Bruck, C., Mammerickx, M. & Burny, A. (1980) Virology, 105, 223-233.
4. Oroszlan, S., Sarngadharan, M.G., Copeland, T.D., Kalyanaraman, V.S., Gilden, R.V. & Gallo, R.C. (1982) Proc. Natl. Acad. Sci. USA 79,1291-1294.
5. Thiry, L., Sprecher-Goldberger, S., Jacquemin, P., De Caluwé, J.P., Burny, A., Clumeck, N., Taelman, H. & Henrivaux, P. (1984) Abstracts XV Meeting European Tumour Virus Group, 62.

A COMPARATIVE STUDY OF

BOVINE LEUKEMIA VIRUS (BLV) DETECTION METHODS

U.T. Banders, J.A. Meldrajs, V.V. Konicheva, V.P. Lozha and R.A. Kukaine

Institute of Microbiology, Latvian SSR Academy of Science, Kleisti 226067 Riga, USSR

Electron Microscopy (EM), Reverse Transcriptase test (RT) , Concurrent Radioimmunoassay (cRIA) for major core protein p-24, and RNA dot-blot hybridization were used for quantitative BLV detection in culture fluids of BLV producing Foetal Lamb Kidney (FLK) cell lines and short term lymphocyte cultures. It was established that for EM studies a probe should contain $5x10^6$ viruses, for the RT test $1x10^7$, for cRIA $1x10^6$ and for RNA dot-blot hybridization $1x10^5$ viruses. The sensitivity of RT and EM methods is limited by the purity of initial material while that of cRIA and RNA dot-blot hybridization are not affected by this factor. We can get quantitative results by all four assays and under standard conditions it is possible to make recalculations between the methods.

For detection of BLV, the etiological agent of enzootic bovine leukosis, various assays are used according to the aim of the experiment and the type of material under study: syncytia formation test, EM, RT, and a number of immunological methods for BLV protein (1,2). The literature, however, reports on the quantitative aspect for cRIA only (3). In the present work the quantitative aspects of four methods for BLV detection are compared: EM, RT test, cRIA and RNA dot-blot hybridization using the same material. Characteristics of initial materials and final results are compared.

Virus-containing material was obtained from culture fluid of FLK(4) and short term lymphocyte cell cultures clarified by centrifugation at 10,000xg, followed by ultracentrifugation through 20% sucrose. The pelleted material was then suspended in buffer (5).

A 150 times concentrated BLV solution was used for EM studies. Virus suspension was sedimented on a 1% agar support by centrifugation in a specially designed 0.1 ml chamber (5). The obtained sediment was prepared for Em examination and virus particles were counted in ultrathin sections from side to side of the sediment according to Brown et al. (6). The thickness of the sediment was measured at a 20,000 magnification from side to side on serial microphotographs.

To obtain the BLV major core protein p-24, virus lysates were purified by chromatography on phosphacellulose, followed by gel chromatography (7). Purified p-24 was labelled with ^{125}I by the chloramine T procedure (8). The specific activity was 5 uCi/ug and 95% of the radioactivity precipitated in TCA. Rabbit anti-p-24 serum diluted 1:8000 precipitated 50% of ^{125}I-p-24. cRIA was conducted according to Strand and August (9).

For the RT test 5- to 200-fold virus concentrates were used. The RT assay with poly(rA)-oligo$(dT)_{10}$ template was conducted in the presence of 3H-TTP with specific activity 3Ci/mmole according to (5). The result was considered positive if the difference between probe and blank was 300 or more cpm in 20 minutes of the reaction.

For preparation of RNA and detection of BLV specific sequences, clarified BLV-containing culture medium was supplemented with: SDS to a 1% concentration, purified rat liver total RNA up to 1-5 ug/ml and heated proteinase K up to 50 ug/ml. The mixture was incubated for an hour at room temperature. RNA was purified through 5.7 M CsCl (10). 4 ul batches of RNA dilutions were applied to a nitrocellulose filter (Millipore, 0.45 u). Dot-blot hybridization was performed according to Thomas (11), using as the hybridization probe a nick-translated ^{32}p-labelled (12) pLV12 plasmid linearized with Sal I which contained BLV genome fragment (13) with a specific activity of $2x10^8$ cpm/ug. Autoradiography was carried out at -70°C for up to two weeks using X-ray film PM-1 (Svema, USSR) and amplifying screen YB-3 (Novosibirsk Chemical Pharmacy Works, USSR). The spots were scanned with a Beckman DU-8B spectrophotometer.

The sensitivity and error of the EM method were determined previously (5) and coincide with the results reported by Brown (6). The minimum amount for quantitative detection was $5x10^6$ viruses in 0.1 ml of sample . In FLK cultures $1x10^9$ virions and in short term lymphocyte cultures $2.5x10^7$ virions were detected per 1 ml culture fluid. 1 ml FLK culture medium makes a sediment of 1 u and 1 ml of short term lymphocyte culture medium makes 0.6 u.of sediment. Thus, the number of virions in the cultures differed 40-fold, while the thickness of the whole layer differed only 1.3-fold, which indicates the presence of cellular debris in viral concentrates of short term lymphocyte culture. This is shown in Figure 1 where in ultrathin sections of the FLK culture sediment only BLV virions are seen (Fig. 1a), while in the sections of short term lymphocyte culture, besides virions, there are also cellular debris (Fig. 1b).

In a previous report (5) we showed that the quantitative RT assay could be used if the probe contained not less than $1x10^7$ viruses with the specific activity of ^{3}H-TTP 3 Ci/mmole. The determination of the RT activities in BLV preparations from FLK and short term lymphocyte cultures showed that viruses from 1 ml of FLK culture medium give 2640 cpm and from short term lymphocyte cultures give 150 cpm in the RT test.

For the quantitative determination of p-24 in BLV preparations a calibrating curve was built. Unlabelled BLV p-24 of a known concentration was used as a competitive agent. The minimum amount of BLV p-24 determined by cRIA was 0.25 ng, which corresponded to 17.2% of ^{125}I BLV p-24

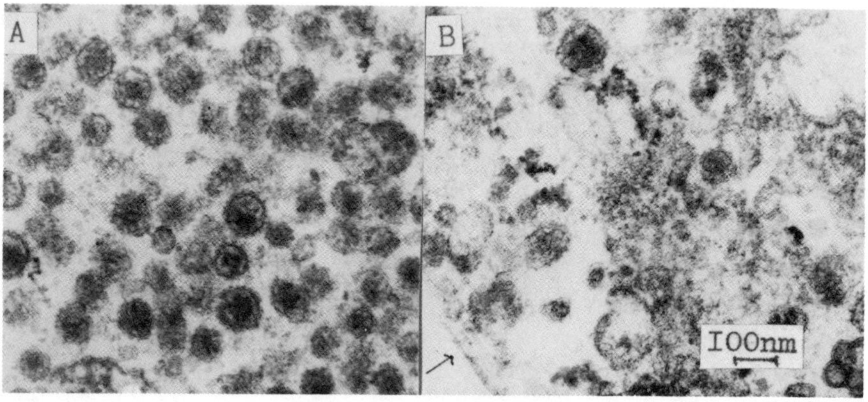

Figure 1. Microphotograph of an ultrathin section of viral sediment. 1A - FLK culture sediment, 1B - Ly culture sediment. The arrow indicates the boundary of the sediment.

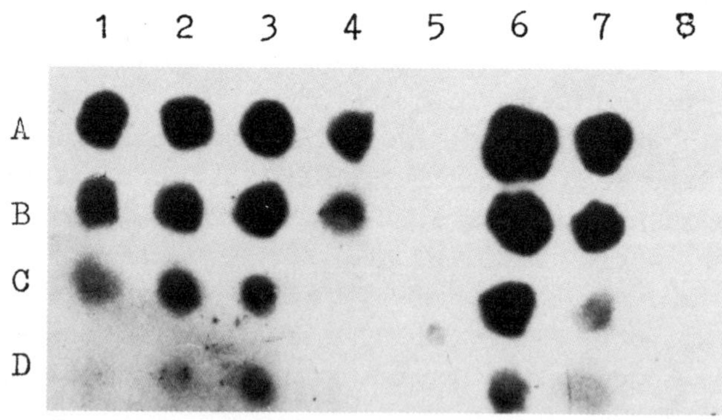

Figure 2. Retention of RNA dotted on the nitrocellulose paper. BLV RNA on spot 1A is from 2.4 ml of Ly culture fluid; 2A is from 0.6 ml of FLK; 3A is from 1.6 ml of FLK; 4A is from 0.8 ml of Ly. On spot B dilution is 1:5, C - 1:25, D - 1:125. On spot 5a 10 ug of total RNA from normal cattle lymphocytes were blotted, 8A - 10 ug of total RNA from normal cattle fibroblasts, while 6A and 7a represent 60 and 2.5 ng of BLV 38 S RNA respectively.

binding inhibition in the reaction.(14). The cRIA determination of the BLV p-24 amount in sediments of culture fluids demonstrated FLK cultures to contain 480 ng of BLV p-24, and lymphocyte cultures - 9.25 ng of BLV p-24 per 1 ml of culture fluid.

To determine the sensitivity of the dot-blot hybridization, BLV 38 S RNA of known concentrations were used. The scanning spectrophotometry revealed that the minimum RNA amount which could be detected by this assay using the probe with specific activity $2x10^8$ cpm/ug corresponded to 10 picograms of BLV 38 S RNA. One microlitre of FLK culture medium contained 16 ng BLV RNA, and lympnocyte culture medium - 0.9 ng (See Fig. 2).

DISCUSSION

To compare the sensitivity of the applied methods, EM data on the virion amount in the initial material were used to express data for RT, cRIA and RNA dot-blot hybridization.

Thus, by EM method it is possible to determine $5x10^6$ virions in a sample, for BLV determination by the RT test $1x10^7$ virions are requird, for cRIA $-1x10^6$ and for the RNA dot-blot hybridization $-1x10^5$ virions. As the quantitative determination in most cases requires concentrated viral material, but the methods vary in the possibilities of analyzing different concentrations, the ratio of the virion amount and cellular debris in the initial material affects the actual sensitivity of a method for the investigation of a culture fluid.

The EM method and RT test, when used to investigate short term lymphocyte culture medium, do not permit concentration of the material more than 100 fold. If the material for the EM investigation is in higher concentrations, it is not possible to count virions through the whole thickness of the sediment, and the determination of RT activity is accompanied by a rise in the nonspecific absorption of ^{3}H-TTp and an absence of linear kinetics of RT reaction can be observed, i.e., if one intends to obtain qualitative results the number of virions per ml in culture medium should not be less that $1x10^7$.

With a purer initial material (FLK, for example) it is possible to raise the degree of concentration and, hence, employ a culture with the virus titre lower than $1x10^7$ virion/ml. The sensitivity of the RT test, employing viruses with insignificant cellular debris, increases due to an increase in the period of linear kinetics up to 20 hours (unpublished data).

For cRIA about 1000-fold concentrated material can be used, which permits quantitative determination of virions from initial material containing $1x10^4$ virion/ml.

The RNA dot-blot hybridization practically does not limit the possibilities of concentrating the initial material and thus this method should be considered to be the most sensitive one.

We can conclude that all the methods permit quantification of BLV under the described conditions, and under standard conditions the amount of virions or their components can be predicted on the basis of one of the methods.

REFERENCES

1. Ferrer, J.F. (1980) in Adv. Vet. Sci. Comp. Med. 24, 1-63.
2. Burny, A., Bruck, C., Chantrenne, H., Cleuter, Y., Dekegel, D., Ghysdael, J., Kettmann, R., Leclercq, M., Leunen, J., Mammerickx, M. and Portetelle, D. (1981). in Viral Oncology, ed. by Klein G. (Raven Press, New York, N.Y.) pp. 231-290.
3. Gupta, P., and Ferrer, J.F. (1980) Int. J. Canc. 25, 663-666.
4. Van der Maaten M.J., and Miller, J.M. (1976) Bibl. Haematol. 43, 360-362.
5. Banders, U.T., Meldrajs, J.A., Ivanova, M.N., Kalnina,

B.A. and Lozha, V.P. (1979) in Reproduction and Biological Properties of Oncornaviruses, ed. Kukaine, R.A. (Zinatne, Riga), 74-81 (In Russian).

6. Brown, R.C., Kostyu, J.A., and Kilgore, A. (1975) Can. Res. 35, 1053-1057.
7. Strand, M., and August, J.T. (1976) J. Biol. Chem. 251, 559-564.
8. Greenwood, F.C., Hunter, W.M., and Glover J.S. (1963) Biochem. J. 89, 114-123.
9. Devare, S.G., Stephenson, J.R., Sarma, P.S., Aaronson, S.A., and Chander, S. (1976) Science 194, 1428-1430.
10. McCandliss, R., Sloma, A., and Pestka, S. (1981) in Methods in Enzymology, eds. Colowick, S. and Kaplan, N. Vol. 79B Interferons, ed. Pestka, S. (Academic Press, Inc. New York, N.Y.), 51-68.
11. Thomas, P.S. (1983) in Methods in Enzymology, eds. Colowick, S., and Kaplan, N. vol. 100B Recombinant DNA, ed. Wu, R., (Academic Press, Inc. New York, N.Y.), 255-266.
12. Maniatis, T., Jeffrey A., and Van de Sande, H. (1975) Biochem. 14, 3787-3794.
13. Tsimanis, A., Bichko, V., Dreilina, D., Meldrajs, J., Lozha, V., Kukaine R., Gren E. (1983) NAR 11, 6079-6087.
14. Konicheva, V.V., and Ilinskaja, T.N. (1982) in Etiology Diagnostics and Epizootology of Bovine Leukosis, ed. Kukaine, R.A. (Zinatne, Riga) 45-49 (in Russian).

STRUCTURAL AND FUNCTIONAL HETEROGENEITY AMONG TYPE D RETROVIRUSES

V. Wunderlich, W. Uckert, J. Denner and D. Bierwolf

Central Institute of Cancer Research, Academy of Sciences, DDR-1115 Berlin, German Democratic Republic.

Tryptic peptide analysis of major internal structural proteins of six type D retroviruses isolated originally from non human primate species (MPMV, LV, SMRV) or from cultured human cells (HeLaV, HEp2V, PMFV) revealed clear differences among these viruses. The p25 peptide maps of MPMV, LV, PMFC and HEp2V were very similar but showed a striking dissimilarity to the p25 map of HeLaV and the p35 map of SMRV. All viruses could be distinguished by peptide maps of at least two of their three low-molecular-weight proteins p10, p12, and pp15. In addition, MPMV and LV contained a minor glycoprotein gp20 that was not detectable in HeLaV, HEp2V and PMFV. This structural diversity correlates in at least one respect with a functional heterogenety. Both intact and disrupted viruses from human cells were able to suppress the response to T-cell mitogens in vitro of lymphocytes from some species, including man, baboon, and rhesus monkey. MPMV, however, was inactive. The suppressive components of high and low molecular weight were identified in PMFV and both were sensitive to heat and proteolytic enzymes. Immunosuppression induced by some type D retroviruses may play an imortant role in immunodeficiency diseases in monkeys and men.

Type D retroviruses (reviewed in 1) have been so far isolated from Old World monkeys (Mason-Pfizer monkey virus -MPMV- and langur virus -LV) and New World monkeys (squirrel monkey retrovirus -SMRV) and from cultures of human cells (HeLa virus -HeLaV-, virus from HEp-2 cells -HEp2V-, and virus from permanent human fibroblasts -PMFV). A role of these viruses in disease, if any, has not yet been demonstrated. Recently, however, outbreaks of siman AIDS in macaques in two different primate centres have been closely associated with a new strain of type D retrovirus related to, but distinct from, MPMV (2,3).

The origin of the type D viruses isolated from continuous human cell lines is unknown. The predominant view is that all these human isolates represent MPMV-contaminants (4). Studies from our and other groups (reviewed in 5), however, indicate both biochemical and immunological differences among MPMV-like viruses. Here we present further evidence from tryptic peptide analysis for heterogeneity of these viruses. In addition, we report that these viruses, with the surprising exception of MPMV, are able to suppress in vitro the mitogen response of lymphocytes from some primate species.

Viruses were usually grown on human A204 rhabdomyosarcoma and sometimes on human Tu197 ovarial carcinoma cells. MPMV, LV, SMRV, and 1204 cells were originally obtained from the Viral Oncology Program, Bethesda, USA. HeP2V was provided by Dr. Ilyin, Moscow, USSR. HeLaV was isolated from HeLa cells strain London. PMFV was originally isolated from a malignant permanent human fibroblast line (6) and shown to be closely related to, but distinct from, MPMV (5). Viruses were purified by sucrose velocity and isopycnic density gradient centrifugation. Viral polypeptides were separated by SDS-PAGE on gradient (7.5 -15%) slab gels and identified by staining techniques or labeling with ^{14}C amino acids, ^{3}H-glucosamine or ^{32}P-phosphoric acid as described (7). Nonglycosylated structural proteins were radioiodinated in the gel and digested with TPCK-trypsin followed by two-dimensional peptide mapping on cellulose-coated thin layer chromatography plates as described (8). Plates were analyzed by autoradiography.

Except SMRV, which is known to possess a quite distinct pattern of structural proteins (1), MPMV and MPMV-like viruses (LV, PMFV, HeLaV, and HEp2V) exhibit a very similar protein pattern with p10, p12, pp15, p25, and gp68 as major internal structural proteins or glycoproteins, respectively (1,7). MPMV and LV contain an additional glycoprotein gp20 that is not detectable in PMFV, HeLaV, and HEp2V regardless of the cell lines in which these viruses are grown (7). Chemical crosslinking studies indicate that the gp20 of MPMV is located in the viral envelope (9).

The tryptic peptide fingerprints of type D retroviruses show a similar genetic polymorphism, as previously demonstrated for murine type B and type C viruses. The fingerprints demonstrate that some of these viruses are derived from similar but distinguishable genes. Our results (8) show a high degree of similarity of the major core proteins p25 of MPMV, LV, PMFV, and HEp2V. They could be distinguished from HeLaV p25 and SMRV p35 although these are functionally related proteins: This was also found when tryptic peptide maps of MPMV and HeLaV p25 were compared.

With respect to the tryptic peptide maps of the three low molecular-weight internal proteins the following results were obtained (8):

- pp15: high similarity of MPMV and PMFV, some dissimilarities to both LV and HEp2V, HeLaV and SMRV completely different,
- p12: MPMV and PMFV identical, LV and HeLaV slightly different, HEp2V clearly distinguishable (SMRV does not contain a p12 protein),
- p10: similar fingerprints for MPMV, PMFV, and HEp2V, somewhat different pattern for LV, HeLaV completey different (p10 of SMRV not analyzed).

Thus, only peptide maps of MPMV and PMFV show nearly

complete identity whereas the other viruses differ from each other at least in two fingerprints. As already mentioned, MPMV and PMFV can be distinguished on the basis of presence or absence of gp20.

Although our data do not exclude the possibility that some of the MPMV-like viruses from human cells represent contaminants we can conclude that such cell lines have not been contaminated recently. The older view that all these human isolates are identical to each other cannot longer be stated. Type D retroviruses probably represent an extended family of viruses, as also concluded from restriction endonuclease maps of the new, simian AIDS-associated type D retroviruses strain (2). Comparative analyses of the genomic sequences of these viruses are therefore highly desirable.

As early as 1980 we reported that the type C virus BaEV and the type D virus PMFV are able to inhibit the in vitro mitogen response of human lymphocytes (10). The existing murine and feline models of retrovirus-induced immunosuppression were thus extended to the human species. Later on we included further viruses and lymphocytes from nonhuman primates in our studies and performed first experiments to characterize the viral immunosuppressive components (11).

Lymphocytes were obtained from blood of normal healthy donors. Lymphocyte blast transformation was induced by T-cell mitogens (Con A, phytohemagglutinin) or during mixed lymphocyte reaction. Assays were performed in microtest plates in quadruplicate with mitogen and cell culture controls as detailed previously (10). Viruses considered as suppressive usually caused, in a dose-dependent manner, more than 50% reduction of control response in amounts as small as 5-10 ug of viral protein per well. Cytotoxic or virus-mitogen binding did not occur. Inhibition of reactivity of mouse lymphocytes by Rauscher murine leukemia virus and of bovine lymphocytes by bovine leukemia virus served as additional controls.

Suppression of mitogen response of lymphocytes from different species was demonstrated with primate retroviruses as follows: BaEV, PMFV, HeLaV, HEp2V (not MPMV) - human lymphocytes; BaEV, PMFV (not MPMV) - baboon lymphocytes (experiments with Dr. Inhjia, Sukhumi, USSR); PMFV (not MPMV) - rhesus monkey lymphocytes. The suppressive effect was therefore not species-specific. Interestingly, even an endogenous virus (BaEV) caused suppression of lymphocytes from its natural host (baboon). Suppression was produced with highly-purified virus both when intact and when disrupted by ether or detergents. Suppressive activity could be copurified with the virus and did not depend on the cell line used for virus propagation. Extracts from virus-producing cells demonstrated suppression whereas extracts from uninfected cells did not.

A rather surprising result of our studies concerns the inability of MPMV to suppress the reactivity of human and rhesus monkey (its natural host) lymphocytes. Even the highest amounts of MPMV tested (60 ug protein per well) did not cause more than 20% reduction of control response, whereas other viruses, e.g. PMFV, produced more than 90% reduction of control response in amounts ranging from 10 to 60 ug protein per well. The reason for these quite different activities is unknown. A related finding may be that early but not late passages of MPMV are able to induce a similar AIDS-like disease in newborn rhesus monkeys (3,12). Thus, during prolonged propagation in vitro MPMV appears to have lost, contrary to MPMV-like isolates from human cells, the property to affect lymphocyte functions.

We have characterized the immunosuppressive components of PMFV in further detail. After Sephacryl S-200 chromatography in a detergent-containing buffer, influence on human lymphocyte activation by Con A was tested from pooled fractions. Activities were essentially found in low molecular weight (about 15K) and high molecular weight (greater than 70K) fractions. the suppressive activity of disrupted PMFV was diminished by heating, freeze-thawing or by treatment with pronase or trypsin, indicating temperature-sensitive proteins as major suppressive components.

These results provide evidence that (i) type D retroviruses constitute an heterogenous group of viruses, (ii) a re-evaluation of a possible role of type D retroviruses in certain human diseases is required, (iii) even closely related viruses may differ in important biological functions of potential significance for their disease-inducing properties, and (iv) type D retroviruses may serve as a model to study immunoregulation in man. Comparative studies of viruses that do or do not block lymphocyte blastogenesis (MPMV-like human isolates versus MPMV) may be helpful to identify those viral sequences which may confer retroviruses the capability to produce an immunodeficiency disease like AIDS.

REFERENCES

1 Fine, D. & Schochetman, G. (1978) Cancer Res. 38, 3123-3139.

2. Daniel, M.D., King, N.W., Letvin, N.L., Hunt, R.D., Sehgal, P.K., & Desrosiers, R.C. (1984) Science 223, 602-605.

3. Marx, P.A., Maul, D.H., Osborn, K.G., Lerche, N.W., Moody, P., Lowenstine, L.J., Hendrickson, R.V., Arthur, L.O., Gilden, R.V., Gravell, M., London, W.T., Sever, J.C., Levy, J.A., Munn, R.J., & Gardner, M.B. (1984) Science 223, 1083-1086.

4. Weiss, R. (1982) in RNA Tumor Viruses, eds. Weiss, R., Teich, N., Varmus, H. & Coffin, J. (Cold Spring Harbor Laboratory, Cold Spring Harbor, NY) pp. 1205-1281.

5. Wunderlich, V., Unckert, W. & Sydow, G. (1983) Arch. Geschwulstforsch. 53, 267-278.

6. Graffi, A., Bierwolf, D., Widmaier, R., Bender, E., Wunderlich, V., Rudolph, M., Mothes, E., Niezabitowski, A. & Papsdorf, G. (1974) Dtsch. Gesundheitswes. 29, 1489-1498.

7. Wunderlich, V. & Uckert, W. (1981) Arch Virol. 70, 43-53.

8. Uckert, W., Hetling, I., & Denner, J. (1984) Arch. Virol. 81, 123-138.
9. Uckert, W., Westermann, P., Hertling, I. & Wunderich, V. (1983) Biomed. Biochim. Acta 42, 177-187.
10. Denner, J., Wunderlich, V. & Bierwolf, D. (1980) Acta biol. med. germ. 39, K19-K26.
11. Denner, J., Wunderlich, V. & Bierwolf, D. (1982) In Abstracts 14th Meeting of the European Tumour Virus Group, Varna, Bulgaria, p. 121.
12. Fine, D.L., Landon, R.J., Pienta, M.T., Kubicek, M.T., Valerio, M.J., Loeb, W.F., & Chopra, H.C. (1975) J. Natl. Cancer Inst. 54, 651-658.

RETROVIRUSES AND ONCOGENES IN THE RAT SARCOMA GALLIERA: AN OLD TUMOR AS A UNIQUE MODEL SYSTEM.

G. Ivaldi[1], P. Pippia[1], S. Rasheed[2], O. Muratore[3], S.P. Raffanti[3], B. Azzarone[4], O.E. Varnier[3].

1. Institute of General Physiology and Biological Chemistry, Sassari, Italy; 2. Department of Pathology, Laboratory of Tumor Biology and Oncogene Research, University of Southern California, Los Angeles, California, USA; 3. Institute of Microbiology, School of Medicine, Genova, Italy. 4. Laboratoire de Pathologie Cellulaire, Villejuif, France.

The Sarcoma Galliera is an old spontaneous tumor of the rat, maintained in vivo since it was first discovered in 1919. Cloned cell lines, which express an endogenous retrovirus, have been screened for in vivo and in vitro parameters of transformation. Cellular oncogenes and endogenous non-transforming retroviruses may play a role in the development of this rare spontaneous sarcoma and thus represent a unique model system.

The Sarcoma Galliera (SG) is a spontaneous solid tumor observed for the first time by Solimano in 1919 in the Galliera strain of the Rattus norvegicus var. albus (1). The tumor has been maintained for over 60 years by inoculation of minced tumoral tissue in the same strain of rats. Non invasive tumors appear in 25-30 days in 90% of the inoculated animals. Histologically the Sarcoma Galliera is a polymorphocellular sarcoma which does not metastasize. The tumor is surrounded by a thick fibrous capsule rich in collagen fibers and has massive non-infiltrative growth characteristics (2).

In 1975 we derived a cell line from the Sarcoma Galliera called **SGS** (Sarcoma Galliera Strain) which is highly tumorigenic (3). Several cultures were obtained from single cell clones and selected for their different cell morphology (4). Cloned cell lines were subsequently screened for different in vitro transformation parameters including substrate adhesion, contact inhibition, saturation density, growth in soft agar (5), plasminogen activator and fibrin clot retractile activity. SGS clones induce tumor formation in 100% of 2-4 months's old male Galliera rats (5) and 4 weeks' old male nude mice (Nu/Nu Swiss) with a very short latency period. Electron microscopy showed the presence of type C particles in SGS cultures which had a high level of reverse transcriptase activity in the supernatant fluids, whereas the normal Galliera rat fibroblasts (FG) showed no activity or viral particles even after chemical induction (4). The virus particles sedimented at a density of about 1.14 g/ml in an equilibrium sucrose gradient and a major protein was cross-reactive with the rat endogenous retrovirus (RaLV) core antigen of about 27,000 D. This retroviral isolate, designated SG-RaLV is poorly infectious to rat cells, but does not replicate in other mammalian cells tested. The virus is capable of rescuing defective sarcoma viruses from both the Kirsten strain of murine sarcoma virus (Ki-MSV) and the Rasheed strain of the rat sarcoma virus (RaSV) transformed non-producer cells. Focus-inducing SG-RaLV pseudotypes (Ki-MSV) were totally neutralized by antiserum made against SD-RaLV. Similar to other endogenous rat retrovirus, this virus does not transform rat cells indicating that it does not carry an oncogene in its genome (4).

Gene transfer experiments showed that DNA from SG tumors contain oncogenic sequences which induce transformation of mouse NIH 3T3 recipient cells (5). The endogenous SG-RaLV may have promoted the expression of a rat cellular oncogene in the SG tumor, since the normal Galliera rat fibroblasts do not release detectable levels of the endogenous rat retrovirus.

DNA transfection studies have shown that the DNA from several human tumors contains oncogenes (6). Several of these transforming sequences are homologus to the transforming genes of two murine sarcoma viruses (MSV), the Harvey and Kirsten strains (7). The oncogenes of these MSV were derived from rat normal cellular sequences during in vivo passage of murine leukemia viruses. Therefore the long in vivo passage history of the Sarcoma Galliera makes this old tumor an unique model system to study the potential interactions of endogenous retrovirses with cellular genes and other enviromental factors.

ACKNOWLEDGMENTS

The work cited was partially supported by grants from the NCI, CA 26246, and from CNR, N. 84.01841, 84.00838, 84.02327 and from NATO, N. 137.80.

REFERENCES

1. Solimano G. (1924) Pathologica 16, 615-619.
2. Cirio L., Macagno F., Nanni G. (1965). Pathologica 52, 1-60.
3. Pippia P., Tilloca G., Vargiu F., Cherchi G.M., Coinu R., Ivaldi G. (1978) Pathologica 70, 19-26.
4. Varnier O.E., Raffanti S.P., Muratore O., Repetto C.M., Pippia P., Tilloca G., Meloni M.A., Ivaldi G., Rasheed S. (1985) Eur. J. Cancer Clin. Oncol. 21, 97-107.
5. Varnier O.E., Ivaldi G., Pippia P., Muratore O., Raffanti S.P., Rasheed S. (1984) In Genetic and Phenotypic Markers of Tumors. Eds. Aaronson SA, Frati

L., Verna R., Plenum Press (New York), 331-335.
6. Krontiris T.G. (1983) New Engl. J. Med. 309, 404-409.
7. Chang E.G., Gonda, M.A.,Ellis R.W., Scolnick E.M., Lowy D.R. (1982) Proc. Natl. Acad. Sci. USA 79, 4848-4852.

3. Retroviruses and Human Pathology

MOLECULAR BIOLOGY OF VIRUSES OF THE HTLV FAMILY

F. Wong-Staal

Laboratory of Tumor Cell Biology, National Cancer Institute, Bethesda, Md., 20205 USA.

Human T-cell leukemia/lymphoma virus (HTLV) consists of three major subgroups: HTLV-I, the etiological agent of adult T-cell leukemia, and HTLV-II, initially obtained also from a patient with a malignant disease, are both capable of transforming T-lymphocytes in vitro; HTLV-III, a cytopathic virus that apparently lacks transforming activity, is the etiological agent of the acquired immunodeficiency syndrome (AIDS). Members of the HTLV family contain genomes with a unique organization. In addition to the replicative genes (gag, pol and env), an additional gene and its product, a 42 kd protein, have been identified for HTLV-I and HTLV-II. This protein is likely to be important in initiation of transformation. Evidence suggests that it functions in transcriptional activation of viral and cellular genes in a manner analogous to some DNA tumor virus proteins. Analysis of the HTLV-III genome is less extensive, but suggests that this virus also has an extra coding sequence at the 3' end. Different isolates of HTLV-III exhibit considerable polymorphism, probably indicative of the highly replicative nature of this virus. In addition, a large amount of viral DNA persists in the unintegrated form both in continuously producing cell lines and in fresh biopsied tissues of AIDS patients. This finding may be relevant to the cytopathic effect of this virus.

INTRODUCTION

Human T-cell leukemia/lymphoma virus (HTLV), a name originally used to designate a retrovirus associated with a form of mature T-cell malignancy, namely adult T-cell leukemia (ALT), now stands for a family of human retroviruses isolated in nature, which preferentially infect a subset of T-lymphocytes (1). In addition to their common cell tropism, viruses of this family share other biological, physiochemical and biochemical properties. However, one major difference in the biological properties of these viruses is directly reflected in their different disease spectrums and transforming capabilities. The virus associated with ATL, renamed HTLV-I, transforms T-cells efficiently in culture. A second virus, HTLV-II, which was obtained initially from cultured T-cells of a patient with Hairy cell leukemia, also has the capacity to transform T-cells in vitro. A third virus subgroup, HTLV-III, lacks transforming activity but is instead highly cytopathic. HTLV-III, has been unambiguously shown to be the etiological agent of the acquired immunodeficiency syndrome (AIDS) (2-5).

Almost all exogenous, pathogenic animal retroviruses belong to one of two categories: the chronic leukemia viruses are replication-competent, require a long latency period for disease induction, and lack transforming activity in vitro. Their genomes contain only the three structural genes (gag, pol and env) that are necessary for virus replication. The acute leukemia or sarcoma viruses are usually replication defective, induce disease rapidly in vivo, and transform appropriate target cells efficiently in vitro. They also carry a cell-derived gene which codes for a product necessary for the initiation and usually also maintenance of the transformed phenotype. Members of the HTLV family form a third distinct category. They are replication-competent, their genomes containing all 3 replicative genes. In addition, there are nucleotide sequences between the env gene and the 3' LTR which contain a long open reading frame (LOR). The LOR sequences

TABLE 1. Properties of the three classes of leukemia viruses

	Acute	Chronic	Subacute (HTLV/BLV)
Disease Induction	Rapid	Slow	Slow
Presence of onc Genes	Yes	No	No
Presence of Gene Coding for Non-Virion Structural Protein	Yes	No	Yes
Clonality of Tumor Cells	Polyclonal	Monoclonal	Monoclonal
Provirus Integration Site	Random	Specific	Random
Transformation In Vitro	Yes	No	Yes
Mechanism of Action	Trans	Cis	(Trans)

are not derived from conserved cellular genes, in contrast to retroviral oncogenes. Even though HTLV-I appears to induce ALT only after long latency periods, along with HTLV-II it can transform T-lymphocytes rapidly and efficiently in vitro. The LOR product of HTLV-I and HTLV-II is believed to be important in initiating transformation by these viruses. The function of the LOR sequences of HTLV-III is less clear. Other retroviruses that fit into this category are the distantly related bovine leukemia virus (BLV) and a primate retrovirus (PTLV-I) which is closely related to HTLV-I. We have proposed to call these the subacute leukemia viruses. Table I summarizes comparisons of leukemogenic transforming properties of viruses in these three categories.

THE GENOMES OF HTLV-I AND HTLV-II

The complete nucleotide sequence of one isolate of HTLV-I (6) and partial sequences of other HTLV-I isolates (unpublished) as well as one of HTLV-II and the several nearly identical isolates of HTLV-I have been revealed from these studies. First, the long terminal repeat (LTR) is unusually long as compared to other retroviruses, with the extra length attributed to the R and U5 sequences. Second, a long, non-coding sequence with multiple stop codons separates the gag and pol genes. Third, there is a region of about 1.6 kb between the carboxy terminus of the env gene and 3'LTR that contains several open reading frames. This region, initially referred to as the pX region, (6) is not closely homologous to celullar sequences of vertebrate cells (10) and therefore is not a typical retroviral oncogene. Deletions and substitutions within the first 0.6 kb of pX found in a variant, HTLV-1b, obtained from an African ATL patient did not affect the transforming capacity of this virus (1), (unpublished with L. Ratner). Comparison of the pX's of HTLV-I and HTLV-II revealed that the first 0.6 kb is nonconserved, but the following 1.0 kb is highly conserved, and contains a single long open reading frame (LOR). (9,12) Splice acceptor consensus sequences are present 5' to LOR which does not initiate with the ATG codon. (9) Therefore, the LOR protein product is likely to be a fused protein containing amino acid residues coded by gag or env. The HTLV-I LOR sequence predicts a protein product of at least 38 kd. Sera of patients positive for HTLV-I recognize a 40-42 kd protein expressed in all HTLV-transformed cells, including non-producer cells that do not synthesize virus or virion structural proteins. Amino acid analysis of cyanogen bromide cleavage fragments of this protein suggests that it is at least in part coded by the LOR sequences (13). Sequence analysis of the BLV genome also reveals the presence of an open reading frame similar in size to HTLV-I LOR in the corresponding region. (14).

POSSIBLE MECHANISM OF TRANSFORMATION AND LEUKEMOGENESIS BY HTLV-I AND HTLV-II

Cells infected by HTLV-I and HTLV-II in vitro are initially polyclonal and go through a growth crisis within 4-6 weeks. Predominantly clonal cells then emerge as immortalized cells (unpublished data). Often, these cells become independent of T-cell growth factor (TCGF), and morphologically resemble the primary leukemic cells. (15). Although the transformed cells are clonal, the site of provirus integration is variable in different clones. The lack of a conserved integration site suggests that these viruses act by a trans mechanism in cellular transformation, i.e. a diffusible viral protein product is directly involved. By analysing expression of different viral structural proteins at different time intervals after infection and clones of transformed cells containing defective proviruses, we have ruled out the expression of gag, pol and env protens to be necessary for the initiation of transformation (unpublished data). The only remaining candidate is the LOR protein, especially in view of the high degree of conservation of this gene between the two transforming HTLV's. Studies on the promoter-enhancer activity of LTRs of HTLV-I and HTLV-II showed that transcription of LTR-linked genes is elevated manifold in infected cells, indicating a trans-acting transcriptional activation phenomen via a viral protein. (16) There is indirect evidence that the LOR protein is responsible for this enhancing activity. Based on these studies, one can construct a model in which the LOR protein can also regulate cellular promoter-enhancer function at distant sites, and that the cellular genes regulated are associated with T-cell proliferation. Therefore, the mechanism of transformation by HTLV is more similar to certain DNA tumor viruses than to other retroviruses. There are already several genes identified that are activated by infection with HTLV-I and HTLV-II, and all these have been linked to T-cell proliferation. Therefore, it is directly testable whether the LOR protein binds to the enhancer-promoter sequences of these genes.

Unlike the in vitro transformed cells, fresh ATL cells frequently contain no detectable viral mRNA or proteins, including LOR (17). In addition, although each of these ATL cell samples is monoclonal, the integration sites of these proviruses vary. So the virus does not seem to function in cis or trans in maintaining the leukemic state. We speculate a two-stage leukemogenesis event, with the early stage being analogous to the in vitro transformation process, resulting in immortalization and enhanced proliferation of the infected cells. This in turn increases the chance for a mutation or gene rearrangement which leads to the progression of the disease. At this late stage, the virus has done its damage and is no longer needed.

MOLECULAR BIOLOGY OF THE HTLV-III, THE ETIOLOGICAL AGENT OF ACQUIRED IMMUNODEFICIENCY SYNDROME (AIDS)

A novel member of the HTLV family designated as HTLV-III has recently been identified as the etiological agent of AIDS, a disease characterized by depletion of the OKT4+ helper T-cells (see chapter by Robert-Guroff and Gallo, this volume). We have cloned the genomes of several isolates of HTLV-III. (18,19). Nucleotide sequence analysis of two of these clones revealed many structural similarities of HTLV-I and HTLV-II, particularly in the presence of a LOR sequence. Since HTLV-III has no apparent transforming activity, the function of LOR is more obscure. Recent experiments indicated that HTLV-III infected cells contained factors that activate transcription of HTLV-III LTR linked genes, (20) suggesting that the LOR of HTLV-III has a similar function in tran-acting transcriptional activation. Either HTLV-III LOR activates a different set of cellular genes from LOR of HTLV-I or -II to account for the cytopathic, rather than immortalizing, effect of the virus, or HTLV-III has a transforming activity which is masked by its profound cytopathic effect.

The HTLV-III genome is completely exogenous and does not carry a conserved cellular gene. Integrated provirus can be detected in infected cell cultures as well as peripheral blood lymphocytes and lymphonode tissue of AIDS and pre-AIDS patients (19). The infected cells are polyclonal with respect to provirus integration ,as expected for a virus that induces cell death rather than clonal expansion of the target cells. Furthermore, a large amount of unintegrated viral DNA persists in both the long term cultured cells and patient tissues, (19) a feature that seems to be characteristic of other cytopathic retroviruses. We also found that very few (less that one in a hundred) cells are infected in a population of lymphocytes from AIDS and pre-AIDS patients, and virus information is not detectable in several Kaposi tumor tissues examined. These results suggest that HTLV-III does not have a direct role in the proliferation of lymphocytes in lymphadenopathy of pre-AIDS patients or in the clonal expansion of endothelial cells of Kaposi tumors. These are secondary syndromes that develop as a consequence of the depletion or impaired function of the helper-inducer T-lymphocytes infected by HTLV-III.

One salient feature emerging from analyses of the genomes of different HTLV-III isolates is the extent of polymorphism among different isolates. So far, all isolates can be distinguishable from each other based on the analyses with five or six restriction enzymes. There is a whole spectrum with respect to the degree of similarity among different isolates. An isolate from a Haitian patient has practically no correspondence of restriction enzyme sites except in the LTR regions (unpublished data with B. Hahn et al.), and probably represents one end of the spectrum. This degree of genetic diversity is not seen with different HTLV-I and HTLV-II isolates, and may be due to the highly replicative nature of HTLV-III as opposed to the cryptic state of the HTLV-I and HTLV-II proviruses in vivo. It will be important to determine if changes in the HTLV-III genomes cluster in any particular regions and if they are significant enough to alter the immunological reactivities of the different isolates.

REFERENCES

1. Wong-Staal, F. & Gallo, R.C. (1984) Blood, in press.
2. Popovic, M., Sarngadharan, M.G., Reed, E., & Gallo, R.C. (1984) Science, 24, 497-500.
3. Gallo, R.C., Salahuddin, S.Z., Papovic, M., Sheared, G.M., Kaplan, M., Haynes, B.F., Palker, Y.J., Redfield, R., Oleske, J., Safai, B., White, F., Foster, P., & Markham, P.D. (1984) Science, 224, 500-503.
4. Sarngadharan, M.G., Popovic, M., Bruch, L., Schupbach, J., & Gallo, R.C. (1984): Science, 224, 506-508.
5. Schupbach, J., Sarngadharan, M.G., & Gallo, R.C. (1984) Science, 224, 607-610.
6. Seiki, M., Hattori, S., Hirayama, Y., & Yoshida, M. (1983) Proc. Natl. Acad. Sci. USA, 80, 3618-3622.
7. Shimotohno, K., Golde, D.W., Miwa, M., Sugimura, T., & Chen, I.S.Y. (1984) proc. Natl. Acad. Sci. USA, 81, 1079-1083.
8. Sodroski, J., Trus, M., Perkins, D., Patarca, R., Wong-Staal, F., Gelmann, E., Gallo, R.C. & Haseltine, W.A. (1984) Proc. Natl. Acad. Sci. USA, 81:4617-4621.
9. Haseltine, W.A., Sodroski, J., Patarca, R., Gribbs, D., Perkins, D., & Wong-Staal, F. (1984) Science, 225, 419-421.
10. Franchini, G., Wong-Staal, F., & Gallo, R.C. (1984) J. of Invest. Dermatology, 83, 063A-066S, Williams and Wilkins Co.
11. Hahn, B.H., Shaw, G.M., Popovic, M., LoMonico, A., Gallo, R.C., & Wong-Staal, F. (1984) Int. J. Cancer, in press;
12. Shaw, G.M., Gonda, M.A., Flickinger, G.H., Hahn, B.H., Gallo, R.C., and Wong-Staal, F. (1984) Proc. Natl. Acad. Sci. USA, 81, 4544-4548.

13. Lee, T.H., Coligan, J.E., Sadroski, J.G., Haseltine, W.A., Salahuddin, S.Z., Wong-Staal, F., Gallo, R.C., & Essex, M. (1984) Science, 226-57-61.
14. Rice, N., Stephens, R.M., Couez, D., Deschamp, H., Keltmann, R., Barny, A., & Gilden, R. (1984) Virology, in press.
15. Gallo, R.C. (1984) In: Cancer Surveys, edited by L.M. Franks, L.M. Wyke, and R.A. Weiss, Oxford University Press, Oxford.
16. Sodroski, J.G., Rosen C.A. & Haseltine, W.A. (1984) Science, 225, 381-385.
17. Franchini, G., Wong-Staal, F. & Gallo, R.C. (1984) Proc. Natl. Acad. Sci. USA, in press.
18. Hahn, B.H., Shaw, G.M., Aryn, S.K., Popovic, M., Gallo, R.C., & Wong-Staal, F. (1984) Nature, in press.
19. Shaw, G.M., Hahn, B.H., Arya, S.K., Groopman, G., Gallo, R.C. & Wong-Staal, Science, in press.
20. Sodroski, J., Rosen, C., Wong-Staal, F., Popovic, M., Arya, S.K., Gallo, R.C., & Haseltine, W.A., Science, in press.

ACTIVATION OF RETROVIRAL GENES IN HUMAN REPRODUCTIVE TISSUES AND TUMORS

A. Vaheri[1], J. Suni[1], A. Narvanen[1], R. Pakkanen[1], and T. Wahlstrom[2]

1. Department of Virology and 2. Department of Pathology, University of Helsinki, Haartmaninkatu 3, SF-00290 Helsinki, Finland

Retroviruses may be classified into two categories: exogenous and endogenous. Naturally occurring pathogenic exogenous retroviruses have been found in a number of vertebrates; in humans the T cell leukemia/lymphoma retroviruses, HTLV I, II and III, have been associated with T-cell leukemias and the acquired immunodeficiency syndrome. Endogenous retroviruses, present in proviral DNA form in the germ line, have been detected in most vertebrate species studied, including chickens, rodents and cats. In addition to proviruses, the murine species carry in the DNA also intracisternal A particle genes (1) and VL30 sequencs (2), for which no extracellular form or protein product have been demonstrated, respectively. Endogenous retroviruses have been isolated in infectious form from several subhuman primates (3,4); the baboon endogenous retrovirus (BaEV), that appears to be relatively readily isolated from placenta and that shows extensive homology with one of the feline endogenous retroviruses RD114 (5,6) is a well known example. To date, human endogenous retroviruses have not been isolated in infectious form and producer cell lines have not been established. There is, however, good evidence for the presence of retroviral sequences in human DNA and also increasing evidence that human retroviral genes are active at the transcriptional and translational levels. In the following we briefly summarize the evidence (see Table 1) and describe our recent results on the activation of retroviral genes in human reproductive tissues and in certain tumors.

Table 1. Evidence for human endogenous retroviral genes and their activation.

Finding	Reference
Retrovirus-like particles in:	
term placentas	7, 8
oocytes	13
cultured teratocarcinoma cells	9,10
psoriasis	14-16
Retrovirus-like reverse transcriptase in:	
placental extracts	11
follicular fluids	13
Inhibitor of the transcriptase in:	
placental extracts	12
Retroviral DNA sequences:	
C-type-related	17-22
MMTV-related	23,24
Retroviral mRNA transcripts:	
Northern blotting	26
in situ hybridization	see text
Retrovirus-related IgG-antibodies in:	
human sera	31
Retrovirus-related polypepide antigen in:	
normal and malignant trophoblastic cells	31,32,34,40
renal cell adenocarinoma tissue and patient urine	14,45
Retrovirus-related Mr 75,000 protein in:	
normal syncytiotrophoblasts	40
cultured choriocarcinoma cells	40
renal cell adenocarcinoma tissue	45

VIRUS PARTICLES AND ASSOCIATED DNA POLYMERASE

Particles closely ressembling animal retroviruses have been seen budding from syncytiotrophoblasts of human placentas (7,8) and from cultured human teratocarcinoma cells (9,10). Both types of particles have an associated reverse transcriptase-like activity (10,11) and a specific Mr 60,000-65,000 inhibitor of the enzyme activity has been partially purified from human placental extracts (12). Larsson and collaborators reported in 1981 on detection of small retrovirus-like particles, measuring 60-80 nm in diameter, in human oocytes and on detection of reverse transcriptase activity in some specimens of follicular fluid (13). Iversen and Dalen have provided evidence for the presence of retrovirus-like particles in psoriatic skin tissue and in urine of patients with fulminant psoriasis (14-16). Obviously there is no direct evidence to associate the above findings specifically with endogenous retroviral sequencs rather than with exogenous retroviruses, if any.

RETROVIRUS-RELATED DNA SEQUENCES AND THEIR TRANSCRIPTION

There is good evidence that human DNA contains retrovirus-related nucleotide sequences. Nucleic acid reassociation studies first revealed that humans and other primates contain multiple baboon endogenous virus (BaEV)-related sequences in their chromosomal DNA (17). A defective, endogenous provirus was recently isolated from a human recombinant DNA library by using as probe an endogenous chimpanzee retroviral pol fragment highly related to that of BaEV (18). This genome, termed HC-20 (or endogenous retrovirus-1, erv-1), has been assigned to human chromosome 18 (19). The erv-1 provirus contains gag and pol genes, which are significantly related to those of both Moloney murine leukemia virus (Mo-MuLV) and BaEV, env-related sequences of the expected length, and a 3' long terminal repeat (LTR), but no 5' lTR (18). Other reports have described the isolation from a human library of retroviral clones or detection of DNA sequences that are related to MuLV (20, 21), BaEV LTR (22), or mouse mammary tumor virus (MMTV) (23,24). Zabarovsky et al. (25) described linkage of retroviral-like sequences to a variant human c-mos proto-oncogene in the human genome. Taken together, the above data indicate that human DNA contains multiple, probably hundreds of copies of endogenous type C and B retroviral DNA sequences, many of which are truncated or defective but some of which appear to represent full length proviral DNAs flanked by LTR elements.

In contrast to this ample evidence on DNA sequences only scattered data exist on retrovirus-related mRNA transcripts. Rabson et al. (26) have reported on a human placental 3.0 kb RNA species that hybridizes to LTR and env DNA probes, a 1.7 kb env-reactive RNA found both in placentas and in a human colon carcinoma cell line and a 6.8 kb RNA species reactive with gag, pol, and env probes in the T-cell acute leukemia cell line 8402 that does not contain HTLV sequences. These authors found no hybridization of poly(A)$^+$ RNA present in placenta to the gag or pol probes used. In contrast using the in situ hybridization procedure, in collaboration with Drs. M. Cohen, S. Pfeifer-Ohlsson and R. Ohlsson, we located retrovirus-related mRNA transcripts to the syncytiotrophoblasts of first-trimester placentas using a HC-20 gag-pol subclone in medium stringency conditions (R.P. et al., manuscript in preparation).

IgG ANTIBODIES IN HUMAN SERA

IgG antibodies capable of inhibiting purified BaEV reverse transcriptase as well as human sperm DNA polymerase have been detected in individual partners from infertile marriages (27). There are also reports on detection of human antibody reacting with retroviral glycoproteins (28). Most of these antibodies, however, probably represent natural antibodies reacting with common carbohydrate moieties in glycoproteins and glycolipids (29,30).

Using a sensitive solid-phase enzyme immunoassay (EIA) we detected IgG antibodies in 118 out of 1540 human cord blood sera (7.7%) on the basis of their cross-reactivity with the feline endogenous retrovirus RD114 (31). Blocking assays with specific antibodies to animal retrovirus p30 proteins, use of control antigen, and immunoblotting experiments indicated that the human antibodies reacted specifically with the p30 protein of RD114 virus. Interestingly, the occurrence of antibodies in cord-blood serum had a highly significant correlation ($p < 0.0005$) to complications during pregnancy and also correlated to the number of previous abortions and stillbirths. More recent studies (J.S. et al., unpublished) have indicated that the occurrence of retrovirus p30-reactive IgG antibodies is not restricted to cord-blood sera but they are also found in nonpregnant women and in men.

RETROVIRUS-RELATED POLYPEPTIDE ANTIGENS IN NORMAL AND MALIGNANT TROPHOBLASTIC CELLS

The close correlation between the p30-reactive IgG antibodies and complicated pregnancy led us to look for a p30-related antigen in placenta. Using antibodies to RD114 p30 by immunperoxidase tissue staining retrovirus, we found p30-related antigen uniformly in sections of all placental specimens studied (early and term pregnancies, blighted ova, hydatidiform moles, destructive moles and choriocarcinomas). In each case the p30-related antigen was largely confined to cells with syncytiotrophoblastic morphology (31; see Table 2). We could thus conclude that retrovirus p30-related antigen is selectively expressed in the highly differentiated syncytiotrophoblasts which in the normal placenta are directly exposed to maternal blood. These findings also led us to suggest that the retrovirus-reactive IgG antibodies in cord blood sera may

Table 2. Reactivity of antibodies with normal and malignant trophoblastic tissues and cultured cells.

Antibody	Immunoperoxidase staining of STP cells	Immunoblotting First trimester STP cells	Immunoblotting Cultured choriocarcinoma cells
Polyclonal anti-RD114 p30	+a	N.D.	N.D.
Monoclonal HPS-1	+a	+c	Mr 130,000
Monoclonal anti-HTLV-1 p19	+b		Mr 28,000
Polyclonal anti-HTLV-I p24	+b		N.D.
Polyclonal anti-synthetic peptide 23	+b	Mr 75,000	Mr 75,000 - doublet at Mr 100,000-110,000

a = Staining of cells with syncytiotrophoblastic morphology in all normal human first-trimester and term placentas, blighted ova, hydatidiform and destructive moles and choriocarcinomas studied. b = As above, but no staining of term placentas. c = Spot immunoblotting. N.D.= not done. STP = syncytiotrophoblastic cells. For references see text.

represent a maternal autoimmune-like response to the p30-related syncytiotrophoblast antigen(s) escaping during cellular damage due to the complictions occurring during pregnancy.

To characterize the retrovirus p30-related antigen(s) further we isolated syncytiotrophoblasts from first-trimester placentas and immunopurified using anti-RD114-p30 IgG Sepharose, from the cell extracts antigen(s) to immunize mice. A monoclonal IgG antibody, designated HPS-1 (Human Placental Syncytiotrophoblast), was selected which reacted in EIA and immunoblotting both with the syncytiotrophoblast antigen and with mammalian retroviruses, but not with an avian retrovirus (32). In immunohistology, HPS-1 gave a pattern fully identical with the one observed for the polyclonal anti-RD114 p30 as summarized in Table 2. Moreover, unlike the polyclonal antibodies, HPS-1 also reacted in immunoblotting with homogenates of cultured JAr choriocarcinma cells and detected an Mr 130,000 polypeptide (32). The HPS-1 reactive antigen has in these cells as well as in cultured renal adenocarcinoma cells (see below) a very conspicuous distribution. It has an apparent affinity to vimentin, an association persisting when vinblastine was used to induce perinuclear coiling of vimentin filaments (33). Work is in progress to characterize biochemically the HPS-1 reactive antigenic polypeptide(s) to determine whether they represent, as is expected, translation products of human endogenous retroviral gene sequences.

Further proof for the concept of oncoplacental activation of human retroviral DNA sequences was obtained when similar experiments were carried out using the anti-HTLV-I p19 monoclonal (34) and with the anti-HTLV-I p24 polyclonal antibodies (unpublished), both kindly provided by Drs. M. Robert-Guroff and R.C. Gallo. These antibodies, as summarized in Table 2, gave a staining pattern identical to that of HPS-1 but, unlike HPS-1, did not react with term placentas. In immunoblotting of cultured choriocarcinma cells (JAr or BeWo) anti-HTLV-I p19 detected a single polypeptide at Mr 28,000. The monoclonal antibody to HTLV-I p19 has also been shown to detect, according to immunofluorescence staining, a human thymic epithelial antigen acquired during ontogeny (35). This antigen appeared in the fetal thymic epithelium in the 15th week of gestation (35), whereas the reactivity we detected disappears from the placental synsytiotrophoblasts around the same time of gestation (34). Since neither the placental nor the thymic antigen has been characterized biochemically, the possibility remains that anti-p19 detects Mr 28,000 due to "molecular mimicry" (36), i.e., the whole polypeptides HTLV-I p19 and Mr 28,000 are unrelated but share short aminoacid sequences giving rise to immunological cross-reactions. Alternatively, proteins encoded by the HTLV-I genome (37) and the gene products of the human endogenous gag sequences (see above) are related to the extent that anti-HTLV-I p19 reacts with both. It should be noted that the previous observations (38) on lack of HTLV-specific gene sequencs in normal cellular DNA do not necessarily exclude this last possibility. The reason is that the minimum requirement for an antigenic cross-reactivity between two proteins is the sharing of only 4-6 amino acids in sequence (39). Such a low degree of homology would not be detected by the methods used in nucleic acid hybridization. Chemical characterization of the p28 polypeptide is needed to distinguish between these and other possibilities.

More recently we have used antibodies to a synthetic peptide, Sp23, the sequence of which (except Cys) was deduced from the cloned HC-20 gag-related DNA sequence (18), apparently corresponding to the p30 region (see Table 3). These antibodies give in immunohistology a strong staining pattern (Fig. 1) identical to that obtained with anti-HTLV-I p19 and detected an Mr 75,000 polypeptide in syncytiotrophoblasts isolated from first-trimester placentas and three different lines of cultured choriocarcinoma cells (Fig. 2). The undecapeptide blocked the reactivity of the antibody (40).

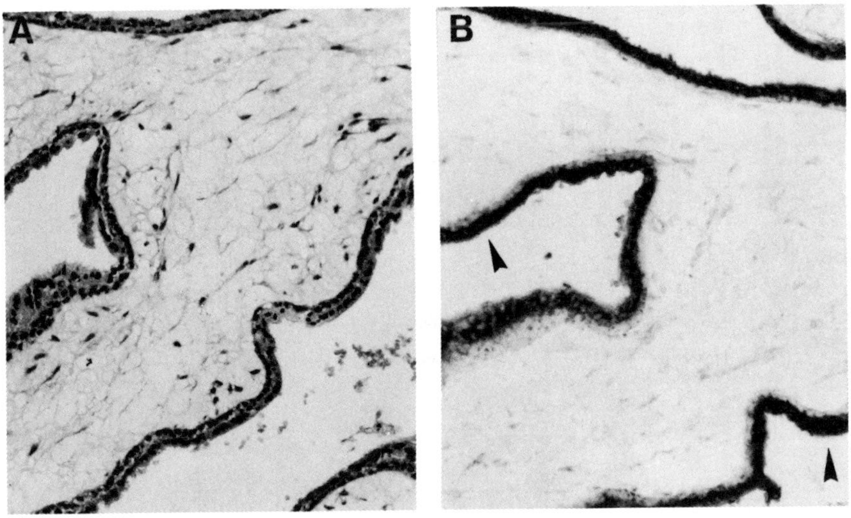

Figure 1. Retrovirus-related antigen in normal human placenta. Frame A shows a normal placenta, gestational age 8 weeks, stained with hematoxylin-eosin. Magnification 160x. Frame B shows an adjacent section stained by the immunoperoxidase method using the anti-Sp23 antiserum. The positive stain reaction is confined to the syncytiotrophoblasts (arrow heads) on the surface of the chorionic villi.

Table 3. Sequence homology of Sp23 undecapeptide with defined retrovirus p24-p30 proteins.

Peptide	
Sp23 (HC-20, human DNA)	Cys-Glu-Asn-Pro-Ser-Gln-Phe-Tyr-Glu-Arg-Leu
MuMV (murine)	-Glu-Ser-Pro-Ser-Ala-Phe-Leu-Glu-Arg-Leu
BaEV (baboon)	-Glu-Ser-Pro-Ala-Ala-Phe-Met-Glu-Arg-Leu
SSAV (woolly monkey)	-Glu-Pro-Pro-Ser-Val-Phe-Val-Glu-Arg-Leu
HTLV (human)	-Glu-Pro-Tyr-His-Ala-Phe-Val-Glu-Arg-Leu

Modified from ref. 40. Homologies with Sp23 are underlined. In the original publications, Leu and Tyr residues in the seventh positions were inadvertedly switched between the human and MuLV sequence. SSAV, simian sarcoma-associated virus.

RETROVIRUS-RELATED Mr 75,000 PROTEIN IN RENAL CELL ADENOCARCINOMA TISSUE

In search for malignant tumors other than destructive moles and choriocarcinoams that would express retrovirus-related markers, we encountered, initially using immunohistochemistry, a uniformly positive reaction in hypernephromas also called renal cell adenocarcinoma (RCC). Most convincingly all 42 individual tumors tested to date have given a positive result and all controls including normal kidneys, Wilms' tumors and adenocarcinomas of uterine corpus, uterine cervix or colon among others have been uniformly negative (41). Notably, a positive staining pattern is obtained with any of the monoclonal (HPS, a-HTLV-I p19) or polyclonal (a-RD114 p30, a-HTLV-I p24, a-Sp23) antibodies reactive with the trophoblastic tissues and cultured cells. Control antibodies (specifically blocked polyclonal antibodies, unrelated monoclonal antibodies or polyclonal antibodies to unrelated synthetic peptides) give a negative result on RCC (41,45). When we found that the retrovirus-related antibodies reacted not only with the RCC tumor cell cytoplasma but also with the lumen or proximal tubuli we searched for retrovirus-related antigen in RCC patient urine. With a radioimmunoassay, using ^{125}I-RD114 p30 and anti-RD114 p30 polyclonal antibodies as reagents, we could demonstrate retrovirus p30-related antigen activity in RCC urine but not in controls and interestingly after nephrectomy this activity tended to disappear unless metastases persisted (41).

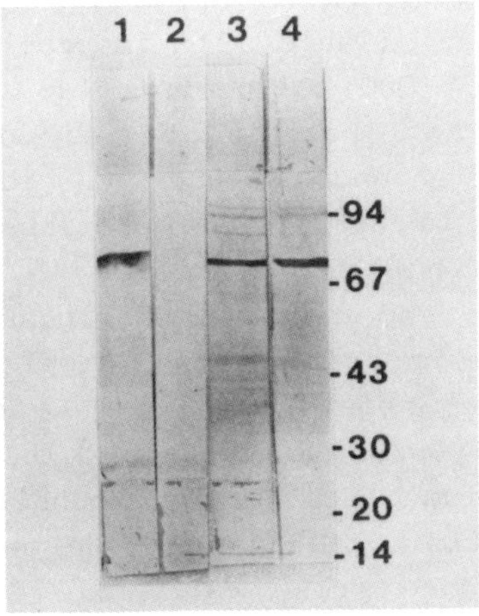

Figure 2. Immunoblotting of JEG-3 choriocarcinoma. Lane 1: staining with rabbit antibody to synthetic peptide Sp23 rabbit serum. Lanes 2-4 demonstrate blocking of anti-Sp23 reactivity with the undecapeptide Sp23. Anti-Sp23 diluted 1:500 was mixed with 2 ug/ml of Sp23 (lane 2), with 200 ng/ml of Sp23 (lane 3), or with 2 ug/ml unrelated didecapeptide (lane 4) and subsequently used in immunoblotting of JEG-3 choriocarcinoma cells. Molecular weights of the marker proteins are indicated in kilodaltons on the right. (from ref. 40, with permission).

We have no plausible explanation for the selective expression of retroviral markers in RCC. As a kidney tumor it is relatively common, and has a propensity to produce only solitary metastases, often in the lungs or the brain. RCC is one of the few tumors which has been reported to respond to interferon treatment (42) and persevering anecdotal knowledge has it that RCC metastases may regress spontaneously after nephrectomy. RCC originates in the mature epithelial cell of the proximal convoluted tubule of the nephron (43), while the other main malignant kidney tumor, Wilms' tumor, has its origin in the metanephric blastema and is composed of both epithelial and mesenchymal elements (44).

After we detected that antibodies to the synthetic undecapeptide Sp23 (Table 3) immunoblotted from RCC extracts and Mr 75,000 polypeptide (45) comigrating with the polypeptide that these antibodies detect in isolated syncytiotrophoblasts and cultured choriocarcinoma cells, we set ourselved to purify the proteins. The Mr 75,000 polypeptides have now been purified to homogeneity both from RCC extracts and cultured choriocarcinoma cells for biochemical and immunochemical characterization

The retrovirus-relatd HC-20 DNA clone from the sequence of which Sp23 was deduced detects, as mentioned above, at medium stringency conditions mRNA in syncytiotrophoblasts of first trimester placentas. However, this cloned probe fails to react with RCC or cultured choriocarcinoma cells in which the Mr 75,000 polypeptide(s) are expressed at a fairly high level (0.05% of total protein). Thus the HC-20 retroviral sequences, which lack the 5' LTR (18), probably do not encode the Mr 75,000 polypeptide. Protein sequencing of the Mr 75,000 is therefore needed not only to establish its relationship to known retroviral polypeptides, but also to clone the Mr 75000 gene(s) from human DNA libraries.

CONCLUSIONS

Human retroviral DNA sequences appear to be selectively expressed in certain reproductive tissues (placental syncytiotrophoblasts and possibly oocytes). Placental tissue contained polyA$^+$ RNA reactive with one of the cloned env probes (26) and in situ hybridization with another gag-pol probe has demonstrated mRNA transcripts in syncytiotrophoblasts of first-trimester placentas (Table 1). As summarized in Table 2, some of the retrovirus gag related antibodies reacted with the syncytiotrophoblasts throughout pregnancy while the reactivity of other antibodies is confined to first-trimester only. Moreover, the different antibodies immunoblotted three distinct polypeptides from cultured choriocarcinoma cells, Mr 28,000, 130,000 and 75,000. These results suggest that in normal and malignant throphoblastic cells a family of retroviral genes may be activated. Of the gene products the Mr 75,000 polypeptide is particularly strongly expressed, and an Mr 75,000 polypeptide similar by several criteria is also strongly expressed in an epithelial kidney tumor, renal cell adenocarcinoma. Clearly we have no explanation for the apparently selective expression of human retrovirus related genes in human syncytiotrophoblasts and in this tumor, and do not know whether this activation has any role in reproductive physiology or tumor pathogenesis. We can conclude, however, that the gene products, the Mr 75,000 protein in particular, appear to provide a very useful tumor marker.

REFERENCES

1. Ono, M., Kitasato, H., Ohishi, H. & Motobayashi-Nakajima, Y. (1984) J. Virol. 50:352-358.
2. Hodgson, C.P., Elder, P.K., Ono, T., Foster D.N. & Getz M.J. (1983) Mol. Cell. Biol. 3:2221-2231.
3. Todaro, G.J. (1980) In: Viruses in Naturally occurring Cancers, eds. Essex, M., Todaro, G. & zur Hausen H.

(Cold Spring Harbor Lab., Cold Spring Harbor, NY), Vol. 7, pp. 709-717.

4. Nooter, K. & Bentvelzen, P. (1980) Biochim. Biophys. Acta 605:461-487.
5. Sherr, C.J., Fedele, L.A., Benveniste, R.E. & Todaro, G.J. (1975) J. Virol. 15:1440-1448.
6. Oroszlan, S. & Gilden R.V. (1980) in Molecular Biology of RNA tumor viruses, ed. Stephenson, J.R. (Academic, New York, NY), pp. 299-344.
7. Kalter, S.S., Helmke, R.J., Heberling, R.L., Panigel, M., Fowler, A.K., Strickland, J.E. & Hellman, A. (1973) J. Natl. Cancer Inst. 50:1081-1084.
8. Dirksen, E.R. & Levy, J.A. (1977) J. Natl. Cancer Inst. 59:1187-1192.
9. Boller, K., Frank, H., Lower, J., Lower, R. & Kurth, R. (1983) J.Gen. Virol. 64:2549-2559.
10. Lower, R., Lower, J., Frank, H., Harzmann, R. & Kurth, R.H (1984) J. Gen. Virol. 65:887-898.
11. Nelson, J., Leong, J. & Levy, J. (1978) Proc. Natl. Acad. Sci. USA 75:6263-6267.
12. Leong, J.C., Wood, S.O., Lyford, A.O. & Levy, J.A. (1984) Int. J. Cancer 33:435-439.
13. Larsson, E., Nilsson, B.O., Sundstrom, P. & Widehn, S. (1981) Int. J. Cancer 28:551-557.
14. Dalen, A.B., Hellgren, L., Iversen, O.J., & Vincent, J. (1983) Acta Path. Microbiol. Immunol. Scand. Sect. B, 91:221-229.
15. Iversen, O.J., & Dalen, A.B. (1983) Acta Path. Microbiol. Scand. Sect. B, 91:343-349.
16. Iversen, O.J., (1983). Acta Path. Microbiol. Scand. Sect. B, 91:407-412.
17. Benveniste, R.E. & Todaro, G.J. (1974) Proc. Natl. Acad. Sci. USA 71:4513-4518.
18. Bonner, T.I., O'Connell, C. & Cohen, M. (1982) Proc. Natl. Acad. Sci. USA 79:4709-4713.
19. O'Brien, S.J., Bonner, T.I., Cohen, M., O'Connell, C. & Nash, W.G. (1983) Nature 303:74-77.
20. Martin, M.A., Bryan, T., Rasheed, S. & Khan, A.S. (1981) Proc. Natl. Acad. Sci. USA 78:4892-4896.

21. Repaske, R., O'Neill, R.R., Steele, .E. & Martin, M.A. (1983) Proc. Natl. Acad. Sci. USA 80:678-682.
22. Noda, M., Kurihara, M. & Takano, T. (1982) Nucl. Acids Res. 10:2865-2878.
23. Callahan R., Drohan W., Tronick S. & Schlom, J. (1982) Detection and cloning of human DNA sequences related to the mouse mammary tumor virus genome. Proc. Natl. Acad. Sci. USA 79:5503-5507.
24. May, F.E.B., Westley, B.R., Rochefort, H., Buetti, E. & Diggelman, H. (1983) Nucl. Acids. Res. 11:4127-4139.
25. Zabarovsky, E.R., Chumakov, I. & Kisselev, L.L. (1983) Gene 23:379-384.
26. Rabson, A.B., Steele, P.E., Garon, C.F. & Martin, M.A. (1983) Nature 306:604-607.
27. Witkin, S.S., Higgins, P.J. & Bendich, A. (1978) Clin. Exp. Immunol. 33:244-251.
28. Kurth, R., Teich, N.M. Weiss, R. & Oliver, R.T.D. (1977) Proc. Natl. Acad. Sci. USA 74:1237-1241.
29. Barbacid, M., Bolognesi, D. & Aaronson, S.A. (1980) Proc. Natl. Acad. Sci. USA 77:1617-1621.
30. Snyder, H.W. Jr. & Fleissner, E. (1980) Proc. Natl. Acad. Sci. USA 77:1622-1626.
31. Suni, J., Wahlstrom, RhT. & Vaheri, A. (1981) Int. J. Cancer 28:559-566.
32. Wahlstrom, T., Nieminen, P., Narvanen, A., Suni, J., Lehtovirta, P., Saksela, E. & Vaheri, A. Placenta (in press).
33. Wahlstrom, T., Narvanen, A., Virtanen, I, Suni, J. & Vaheri, A. in Gene Expression During Normal and Malignant Differentiation, eds. Andersson, L., Ekblom, P. & Gahmberg, C.G. (Academic), in press.
34. Suni, J., Narvanen, A., Wahlstrom, T., Lehtovirta, P. & Vaheri, A. (1984) Int. J. Cancer 33:293-298.
35. Haynes, B.F., Robert-Guroff, M., Metzgar, R.S., Franchini,G., Kalyanaraman, V.S., Palker, T.J., & Gallo, R.C. (1983) J. Exp. Med. 157:907-920.
36. Fujinami, R.S., Oldstone, M.B.A., Wroblewska, Z., Frankel, M.E. & Koprowski, H. (1983) Proc. Natl. Acad. Sci. USA 80:2346-2350.

37. Seiki, M., Hattori, S., Hirayama, Y. & Yoshida, M. (1983) Proc. Natl. Acad. Sci. USA 80:3618-3622.
38. Reitz, M.S. Jr., Poiesz, B.J., Ruscetti, F.W. & Gallo, R.C. (1981) Proc. Natl. Acad. Sci. USA 78:1887-1891.
39. Walter, G. & Doolittle, R.F. (1983) in Genetic Engineering, eds. Setlow, J.K. & Hollaender, A. (Plenum, New York, NY), Vo2l. 5, pp. 61-91.
40. Suni, J., Narvanen, A., Wahlstrom, T., Aho, M., Pakkanen, E., Vaheri, A., Copeland, T., Cohen, M. & Oroszlan, S. Proc. Natl. Acad. Sc. USA (in press).
41. Wahlstrom, T., Suni, J., Nieminen, P., Narvanen, A., Lentonen, T. & Vaheri, A. Lab. Invest. (submitted).
42. Quesada, J.R. Swanson, D.A., Trindade, A. & Gutterman, J.V. (1983) Cancer Res. 43, 940-943.
43. Oberling, C., Riviere, M., & Haguenau, F. (1960) Nature (Lond.) 186, 402-403.
44. Knudson, A.G. & Strong, L.C. (1972) J. Natl. Cancer Inst. 48, 313-324.
45. Wahlstrom, T., Narvanen, A., Aho, M., Suni, J., Vaheri, A., Copeland, T., Cohen, M. & Oroszlan, S. Nature (submitted).

RETROVIRUS AND AIDS

J.C. Chermann, F. Barre-Sinoussi and L. Montagnier

Unité d'Oncologie Virale, Institut Pasteur, 25, rue du Dr. Roux, 75724 Paris Cédex 15, France

Lymphadenopathy Associated Virus (LAV) is one prototype viral isolate of the virus proposed as the cause of AIDS. In all cases of AIDS, it was possible to isolate LAV: sexually active male homosexuals, intravenous drug users, recipients of blood transfusions, hemophiliacs, Africans and Haitians. All isolates have the characteristics of a retrovirus. LAV is T_4 lymphotropic and cytopathic for the T_4 helper-inducer subset. The T_4 molecule is involved in the cellular receptor for the virus. The seroepidemiological study shows a prevalence of IgG antibodies to LAV in patients with AIDS related complexes or AIDS. LAV was shown to be infectious for chimpanzees. The inactivation of LAV by chemical and physical agents is reported. LAV reverse transcriptase is strongly inhibited by an inhibitor of murine retroviruses, the ammonium 21 tungsto 9 antimoniate.

The epidemiological pattern of Acquired Immunodeficiency Syndrome (AIDS) strongly suggests that the disease is transmitted by an infectious agent, most likely a virus. The disease appeared first in young homosexual males and was manifested by <u>Pneumocystis carinii</u> (PCP), other opportunistic infections and/or Kaposi's sarcoma (KS) (1, 2). It has been observed that numerous apparently healthy homosexual men were presenting with a syndrome of persistent generalized lymphanopathy (PGL) of unknown cause (3, 4). AIDS is associated with a depletion of T cells, especially the helper/inducer subset (T_4 lymphocytes) resulting in an inverted helper/suppressor ratio (5-9) B-lymphocyte function is also abnormal in patients with AIDS as evidenced by polyclonal B-cell activation with elevated levels of serum immunoglobulins, and circulating immune complexes (10, 11).

Most cases of AIDS have occured in defined populations such as sexually active homosexual men (12), intravenous drug users (13), recipients of certain blood products (14), Haitians (15) and Africans (16, 17). Since a profound depression of cellular immunity involving T-lymphocytes has been described, the putative viral agent must be T-lymphoctropic. Some retroviruses such as feline leukemia viruses are known to cause a severe immune impairment in infected cats (18). The identification of a protein called T-cell-growth-factor (TCGF or IL_2 interleukin 2) permits the long term culture of human T-lymphocytes (19) and the isolation of human retroviruses, the human T-leukemia/lymphoma viruses (HTLV I) (20, 21) and HTLV II (22). The hypothesis that AIDS is caused by a retrovirus had been reported indirectly a few years ago (23). But with the use of antibodies to interferon (24) we were able to isolate another new lymphotrophic retrovirus. Lymphadenopathy Associated Virus (25, 26) and there is now strong evidence suggesting that this virus is the cause of AIDS.

The first isolate of LAV was from a non-immunodepressed homosexual patient with persistent generalized lymphadenopathy (25, 26) and the following isolates were from patients with frank AIDS (27, 28, 29, 30). A model for the role of LAV in the pathogenesis of AIDS was previously reported (27, 31).

Similar viruses were isolated from US patients and called HTLV III (32, 33, 34, 35) or ARV (AIDS related viruses) (36).

VIRAL ISOLATES

The procedure of LAV isolation was previously described from a lymph node biopsy of a homosexual male (25) and applied for patients with prodrome of frank AIDS. To this date, 25 isolates of LAV have been obtained -- 19 from frank AIDS, 5 from PGL, 1 from an asymptomatic carrier (hemophiliac B) and 0 from normal control population. They were from caucasian, Hatian or African patients. In all cases of AIDS it was possible to isolate the virus: i.v. drug addicts (unpublished results), transfusion-AIDS cases (donor and recipient) (37), hemophilics (28), Zairians (29), Haitians, bone marrow transplants recipients (unpublished results), and homosexuals with Kaposi's sarcoma or/and opportunistic infections (27, 31). LAV has the characteristics of a retrovirus by the classical criteria (density 1.16 in a sucrose gradient, Mg^{++} dependent reverse transcriptase, high molecular weight RNA, and morphogenesis by budding at the cell surface). All isolates have in common the inability to transform T-lymphocytes and a T_4 lymphocytopathogenic effect. All isolates have the same morphology revealed by electron microscopy studies. The p25 major internal core protein is antigenically identical from all different isolates as reported by F. Barré-Sinoussi in this book.

VIRAL LYMPHOTROPISM FOR THE HELPER/INDUCER T-LYMPHOCYTE SUBSET AND INDUCTION OF A CYTOPATHIC EFFECT

Since a profound depression of cellular immunity, involving T-lymphocytes of helper type, was described in AIDS patients, the putative agent must be lymphotropic. LAV replicated in an unfractionated T-lymphocytes population as early as 9 days after its infection and declined thereafter. Comparable results were obtained when T-lymphocytes from normal donor were first fractionated in two populations: T_4 (helper/inducer) and T_8 (cytotoxic/

suppressor); only a T_4+ lymphocyte subset was infected and replicated LAV whereas no virus was released by T subset. The same tropism is observed "in vivo": only "AIDS" patients stimulated T_4-lymphocytes released the virus and only a subset of T_4-lyphocytes (10 per cent) expressed the virus as ascertained by immunofluorescence. No virus was released by T_8-lymphocytes (27, 31, 38). Comparing the T_4 antigen in the course of LAV infection, a decrease of this marker at the cell surface is observed during and after virus production (31). Thus, it was recently shown that the T_4 molecule could be involved in the receptor of T_4-lymphocytes for LAV (D. Klatzmann et al., personal communication, and T. Cheingsons-Popov, this book). LAV is cytopathic for the T_4 helper lymphocytes (27, 38) and kills the same cells as those disappearing in AIDS: when no virus is isolated from AIDS patients, one can say that they have no more cells susceptible to LAV infection. The virus can infect lymphocytes, but only stimulated T_4-lymphocytes replicate LAV.

SEROEPIDEMIOLOGICAL STUDIES

The seroepidemiological studies (39, 40, F. Brun-Vezinet, this book) showed a prevalence of IgG antibodies to LAV in patients with AIDS, AIDS-related complexes or at risk, compared to a control group.

MOLECULAR CLONING OF LAV

The integrated proviral DNA of LAV has been molecularly cloned from infected T-lymphocytes from a healthy donor by M. Alizon and S. Wain-Hobson. No relationshp between LAV and the known HTLV I or II was found by hybridization (M. Alizon et al., in preparation). The molecular clone will provide a very useful tool for determining the origin of the virus and its evolution.

INFECTION OF CHIMPANZEES WITH LAV

Two chimpanzees were inoculated with LAV and infection was documented by repeated isolation of virus from peripheral blood lymphocytes and by detection of antibodies to LAV p25 in serum. The two chmpanzees presented an inverted T_4/T_8 ratio six months after LAV inoculation (D. Francis et al., unpublished results).

INACTIVATION OF LAV BY CHEMICAL DISINFECTANTS

We have examined the inactivation of LAV by several commonly used chemical disinfectants, using the reverse transcriptase assay as a marker of viral inactivation. From this study (41) it appears that LAV is inactivated by a contact with a solution of 25 percent of ethanol, 0.2 percent of sodium hypochloride and 1 percent glutaraldehyde.

INACTIVATION OF LAV BY PHYSICAL AGENTS

LAV is inactivated at 56°C 30 minutes in aqueous solution, and resistant for the dosage of UV irradiation or gamma irradiation usually employed for sterilization (B. Spire et al., in preparation).

LAV REVERSE TRANSCRIPTASE IS INHIBITED BY SODIUM$_{21}$ TUNGSTO$_9$ ANTIMONIATE (HPA$_{23}$)

LAV purified reverse transcriptase (42) is competitively inhibited by HPA$_{23}$, an "in vivo" inhibitor of the replication of some retroviruses (43) (44). This compound is one of the products which is actually tested as an anti-retroviral drug in human AIDS patients (D. Dormont et al. unpublished results).

REFERENCES

1. Gottlib, M.S., Schanker, H.M., Fant, P.T. et al. 1981. Morbid Mortal Weekly Rep. 30, 250-252.
2. Friedman-Kien, A., Laubenstein, L., Marmor, M., et al. (1981) Morbid Mortal Weekly Rep. 30, 305-308.
3. Mildvan, D., Mathur, U., Enlow, R.W. et al. (1982) Morbid Mortal Weekly Rep. 31, 249-251.
4. Mathur, U., Enlow, R.W., Spigland, I., William, D.C., Winchester, R.J., & Mildvan, D. (1982) Program and Abstracts of the 22nd Interscience Conference on Antimicrobial Agents and Chemotherapy, Miami Beach, Florida (abst. 853).
5. Komfeld, H., Stouwe, R.A., Lange, M., Reddy, M.M.,& Grieco M.H. (1982). N. Engl. J. Med. 307, 729-731.
6. Goldsmith, J.C., Moseley, P.L., Monick, M., Brady, M.,& Hunninghake, G., 1983. Ann. Int. Med. 98, 294-296.
7. Lederman, M.M., Ratnoff, O.D., Scillian, J.J., Jones, P.K., & Schacter B. (1983) New Engl. J. Med. 308, 79-83.
8. Stahl, R.E., Friedman-Kien, A., Dubin, R., Marmor, M., & Zolla-Pazner, S. (1982) Am. J. Med. 73, 171-178.
9. Moll, B., Emerson, E.E., Small, C.B., Friedland, G.H., Klein, R.S., & Spigland, I (1982) Clin. Immunol. Immnopathol. 25, 417-423.
10. Stahl, R.E., Friedman-Kien, A., Dubin, R., Marmor, M., & Zolla-Pazner, S. (1982) Amer J. Med. 73, 171.
11. Hersh, E.M., Reuben, J.M., Rios, A., Mansell, P.W.A., Newell, G.R., McClure, J.E. & Goldstein, A.L. (1983) N. Engl. J. Med. 305, 45.
12. Mildvan, D., Mathur, U., Enlow, R.W. et al. (1982) Ann. Intern. Med. 96, 700-704.
13. Gold, K., Thomas, D. & Garrett, T.J. (1982) N. Engl. J. Med. 307, 498.
14. Pneumocystis Carinii Pneumonia among persons with hemophilia A. (1982) M.M.C.R. 31, 365-367.
15. Vieira, J., Frank, E., Spira, T.J. & Landesman, S.H. (1983) N. Engl. J. Med. 308, 125-129.

16. Clumeck, N., Mascart-Lemone, F., De Maulbeuge, J., Brenez, D. & Marcellis L. (1983) The Lancet i:642.
17. Vandepitte, J., Verwilghen, R. & Zachee P. (1983) The Lancet i: 925-926.
18. Training, Z., Wenicke, D., Ungar-Waron, H. & Essex, M. (1983) Science 220, 858-859.
19. Morgan, D.A., Ruscetti, F.W. & Gallo, R.C. (1976) Science 193, 1007-1008.
20. Piesz, B.J., Ruscetti, F.W., Hazdar, A.F., Bunn, P.A., Minna, J.D. & Gallo, R.C. (1980) Proc. Natl. Acad. Sci. USA 77, 7415-7419.
21. Yoshida, M., Miyoshi, I. & Hinuma, Y. (1982) Proc. Natl. Acad. Sci. USA 79, 2031-2035.
22. Kalyanaraman, V.S., Sarngadharan, M.G., Robert-Guroff, M., Blayney, D., Golde, D. & Gallo R.C. (1982) Science 218, 571-573.
23. Essex, M., McLane, F., Lee, T.H. et al. (1983) Science 220, 859-862.
24. Barre-Sinoussi, F., Montagnier, L., Lidereau, R., Sisman,J., Wood, J. & Chermann, J.C. (1979) Ann. Microbiol. (Inst. Pasteur) (130B) 349-362.
25. Barre-Sinoussi, F., Chermann, J.C., Rey, F., Nugeyre, M.T., Chamaret, S., Gruest, J., Dauguet, C., Axler-Blin, C., Vezinet-Brun, F., Rouzioux, C., Rozenbaum, W. & Montagnier, L. (1983) Science 220, 868-871.
26. Chermann, J.C., Barre-Sinoussi, F., Dauguet, C., Brun-Vezinet, F., Rouzioux, C., Rozenbaum, W. & Montagnier, L. (1984) Antibiotics and Chemotherapy 32, 48-53.
27. Montagnier, L., Chermann, J.C., Barre-Sinoussi, F., Chamaret, S., Gruest, J., Nugeyre, M.T., Rey, F., Dauguet, C., Axler-Blin, C., Vezinet-Brun, F., Rouzioux, C., Saimot, A.G., Rozenbaum, W., Gluckman, J.C., Klatzmann, D., Vilmer, E., Griscelli, C., Gazengel, C. & Brunet, J.B. (1984) Cold Spring Harbor Laboratory New York, 363-379.
28. Vilmer, E., Barre-Sinoussi, F., Rouzioux, C., Gazengel, C., Vezinet-Brun, F., Dauguet, C., Fischer,

A., Manigne, P., Chermann, J.C., Griscelli, C. & Montagnier, L. (1984) Lancet ii, 753-757.
29. Ellrodt, A., Barre-Sinoussi, F., Le Bras, P.H., Nugeyre, M.T., Palazzo, L., Rey, F., Brun-Vezinet, F., Rouziouz, C., Segond, P., Caquet, R., Montagnier, L. & Chermann, J.C. (1984) Lancet i, 1383-1385.
30. Barre-Sinoussi, F., Chermann, J.C. & Montagnier, L. (1984) Manipulation of host defense mechanisms Ed. Tadao Aoki (Japan), in press.
31. Chermann, J.C., Barre-Sinoussi, F. & Montagnier, L. (1984) UCLA Symposia on Molecular and Cellular Biology. New Series, eds. Michael S. Gottlieb and Jerome E. Groopman (Alan R. Liss, Inc. New York) 16, 31-46.
32. Gallo, R.C., Salahuddin, J.Z., Popovic, M. et al. (1984) Science 224, 500-503.
33. Sarngadharan, M.G. Popovic, M., Bruch, L., Schupbach, J. & Gallo, R.C. (1984) Science 224, 506-508.
34. Popovic M., Sarngadharan, M.G., Read, E. & Gallo, R.C. (1984) Science 224, 497-500.
35. Schupbach, J., Popovic, M., Gilden, R.V. et al. (1984) Science 224, 503-505.
36. Levy J.A., Hoffman, A.D., Kramer, S.M., Landis, J.A., Shimabukuro, J.M. & Oshiro, L.S. (1984) Science 225, 840-843.
37. Feorino, M.P., Kalyanaraman, V.S., Haverkos, H.W., Cabradilla, C.D., Warfield, D.T., Jaffe, H.W., Harrison, A.K., Goldringer, D., Gottlieb, M.S., Chermann, J.C. , Barre-Sinoussi, F., Spira, T.J., McDougal, J.C., Curran, J.W., Montagnier, L., Murphy, F.A. & Francis, D.P. (1984) Science 225, 69-72.
38. Klatzmann, D., Barre-Sinoussi, F., Chermann, J.C., Nugeyre, M.T., Dauguet, C., Vilmer, E., Brun-Vezinet, F., Griscelli C., Rouzioux, C. & Montagnier, L. (1984) Science 225, 59-63.
39. Brun-Vezinet, F. & Rouzioux, F., (1984) Acquired Immunodeficiency Syndrome, UCLA, Symposia on Molecular and Cellular Biology New Series, Eds. Michael Gottlieb and Jerome E. Groopman (Alan R. Liss. Inc. New York)

16, 83-90.

40. Brun-Vezinet, F., Rouzioux, C., Barre-Sinoussi, F., et al. (1983) Lancet i, 1253-1256.
41. Spire, B., Barre-Sinoussi, F., Montagnier, L. & Chermann, J.C. (1984) Lancet ii, 899-901.
42. Rey, M.A., Spire, B., Dormont, D., Barre-Sinoussi, F., Montagnier, L. & Chermann, J.C. (1984) Biochem. Biophys. Res. Comm. 121,126-133.
43. Chermann, J.C., Sinoussi, F., & Jasmin, C. (1975) Biochem. Biophys. Res. Comm 65, 1229-1236.
44. Jasmin, C., Chermann, J.C., Herve, G., Teze, A., Souchay, P., Boy-Loustau, C., Raybaud, N., Sinoussi, F. & Raynoud M. (1974) Journal of the National Cancer Institute 53, 469-474.

HUMAN T-CELL LEUKEMIA (LYMPHOTROPIC) RETROVIRUSES: THE HTLV FAMILY AND THEIR ROLE IN LEUKEMIAS, LYMPHOMAS AND AIDS

M. Robert-Guroff and R. C. Gallo

Laboratory of Tumor Cell Biology, Developmental Therapeutics Program, Division of Cancer Treatment, National Cancer Institute, Bethesda, Md. 20205.

The human T-cell leukemia/lymphoma (lymphotrophic) viruses comprise a family of human retroviruses whch exert disparate effects on human T-cells and which are associated with at least two forms of disease. HTLV-I and -II exert proliferative effects on T-cells, while the predominant effect of HTLV-III is a cytopathic one. Evidence for the association of HTLV-I with adult T-cell leukemia and for the association of HTLV-III with the acquired immunodeficiency syndrome is reviewed here. Current thoughts on possible mechanisms of these viral pathogenic effects are discussed.

THE HTLV FAMILY

The human T-cell leukemia/lymphoma viruses (HTLV) comprise a family of type C retroviruses, so far limited to three members, but possessing two and probably several more variants and/or additional sub-types. HTLV-I, the prototype virus, was isolated and characterized in 1980 (1) and until recently was probably the best characterized. The current intense interest in HTLV-III, isolated in 1984 (2,3) and undoubtedly the cause of the acquired immunodeficiency syndrome (AIDS), has temporarily superseded HTLV-I in importance and is now almost equally well characterized. Studies on HTLV-II, described in 1982 (4), have contributed a great deal of basic information on the biochemistry and molecular biology of HTLV in general, however, as the type II isolate has yet to be associated with a particular disease, research interest has focused on the other sub types. Both HTLV-I and -III clearly cause disease, although the mechanisms by which they do so are at once baffling and intriguing. While closely related and homologous in many respects, HTLV-I causes a lymphoproliferative effect, while HTLV-III kills cells it infects. We will explore here some of the current concepts offered to explain these disparate effects, and to combat or control them. First, however, we will summarize briefly the basic information on the viruses, necessary to understand directions future research endeavors will take.

The HTLV isolates, I, II and III, as well as two fairly distinct variants, HTLV-Ib (Hahn et al., Int. J. Cancer, in press), and a recent HTLV-III variant (Shaw et al., in preparation), comprise a family because of their striking biochemical and immunological relationships. All HTLV members possess a similar genomic organization resembling other retroviruses in having gag, pol, and env genes (5-7). Unlike other retroviruses, however, all HTLV family members possess an uncharacterized genetic region designated pX, originally thought to encode from 1 to 4 proteins (5). It is the pX region which is believed to contribute to the transforming and cytopathic effects of the viruses. The protein products of these genes are remarkably similar among all 3 viruses. The gag gene products are processed from a precursor of approximately 54,000 to 55,000 molecular weight (8) to mature viral structural proteins of 19,000 (p19), 24,000 (p24), and 15,000 (p15) in HTLV-I and -II isolates (4,9-11). HTLV-III varies in the molecular weights of the smaller gag proteins, although it also posesses a major core protein, p24 (8,12). The env gene products of the three subgroups are also similar, with precursor molecules of approximately 61,000 to 67,000 molecular weight and mature envelope glycoproteins of 41,000 to 46,000 (gp41, gp46) molecular weight in HTLV-I and -III and a glycoprotein of 52,000 (gp52) in HTLV-II (8,13,14). As for the protein product of the pol gene, only the reverse transcriptase of the prototype HLTV-I has been extensively characterized (15). It posseses a molecular weight of approximately 100,000, and prefers Mg^{2+} as cation unlike the reverse transcriptases of most mammalian retroviruses, but similarly to the enzymes of bovine leukemia virus (BLV) and avian myeloblastosis virus (AMV). The enzymes of HTLV-II and -III have not been purified, but they also prefer Mg^{2+} to Mn^{2+} as cation. The protein product(s) of the px genetic sequence has recently been identified as a molecule of between 38,000 to 42,000 molecular weight in HTLV-I and -II (16-18). This size range agrees with the suggestion of Haseltine and his colleagues who sequenced a portion of the px region of HTLV-II and found a long open reading frame (LOR) which could encode a protein of 38,000 molecular weight (19). The sequence obtained in this region was closely related to that of the similar region in HTLV-I. A LOR sequence is also present in HTLV-III (see chapter by Wong-Staal, this volume).

Aside from obvious homologies in structure, the HTLV family members also share immunologic relationships. These are strongest between HTLV-I and -II and between subgroups II and III. HTLV-I and -III show the least immunologic relationship (8, Sarngadharan et al., submitted). It was, however, the detection of low titer antibodies to the precursor protein (p61) of the HTLV-I envelope protein in sera of AIDS patients which gave the strongest initial evidence for an involvement of HTLV-I or an HTLV variant in the disease (20), and which provided a continued impetus for the search for an AIDS-related isolate, culminating in the detection of HTLV-III.

The HTLV family members share other common features, including T-cell tropism and morphologic features typical of type C retroviruses. Although not unique for a retrovirus, HTLV-III does exhibit the unusual appearance by electron microscopy of a collapsed cylindrical core (8), while HTLV-I and -II present a more usual picture. Nevertheless, while the similarities of the HTLV family members are interesting and allow a grouping of the various isolates and a determination of their possible origin and evolutionary relationships, it is the differences among the isolates which provide the greatest interest. By far the most profound difference is a biological one. While all family members cause some cytopathic effect in the cells they infect, for example, syncytial formation or cells which lobulated nuclei, more profound effects also occur. The HTLV-I and -II subgroups clearly cause proliferation of the cells they infect. HTLV-III isolates cause cell killing in all but the most unusual of infected cells. It is these properties which presumably lead to disease in infected individuals.

HTLV AS HUMAN PATHOGENIC AGENTS

HTLV-I was initially isolated from a patient diagnosed with cutaneous T-cell lymphoma (CTCL), a malignancy of mature T-cells of adults (1). While the detection of natural antibodies to HTLV proteins in sera of two patients with similar disease first suggested an association of the virus with CTCL (21,22), more extensive serologic studies of patients with this disease failed to indicate a further association (23). It was Catovsky et al. (24) who subsequently pointed out the resemblance of the disease of the prototype patient to what was termed T-cell lymphosarcoma cell leukemia observed in Caribbean Blacks and adult T-cell leukemia seen in Japanese patients. Extensive seroepidemiological studies which followed clearly established an association of HTLV with these malignancies of mature T-cells, and HTLV-I is now considered to be casually related to ATL. The observations which led to this conclusion and implicated HTLV as an infectious, horizontally transmitted virus include the following: 1) Approximately 90% of patients with ATL have demonstrable serum antibodies to HTLV proteins, whereas antibodies are not detected in numerous other malignancies of the hematopoietic system, or of other tissues, or in sera of non-malignant individuals (23,25,26). 2). Relatives and close contacts of ATL patients are approximately 4 times more likely to possess HTLV-specific antibodies compared to the random healthy population (27). 3) In regions where ATL cases have been shown to cluster, such as th southwestern Japanese islands of Kyushu and Shikoku, HTLV is endemic in the population as indicated by a higher antibody prevalence in the healthy population compared to areas where ATL is not frequent (27). 4) In regions such as the Caribbean where the healthy population exhibits a significant antibody prevalence, adult T-cell malignancies with features similar to ATL comprise a spectrum of disease associated with the virus (28,29). Features of HTLV-I associated disease are summarized in Table 1.

The existence of an HTLV variant etiologically associated with AIDS was postulated based on two observations. The first was the known immune suppressive effects of retroviruses, particularly in the feline leukemia virus system (30). The second, as mentioned above, was the continued detection of antibodies of low titer to an HTLV-I envelope precursor molecule in sera of AIDS patients and associated risk groups (20), while antibodies to HTLV-I core proteins were rarely observed (31). In 1983, reports of HTLV-I in cells of a patient with AIDS (32) and of lymphadenopathy associated virus (LAV) in cells of a patient with lymphadenopathy (33) appeared. The former isolate was most probably an opportunistic infection, but continued to support the hypothesis of HTLV involvement in the disease. The LAV isolate was difficult to evaluate because it remained uncharacterized for some time, apparently due to the poor viral production and poor viability of cultured patient material. In 1984 our series of papers on the isolation,

Table 1. Epidemiological, clinical, and laboratory features of patients with HTLV-I associated disease*

Features	Japan	Caribbean	U.S.A.
Diagnosis	ATL	TLCL	Peripheral T cell lymphoma or Sezary's syndrome
Median Age (yrs)	56	46	34
Sex (M/F)	14/11	3/10	8/4[§]
Race	Oriental	Black	...[o]
Birthplace	Kyushu, Shikoku	Caribbean islands	...
Thymus	Normal	Normal	Normal
Skin involvement (%)	50	30	60
Node involvement (%)	100	100	50
Liver/spleen enlargement (%)	50-60	40	50
Leukemia (%)	76	100	100
Median survival (months)	10	8	12
Cytology	Pleomorphic	Pleomorphic	Somewhat pleomorphic
White blood cells (per mm^3)	39,000-310,000	17,000-435,000	6,800-27,700
Immunoglobulin level	Increased IgA and IgM	Normal	Normal
Hypercalcemia (%)	24	50	70
Erythrocyte rosetting (%)	100	100	100
OKT	T4+; NP; T8-; T3+; T10+	T4+; T6-; T8-; T3+; T10+/-; T11-	T4+; NP; T8-; T3+;
Functional Phenotype	Suppressor	Suppressor	Suppressor
TdT	Negative	Negative	Negative

Table 1. continued

Features	Japan	Caribbean	U.S.A.
Antibody, antigens and/or viral particles	40/60	10/10	10/10

* From reference 60.

§ Four blacks, two Hispanics, three whites, one Aleutian and one Oriental.

° Southeastern United States (four); Massachusetts (one); Alaska (one); Brazil (one), Ecuador (one); Israel (one) and Japan (one).

NOTE: ATL = adult T-cell leukemia; TLCL = T-cell lymphosarcoma; NP = not performed; and TdT = terminal deoxynucletidyltransferase.

characterization, and association of a new human retrovirus, HTLV-III, with AIDS appeared and presented overwhelming evidence for a viral etiology of AIDS (2,3,8,12). In view of isolates of HTLV-III from cells of 48 different patients, reproducibility of the phenomenon could not be denied. Other than detection and isolation of HTLV-III itself, the most important finding was a cell line capable of producing HTLV-III to high titer while somehow withstanding fatal cytopathic effect (2). As a result, virus could be produced in large quantity for analysis and for generation of immunologic reagents and molecular probes for further studies. Extensive seroepidemiologic studies have quickly established the association of AIDS with HTLV-III. Table 2 summarizes these results in some detail. Most notably is the finding of antibodies to HTLV-III in up to 100% of AIDS patients (34) and significant antibody prevalence in every group at risk of acquiring the disease.

Table 2. Antibodies to HTLV-III in sera of patients with AIDS and AIDS related complex

Patients/Donors	Number Positive / Number Tested	(%)
Patients with AIDS	288/297	(97)
Patients with AIDS Related Complex	327/360	(91)
Asymptomatic Homosexual Men	96/235	(41)
High Risk Blood Donors	9/9	
Renal Transplant Recipient from High Risk Donor	1/1	
Controls		
Random Normal Donors	0/238	
Black Women from Baltimore (1962 collection)	0/100	
Healthy Japanese from HTLV-I Endemic Regions	0/123	
Patients with Leukemias and Other Malignancies from HTLV-I Endemic Areas	0/34	
Healthy Surinamese (Methadone Treatment Group)	0/54	
Schizophrenics	0/30	
Hodgkins Patients and Siblings	0/160	
Renal Transplant Recipients	0/24	
Other Immunosuppressed Cases	0/34	
Miscellaneous Patients*	0/84	

* These include heavily transfused patients and those with: Hepatitis B virus infection, primary stage Syphilis, Rheumatoid arthritis, Systemic lupus erythematosus, Acute monoucleosis, Lymphatic leukemias, B- and T-cell lymphomas, Alopacia areata, and Idiopathic splenomegaly.

DISTRIBUTION AND TRANSMISSION OF HTLV

Once clear associations of HTLV-I and -III with ATL and AIDS respectively were established, continued serologic studies have focused on questions important with regard to treatment and prevention of the diseases. These questions include the geographic distribution of the viruses in order to determine populations at risk, the age at first infection of susceptible individuals, identification of a benign disease associated with initial infection, and identification of routes of transmission and possible vectors. Studies of this nature have proceeded more rapidly with HTLV-III and AIDS because of the shorter latent period from infection to appearance of disease. Nevertheless progress has been made in both areas. We will summarize each separately.

To date HTLV-I has been detected serologically almost everywhere it has been sought, although clear endemic areas exist. These include, in addition to the already mentioned southwestern Japan and the Caribbean region, portions of Africa (35-37), and the southeastern United States (38). The endemic Caribbean region extends broadly to South and Central American countries bordering on the basin (39; Merino et al., Int. J. Cancer, in press; Saxinger, in preparation). An interesting observation appearing in these geograhical surveys is the rather discrete pockets or local areas where HTLV antibody prevalence may be quite high bordering on areas with extremely low antibody prevalence. The reasons for this restricted distribution are not known, but it has been observed in Venezuela, Japan, Alaska, and Africa. It suggests the role of microenvironmental factors, in addition to possibly social or genetic influences in viral transmission. While HTLV-I infection was first thought to occur mainly in adults (23), recent evidence suggests young children are also susceptible to infection (Merino et al., Int. J. Cancer, in press). Both antibody titer and prevalence increase with age, indicating continued exposures occur throughout life, either from external sources, or continued viral replication in vivo. While family studies have shown that HTLV-I is transmitted by close contact, other routes of transmission have not been so thoroughly pursued. The identification of healthy virus carriers (40-42) and an increased antibody prevalence in recipients of multiple blood transfusions indicate that transmission by blood is likely to occur (36,43, Gazzolo et al., submitted).

Studies on transmission routes of HTLV-III have proceeded quickly because of the public health aspects of AIDS, because of the nature of the groups at risk for acquiring the disease, and because prior knowledge of the HTLV-I system suggested probable avenues. Two of the AIDS risk groups, hemophiliacs and intravenous drug users, have blood as a common focus. Hemophiliac recipients of certain blood products, namely factor VIII, have a high HTLV-III antibody prevalence, as much as 70% (44, Goedert et al., submitted; Tsoukas et al., submitted). The fact that HTLV-III is rare among individuals with no risk factors, suggests it is not readily transmitted by aerosols or casual contact. Both homosexual and heterosexual contact with AIDS patients however, may result in infection with the agent, as evidence by serologic studies of homosexuals at risk and of heterosexual partners and prostitutes (Goedert et al., submitted; Harris et al., in preparation). Both these routes require intimate contact. Studies of blood donor and recipient pairs have also illustrated transmission of HTLV-III by blood tranfusion (45,46; Groopman et al., N. Engl. J. Med., in press). The recent findings that HTLV-III is present in both semen (47,48) and saliva (49) of infected individuals suggests that transmission of this agent may be much less difficult than HTLV-I and -II. Whether potential recipients have natural defense mechanisms against infections by these routes remains to be seen.

Geographically, the only population to date where HTLV-III seems to be endemic is Haiti (Gazzolo et al., N. Eng. J. Med., in press), which explains why Haitians are at risk for acquiring the disease (58). Other areas endemic for HTLV-I lack evidence of HTLV-III prevalence suggesting the two viruses have a different epidemiologic pattern (Gazzolo et al., N. Engl. J. Med., in press; Clark et al., in preparation). This pattern may come together in Africa, where HTLV-I is thought to have originated (51), and where we believe HTLV-III originated as well. Evidence for HTLV-III in Africa includes a prevalence among Zairian AIDS patients and prostitutes (52; Clumeck et al., in preparation), a significant prevalence among healthy Zairian normal individuals (Gazzolo et al. in preparation), and evidence for low titer antibody to HTLV-III or to a cross reacting variant in Ugandan children (Saxinger et al., submitted).

MECHANISMS OF HTLV PATHOGENESIS

The HTLV family comprises a new class of retrovirus, including BLV and the related primate T-cell leukemia viruses (53), which produce monoclonal tumors after a long latent periods, and do not contain a cellular derived onc gene. However, unlike conventional chronic leukemia viruses, they are capable of transforming primary human T-cells in vitro. For this reason, interest has focused on the protein product of the pX region as possibly involved in the mechanism of this transformation and in pathogenesis in vivo as well. Current hypotheses involving this protein are discussed in the chapter by Wong-Staal (this volume).

Other mechanisms proposed for HTLV-I and -II induced transformation of T-cells invoke the TCGF-receptor system. While an "autochrine mechanism" of T-cell transformation in which HTLV-infected T-cells would both produce and respond to their own TCGF has been ruled out based on the lack of TCGF production by most HTLV-infected cells as well as their failure to transcribe TCGF message RNA (54), it is likely that the TCGF responsive system is involved in some way. All T-cells infected with HTLV express an antigen defined by the monoclonal antibody, "anti-Tac"

(55,56) on their surface (57). If the Tac antigen is normally expressed on particular cells, its expression is enhanced following viral infection. The Tac antigen has been characterized as the cell receptor for TCGF (58) Three possibilities have been suggested for its possible involvement in unrestrained T-cell proliferation (59). First, T-cells which acquire a greater cell density of TCGF receptors would then have a growth advantage as well. They would be better able to compete for available TCGF both in vitro and in vivo. Second, if the TCGF receptor present on HTLV-infected cells were slightly altered, it might have a greater affinity for TCGF and be able to compete more effectively for its growth-promoting activity. Third, again if the receptor were slightly altered, it might be able to be triggered by other molecules with or without growth-promoting activity for T-cells normally, thus leading to events culminating in T-cell growth. The possibilities are now all under investigation.

CONCLUDING REMARKS

Continued molecular, biochemical, and immunologic studies will further elucidate various aspects of the biology of HTLV. Synthesis of peptides based on the nucleotide sequence of specific viral genes and subsequent preparation of specific antisera are providing valuable new reagents for further probing the virus and cells that are infected. Hopefully these approaches will soon lead to production of appropriate vaccine materials and also to sufficient insight into the most effective therapies.

REFERENCES

1. Poiesz, B.J., Ruscetti, F.W., Gazdar, A.F. Bunn, P.A., Minna, J.D. & Gallo, R.C. (1980) Proc. Natl. Acad. Sci. USA 77, 7415-7419.
2. Popovic, M., Sarngadharan, M.G., Read, E. & Gallo, R. C. (1984) Science 224, 497-500.
3. Gallo, R.C., Salahuddin, S.Z., Popovic, M., Shearer, G.M., Kaplan, M., Haynes, B.F., Palker, T.J., Redfield, R., Oleske, J., Safai, B., White, G., Foster, P. & Markham, P.D. (1984) Science 224, 500-503.
4. Kalyanaraman, V.S., Sarngadharan, M.G., Robert-Guroff, M., Miyoshi, I., Blayney, D., Golde, D. & Gallo, R.C. (1982) Science 218, 571-573.
5. Seiki, M., Hattori, S., Hirayama, Y. & Yoshida, M. (1983) Proc. Natl. Acad. Sci. USA, 80, 3618-3622.
6. Shaw, G.M., Gonda, M.A., Flickinger, G.H., Hahn, B.H., Gallo, R.C. & Wong-Staal, F. (1984) Proc. Natl. Acad. Sci. USA 81, 4544-4548.
7. Arya, S.K., Gallo, R.C., Hahn, B., Shaw, G., Popovic, Salahuddin, S.Z. & Wong-Staal, F. (1984) Science 225, 927-930.
8. Schupbach, J., Popovic, M., Gilden, R.V., Gonda, M.A., Sarngadharan, M.G. & Gallo, R.C. (1984) Science 224, 503-505.
9. Kalyanaraman, V.S., Sarngadharan, M.G., Poiesz, B.J., Ruscetti, F.W., & Gallo, R.C. (1981) J. Virol. 38, 906-915.
10. Copeland, T.D., Oroszlan, S., Kalyanaraman, V.S., Sarngadharan, M.G. & Gallo, R.C. (1983) FEBS Ltrs. 162, 390-395.
11. Kalyanaraman, V.S., Jarvis-Morar, M., Sarngadharan, M.G. & Gallo, R.C. (1984) Virology 132, 61-70.
12. Sarngadharan, M.G., Popovic, M., Bruch, L., Schupbach, J. & Gallo, R.C. (1984) Science 224, 506-508.
13. Lee, T.H., Coligan, J.E., Homma, T., McLane, M.F., Tachibana, N. & Essex, M. (1984) Proc. Natl. Acad. Sci. USA 81, 3856-3860.

14. Sodroski, J., Patarca, R., Perkins, D., Briggs, D., Lee, T.H., Essex, M., Coligan, J., Wong-Staal, F., Gallo, R.C. & Haseltine, W.A. (1984) Science 225, 421-424.
15. Rho, H.M., Poiesz, B., Ruscetti, F.W., & Gallo, R.C. (1981) Virology, 112, 355-360.
16. Miwa, M., Shimotohno, K., Hoshino, H., Fujino, M. & Sugimura, T. (1984) Gann 75, 752-755.
17. Slamon, D.J., Shimotohno, K., Cline, M.J., Golde, D.W. & Chen, I.S.Y. (1984) Science 226, 61-65.
18. Lee, T.H., Coligan, J.E., Sodroski, J.G., Haseltine, W.A., Salahuddin, S.Z., Wong-Staal, F., Gallo, R.C. & Essex, M. (1984) Science 226, 57-61.
19. Haseltine, W.A., Sodroski, J., Patarca, R., Briggs, D., Perkins, D. & Wong-Staal, F. (1984) Science 225, 419-421.
20. Essex, M., McLane, M.F., Lee, T.H., Falk, L., Howe, C.W.S., Mullins, J.I., Cabradilla, C. & Francis, D.P. (1983) Science 220, 859-862.
21. Posner, L.E., Robert-Guroff, M., Kalyanaraman, V.S., Poiesz, B.J., Ruscetti, F.W., Fossieck, B., Bunn, P.A., Jr., Minna, J.D., & Gallo, R.C. (1981) J. Exp. Med. 154, 333-346.
22. Kalyanaraman, V.S., Sarngadharan, M.G., Bunn, p.A., Minna, J.D. & Gallo, R.C. (1981) Nature 294, 271-273.
23. Gallo, R.C., Kalyanaraman, V.S., Sarngadharan, M.G., Sliski, A., Vonderheid,E.C., Maeda, M., Nakao, Y., Yamada, K., Ito, Y., Gutensohn, N., Murphy, S., Bunn, P.A. Jr., Catovsky, D., Greaves, M.F., Blayney, D.W., Blattner, W., Jarrett, W.F.H., zur Hausen, H., Seligmann, M., Brouet, J.C., Haynes, B.F., Jegasothy, B.V., Jaffee, E., Cossman, J., Broder, S., Fisher, R.I., Golde, D.W. & Robert-Guroff, M. (1983) Cancer Res. 43, 3892-3899.
24. Catovsky, D., Greaves, M.F., Rose, M., Galton, D.A.B., Goolden, A.W.G., McCluskey, D.R., White, J.M., Lampert, I., Bourikas, G., Ireland, R., Brownell, A.I., Bridges, J.M., Blattner, W.A. & Gallo, R.C. (1982) Lancet 1, 639-643.

25. Robert-Guroff, M., Nakao, Y., Natake, K., Ito, Y., Slisku, A. & Gallo, R.C. (1982) Science 215, 975-978.
26. Kalyanaraman, V.S., Sarngadharan, M.G., Nakao, Y., Ito, Y., Aoki, T. & Gallo, R.C. (1982) Proc. Natl. Acad. Sci. USA 79, 1653-1657.
27. Robert-Guroff, M., Kalyanaraman, V.S., Blattner, W.A., Popovic, M., Sarngadharan, M.G., Maeda, M., Blayney, D., Catovsky, D., Bunn, P.A., Shibata, A., Nakao, Y., Ito, Y., Aoki, T. & Gallo, R.C. (1983) J. Exp. Med. 157, 248-258.
28. Blattner, W.A., Kalyanaraman, V.S., Robert-Guroff, M., Lister, T.A., Galton, D.A.G., Sarin, P.S., Crawford, M.H., Catovsky, D., Greaves, M. & Gallo, R.C. (1982). Int. J. Cancer 30, 257-264.
29. Blattner, W.A., Gibbs, W.N., Saxinger, C., Robert-Guroff, M., Clark, J., Lofter, W., Hanchard, B., Campbell, M. & Gallo, R.C. (1983) Lancet ii, 61-64.
30. Trainin, Z., Wernicke, D., Ungar-Waron, H. & Essex, M. (1983) Science 220, 858-859.
31. Robert-Guroff, M., Balyney, D.W., Safai, B., Lange, M., Gelman, E.P., Gutterman, J.W., Mansell, P.W.A., Goedert, J.L., Groopman, J.E., Steigbigel, N.H., Sidhu, G.S., Johnson, J.M., Friedman-Kien, A.E., Downing, R., Bayley, A.C. & Gallo, R.C. (1984) Lancet ii, 129h8-131.
32. Gallo, R.C., Sarin, P.S., Gelmann, E.P., Robert-Guroff, M., Richardson, E., Kalyanaraman, V.S., Mann, D., Sidhy, G.D., Stahl, R.E., Zolla-Pazner, S., Leibowitch, J. & Popovic, M. (1983) Science 220, 865-867.
33. Barre-Sinoussi, F., Chermann, J.C.,Rey, F., Nugeyre, M.G., Charmaret, S., Gruest, J., Dauguet, C., Axler-Blin, C., Vezinet-Brun, F., Rouzioux, C., Rozenbaum, W. & Montanier, L. (1983) Science 220, 868-871.
34. Safai, B., Sarngadharan, M.G., Groopman, J.E., Arnett, K., Popovic, M., Sliski, A., Schupbach, J. & Gallo, R.C. (1984) Lancet, i, 1439-1440.

35. Hunsmann, G., Schneider, J., Schmitt, J. & Yamamoto, N.,(1983) Int. J. Cancer, 32, 329-332.

36. Saxinger, W., Blattner, W.A., Levine, P.H., Clark, J., Biggar, R., Hoh, M., Moghissi, J., Jacobs, P., Wilson, L., Jacobson, P., Crookes, R., Strong, M., Ansari, A.A., Dean, A.G., Nkrumah, F.K., Mourali, N. & Gallo, R.C. (1984) Science 225, 1473-1476.

37. Biggar, R.J., Saxinger, C., Gardner, C., Collins, W.E., Levine, P.H., Clark, J.W., Nkrumah, F.K. & Blattner, W.A. (1984) Int. J. Cancer 34, 215-219.

38. Blayney, D.W., Blattern, W.A., Robert-Guroff, M., Jaffe, E.S., Fisher, R.I., Bunn, P.A., Jr., Patton, M.G., Rarick, H.R., & Gallo, R.C. (1983) J. Am. Med. Asso., 250, 1048-1502.

39. Robert-Guroff, M., Boutinho, R.A., Zadelhoff, A.W., Vyth-Dreese, F.A. & Rumke, P. (1984) Leuk. Res. 8, 501-504.

40. Sarin, P.S., Aoki, T., Shibata, A., Ohnishi, Y., Aoyagi, Y., Miyakoshi, H., Emura, I., Kalyanaraman, V.S., Robert-Guroff, M., Papovic, M., Sarngadharan, M., Nowell, P.C. & Gallo, R.C. (1983). Proc. Natl. Acad. Sci. USA, 80, 2370-2374.

41. Vyth-Dreese, F.A., Rumke, P., Robert-Guroff, M., de Lange, G. & Gallo, R.C. (1983) Int. J. Cancer 32, 337-342.

42. Gotoh, Y., Sugamura, K., & Hinuma, T. (1982) Proc. Natl. Acad. Sci. USA 79, 4780-4782.

43. Shimoyama, M., Minato, K., Tobinai, K., Horikoshi, N., Ibuka, T., Deura, K., Nagatani, T., Ozaki, Y., Inada, N., Komoda, H. & Hinuma, Y. (1982) Jpn. J. Clin. Oncol. 12, 109-116.

44. Ramsey, R.B., Palmer, E.L., McDougal, J.S., Kalyanaraman, V.S., Jackson, D.W., Chorba, T.L., & Holman, R.C. (1984) Lancet ii, 397-398.

45. Jaffe, H.W., Francis, D.P., McLane, M.F., Cabradilla, C., Curran, J.W., Kilbourne, B.W., Lawrence, D.N., Haverkos, H.W., Spira, T.J., Dodd, R.Y., Gold, J., Armstrong, D., Ley, A., Groopman, J., Mullins, J., Lee, T.H. & Essex, M. (1984) Science 223, 1309-1312.

46. Feorino, P.M., Kalyanaraman, V.S., Haverkos, H.W., Cabradilla, C.D., Warfield, D.T., Jaffe, H.W., Harrison, A.K., Gottlieb, M.S., Goldfinger, D., Chermann, J.C., Barre-Sinoussi, F., Spira, T.T., McDougal, J.S., Curran, J.W., Montagnier, L., Murphy, F.A. & Francis, D.P. (1984) Science 225, 69-72.
47. Zagury, D., Bernard, J., Leibowitch, J., Safai, B., Groopman, J.E., Feldman, M., Sarngadharan, M.G. & Gallo, R.C. (1984). Science 226, 449-551.
48. Ho, D.D., Schooley, R.T., Rota, T.R., Kaplan, J.C., Flyn, T., Salahuddin, S.Z., Gonda, M.A. & Hirsch, M.S. (1984) Science 226, 451-453.
49. Groopman, J.E., Salahuddin, S.Z., Sarngadharan, M.G., Markhan, P.D., Gonda, M., Sliski, A. & Gallo, R.C. (1984) Science 226, 447-449.
50. Vieira, J., Frank, E., Spira, T.J., & Landesman, S.H. (1983) New Engl. J. Med. 308, 125-129.
51. Gallo, R.C., Sliski, A. & Wong-Staal, F. (1983) Lancet ii, 962-963.
52. Brun-Vezinet, F., Rouziouw, C., Montagnier, L., Chamaret, S., Gurest, J., Barre-Sinoussi, F., Feroldi, D., Chermann, J.C., McCormick, J., Mitchell, S., Piot, P., Taelman, H., Mirlangu, K.B., Wobin, O., Mbendi, N., Mazebo, P., Kalambayi, K., Bridts, C., Desmyter, J., Feinsod, F.M. & Quinn, T.C. (1984) Science 226, 453-456.
53. Guo, H.G., Wong-Staal, F. & Gallo, R.C. (1984) Science 223, 1195-1197.
54. Arya, S.K., Wong-Staal, F. & Gallo, R.C. (1984) Science 223, 1086-1087.
55. Uchiyama, T., Broder, S. & Waldmann, T.A. (1981) J. Immunol. 126, 1393-1397.
56. Uchiyama, T., Nelson, D.L., Fleisher, T.A. & Waldmann, T.A. (1981) J. Immunol. 126, 1398-1403.
57. Mann, D.L., Popovic, M., Murray, C., Neuland, C., Strong, D.M., Sarin, P., Gallo, R.C. & Blattner, W.A. (1983) J. Immunol. 131, 2021-2124.
58. Leonard, W.J., Depper, J.M., Uchiyama, T., Smith, K.A., Waldmann, T.A. & Greene, W.C. (1982) Nature 300,

267-269.

59. Gallo, R.C. (1984) In: Franks, L.M., Wyke, L.M. and Weiss, R.A. (eds), Cancer Surveys, Vol. 3, Oxford University Press, Oxford, pp. 113-160.

60. Blattner, W.A., Blayney, D.W., Robert-Guroff, M., Sarngadharan, M.G., Kalyanaraman, V.S., Sarin, P.S., Jaffe, E.S. & Gallo, R.C. (1983) J. Infect. Diseases 147, 406-416.

THE ORGANIZATION OF MOUSE MAMMARY TUMOR VIRUS RELATED SEQUENCES IN HUMAN CELLULAR DNA

R. Callahan, I. Ali, J. Fetherston, T. Horn, and J. Schlom

Laboratory of Tumor Immunology and Biology, National Cancer Institute, National Institutes of Health, Bethesda, Md. 20205.

We have established the existence of two major pol gene families in the evolution of retroviruses, using low stringency blot hybridization and nucleotide sequence analysis. One family consists of mammalian type C viruses. The second pol gene family consists of type A,B,D, and avian type C viruses. In this article we review the evidence for mouse mammary tumor virus related sequences in human cellular DNA and summarize our results which establish this class of human retroviral genomes as members of the second pol gene family.

Several factors have been implicated in the etiology of human breast cancer. The potential involvement of members of the Retroviridae family of viruses has represented a major focus of investigation (1 for review). This is primarily a result of studies of mammary cancer in laboratory mice, where infectious type-B retroviruses (mouse mammary tumor virus, MMTV) have been shown to be associated with a high incidence of mammary tumors. With the exception of species of the genus Mus (2,3) and Rattus (4), attempts to identify DNA sequences related to the MMTV genome in DNAs of all other mammalian species tested have not been consistently successful (5,6). Other studies

(7,8), using liquid hybridization and MMTV cDNA probes, reported the presence of RNA species, in human mammary tumors, related to the viral genome. The lack of uniform probes, the potential for contamination of cDNA preparations with cellular DNA or RNA, and the relative lack of sensitivity of liquid hybridization techniques made these findings difficult to interpret.

MMTV RELATED SEQUENCES IN HUMAN CELLULAR DNA

The availability of molecularly cloned MMTV genomic DNA and the increased sensitivity of the blot-hybridization technique for analysis of restriction endonuclease digests of DNA led us to reexamine the possibility of MMTV related sequences in human cellular DNA (9). Preliminary attempts to detect MMTV related sequences in PstI, EcoRI, and BamHI restricted human cellular DNA using stringent conditions for blot-hybridization were unsuccessful. Using less stringent hybridization conditions, labeled MMTV proviral DNA (representing the entire genome) detected four major bands (3.7, 3.5, 2.9, and 1.9 kbp), as well as other less intense bands (2.1,1.8, 1.6 and 1.4 kbp) in EcoRI restricted human breast tumor and normal cellular DNAs. Restricted cellular DNA from other mammalian species each contained a unique pattern of MMTV related fragments.

The specific regions of the MMTV provirus represented in the discrete EcoRI human bands were evaluated using as probes subgenomic fragments corresponding to the gag-pol, and env regions of the viral genome. The gag-pol probe reacts primarily with the 3.7 and 3.5kbp bands, and to a lesser extent with the 2.9 and 1.9 kbp bands. The env probe reacts with five (2.1, 1.9, 1.8, 1.6 and 1.4 kbp) restriction bands. The thermal stability of the hybrids formed with the MMTV env probe was assessed to determine the extent of base pair mismatch. The results suggest that the Tm of MMTV proviral-human DNA hybrids is between 54 and 60°C (in 3XSSC) or 30 to 40 % mismatch. Neither of the subgenomic MMTV probes reacted with salmon sperm DNA.

These observations have been confirmed by May et al. (10) and Sweet et al. (personal communication) using similar blot hybridization conditions. Recently, we (unpublished observations) and May et al. (10) have also detected sequences related to the long terminal repeat region (LTR) of the MMTV genome in restricted human cellular DNA. This is of particular interest since the MMTV LTR contains sequences which bind the glucocorticoid receptor protein making expression of the viral genome hormone dependent. The significance of this observation and its relevance to the known hormone responsiveness of many human breast tumors must await the isolation of recombinant DNA clones containing these sequences.

A library of human fetal liver cellular DNA (11) in lambda Charon 4A (12), was screened for the presence of MMTV related sequences. The use of low stringency hybridization conditions led to the identification of 55 plaques, out of $5x10^5$ plaques screened, which reacted specifically with labeled MMTV proviral DNA. One of these clones, designated HLM-2, was chosen for further study. A partial restriction map of HLM-2 DNA is shown in Figure 1. EcoRI restriction fragments (8.2, 3.7, 1.8, and 1.4 kbp) of HLM-2 DNA were hybridized with labeled DNA probes representing the gag, pol, env, and LTR regions of the MMTV genome. Most striking was the intensity with which the MMTV pol probe hybridized with the 3.7 kbp EcORI fragment. Upon longer exposure, sequence homology was detectable between the MMTV gag probe and the 3.7 kbp EcoRI fragment and between the MMTV env probe and the 8.2 and 1.8 kbp EcoRI fragments. The MMTV LTR probe did not hybridize specifically with HLM-2 DNA, nor with several other recombinant clones which did hybridize with MMTV proviral DNA.

The organization of the MMTV related sequences in HLM-2 DNA has been defined by additional restriction enzyme mapping using the MMTV gag, pol, and env probes, and is summarized in Figure 1. Two unexpected observations emerged from this analysis. First, two regions at the

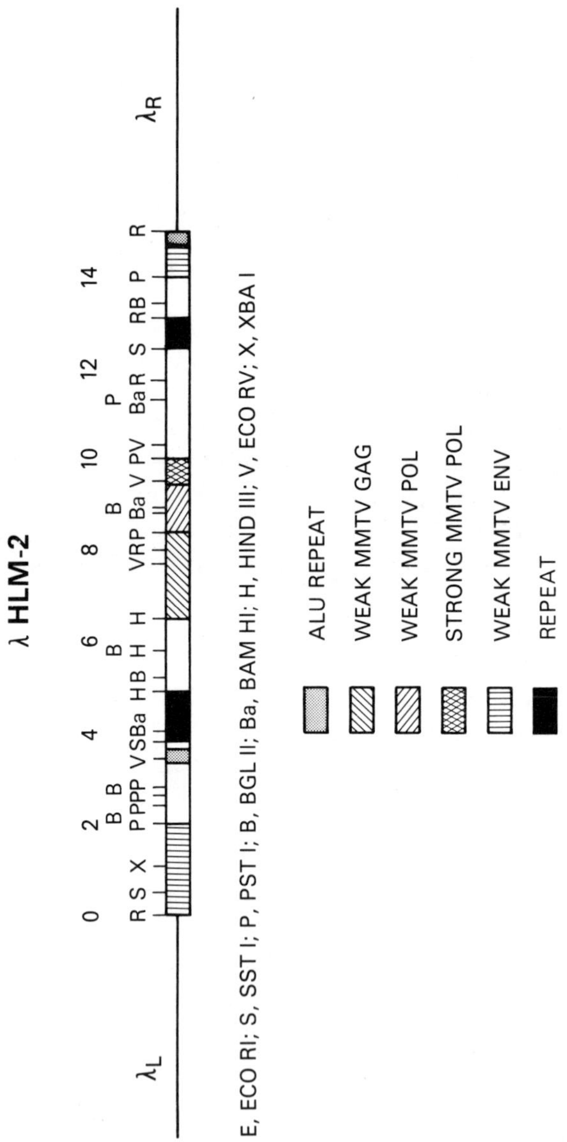

Figure 1. A partial restriction enzyme map of human recombinant clone HLM-2. The symbols λ_L and λ_R designate respectively the long and short arms of lambda Charon 4A. The restriction sites and regions of HLM-2 which contain MMTV related sequences are indicated.

opposite ends of the HLP-2 DNA contain MMTC env related sequences. Second, the MMTV pol and env related sequences are interrupted by non-MMTV related sequences (between map position 12 and 13) which are repeated between map position 4 and 5 in the HLM-2 DNA. Nucleotide sequence analysis has shown that these repeats are approximately 100 base pairs long, and 88% related (unpublished observations).

Recently, we have analyzed several more MMTV related human recombinant clones by restriction enzyme and heteroduplex analysis (Callahan et al., manuscript in preparation). Two relevant observations emerged from these studies. First, the human MMTV related sequences defined in HLM-2 are members of a highly diverged family of retroviral related sequences in human cellular DNA. This was demonstrated by the large number of restriction site polymorphisms observed between different clones and by heteroduplex analysis. Under stringent spreading conditions several combinations of recombinant clones showed no heteroduplex formation. As the spreading conditions were relaxed long stretches of homology were observed. In some cases deletion or insertion loops could be observed within a heteroduplex. The large sequence diversity of the different recombinant clones suggests that in evolutionary terms, this family of retroviral genes was not recently introduced into the human cellular genome. Second, each of the recombinant clones contained the repeat sequence observed in HLM-2. The sequence shares no homology with the alu family of repetitive cellular DNA sequences and was always found flanking the MMTV gag-pol related sequences. Based on these and other results we have speculated that the MMTV gag and pol related sequences in the human recombinant DNA clones are organized in a manner expected for a genetically transmitted or endogenous proviral genome. The repeated sequences which bound the gag-pol related sequences correspond to proviral long terminal repeat (LTR) sequences. Since the 3' end of the MMTV pol gene hybridizies to a EcoR-Pstl restriction fragment at 9.5-10

HLM-2 map units (Figure 1), the region between 10 to 12.5 map units could correspond to an env gene which is unrelated to that of MMTV.

The organizational relationship between MMTV gag-pol and MMTV env related human DNA remains unclear. We have determined the nucleotide sequence of the MMTV env related 1.8 kbp EcoRI fragment (13 to 15 map units, Figure 1) of HLM-2 (unpublished data). Weak nucleotide sequence homology between the gp52 region of the MMTV env gene and the region between 14 and 14.6 HLM-2 map units could be detected. However, it is in the opposite orientation relative to the MMTV gag-pol related sequences and there is no significant open reading frame for peptide synthesis. No homology with the gp36 portion of MMTV env was observed. More recently, we have begun to characterize another human recombinant clone (HLM46A) which was initially detected using the entire MMTV genome as a probe. HLM46A contains only MMTV env related sequences and shares no homology with the human MMTV gag-pol related proviral genome. By the criteria of blot hybridization, HLM64A shares more extensive sequence homology with the MMTV env gene than do the corresponding sequences in HLM-2. However, like HLM-2 the region of homology in HLM46A corresponds to the gp52 portion of the MMTV env. Although recombinant clones containing continuous MMTV gag-pol and env related sequences have not been found, their potential existence cannot as yet be excluded.

We have begun to assess the organization of the human MMTV gag-pol related proviral sequences in human cellular DNA. Consistent with the restriction site polymorphism noted in the analysis of the recombinant clones, families of discrete restriction fragments containing sequences related to the HLM-2 3.7 kpb EcoRI fragment were detected. Significantly, the pattern of major EcoRI related fragments (3.7, 3.5, 2.9 and 1.9 kbp) is similar to that observed using the entire MMTV genome as a probe under low stringency blot hybridization conditions. The use of other restriction enzymes revealed the presence of major related cellular DNA fragments which are identical in size to those found in different human recombinant clones. This suggests that our collection of MMTV gag-pol related human recombinant clones is representative of the major families of viral related restriction fragments observed in human cellular DNA. The frequency of these clones in the human recombinant DNA library suggests that there are several copies of these sequences in human cellular DNA. Quantitative dot blot analysis of human cellular DNA with HLM-2 probes is consistent with 200 copies of the pol and 2000 copies of the LTR sequences in human cellular DNA. This result raises the possibility that a significant number of the LTR-like elements are not associated with retroviral related structural genes. What is the origin of these highly reiterated LTR related sequences? One possibility is that during the evolution of the species, the LTR elements were separated from viral structural genes by cellular recombination events and then subsequently amplified. Such a mechanism seems likely for the origin of "solitary" type C viral LTR elements in murine cellular DNA (13). Another possibility is that inappropriately spliced RNA was inserted after reverse transcription into the germ line. A similar phenomenon may have occurred with the MMTV LTR in the Balb/c strain of mice (14,15).

To determine whether there are tumor specific amplifications of the HLM-2 proviral sequences and how conserved these sequences are between individuals, we have begun to screen cellular DNA from normal and breast tumor tissue. Our results to date provide no evidence for the amplificiation of proviral sequences in primary breast tumor DNA. This may reflect the limited number of tumors tested or the variability in the fraction of the material which are tumor cells. In this connection May et al. (10) have shown that the MCF-7 human breast tumor cell line contains two MMTC related EcoRI restriction fragments not seen in a normal human placenta cellular DNA. The significance of this finding is difficult to assess since the karyotype of the MCF-7 cell line is very different from that of normal cells; indicating several genetic rearrangements which may have been incurred during passage in tissue culture. In addition, we have observed several restriction site polymorphisms in cellular DNA from normal human tissues. Whether these polymphorphisms reflect the presence or absence of specific proviral gonomes in individual cellular DNAs or the highly diverged nature of this family of proviral genomes will require further study.

EVOLUTIONARY RELATIONSHIPS BETWEEN DIFFFERENT CLASSES OF RETROVIRUSES

Retroviruses (16) have been classified on the basis of their morphological properties (17,18). While four different genera (type A,B,C and D) are recognized, viruses within the type A,B, and D virus genera share certain morphogenic and biochemical properties. Initially, defective intracisternal type A viral particles were observed in early mouse embryos and in certain murine tumors (19-23). Later studies revealed the existence of infectious retroviruses containing extensive homology to the A particle genome (24). Type C viruses, which are widely distributed among birds and mammals, have been shown to cause leukemia and other tumors. The most recently described type D retroviruses appear limited to primate species, and their oncogenicity remains to be established (25). Earlier studies have shown that the major structural proteins encoded within the gag gene of type C and D retroviruses share antigenic determinants, as do the major proteins of type B, and D retroviruses (26). Moreover, certain mammalian type C, and type D retroviruses share common determinants in the env coded gp70 protein (27-28) as well as sequence homology in their p15E coding region (29). These patterns of homology indicate that the evolution of recent retrovirus groups involved genetic interactions among their progenitors.

We have analyzed the genetic relatedness of retroviruses using low stringency blot hybridization conditions (30). Reciprocal relations were observed among each class of retroviruses. A major region of homology could be demonstrated in the pol genes of type A, B, and D and avian type C retroviruses. These findings strongly imply genetic relatedness between the pol genes of representatives of the four major retrovirus genera. In contrast, when analogous studies were performed using mammalian type C viral DNAs, no pol gene holomologies were observed. To precisely assess the extent of homology between the pol genes of these retroviruses, we undertook comparative nucleotide sequence analysis (30). The results of these studies establish that the pol genes of prototype type A, type B, avian type C, and type D retrovirus genera are all geneticly related.These findings correlate well with the known functional similarities in the reverse transcriptases coded for by their pol genes. These enzymes exhibit similar template and cation preferences which differ markedly from those of mammalian type C viruses (31-33). In contrast, this analysis detected no comparable homology type at either the nucleotide or amino acid sequence levels between any of these pol genes and that of M-MuLV. Thus, our studies provide strong support for the concept of two major pol gene progenitors, one for mammalian type C viruses and the other for types A, B, D and avian type C retroviruses.

Since infectious type B retroviruses (MMTV) have only been isolated from murine species, we have explored the possibility that infectious members of other classes of retroviruses might also share homology with the human recombinant clone HLM-2 (Callahan et al., manuscript in preparation). A major region of homology between the type A, B, and D retroviral genomes and HLM-2 DNA corresponds to their respective pol genes (Figure 2). In the case of SMRV (type D, squirrel monkey retrovirus) the homology spans the 3' half of the gag gene through the entire pol gene. In addition, the SMRV LTR also hybridizes weakly with the HLM-2 LTR and the M432 viral genome (murine type A related retrovirus) hybridizes to a region of HLM-2 immediately adjacent to the 3' LTR. No homology was

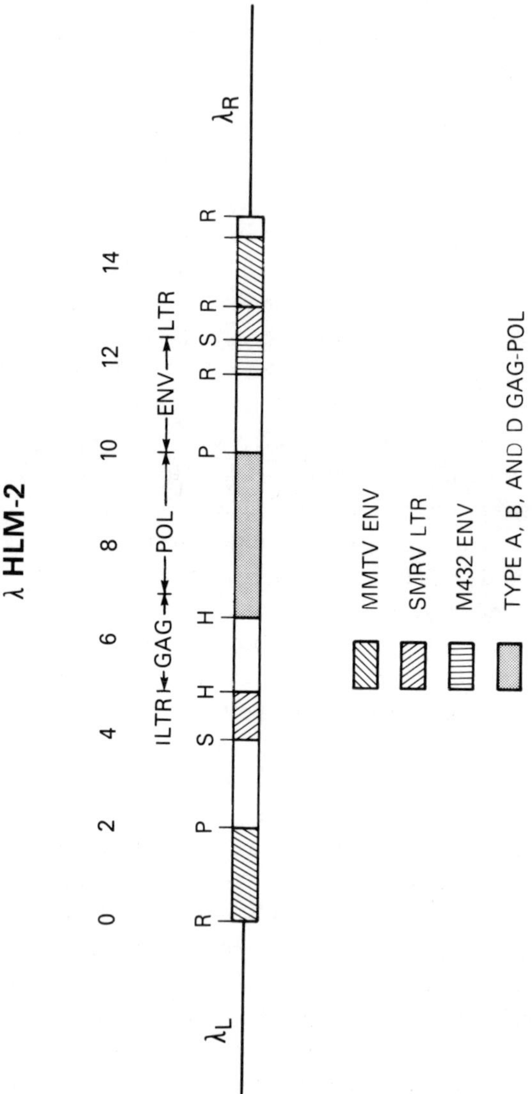

Figure 2. Homology regions between human recombinant HLM-2 and prototypes of different retroviral genera. The regions of homology were determined by reciprocal low strigency blot hybridization of restricted HLM-2 and proviral DNA (Callahan et al., manuscript in preparation).

detected with a number of different mammalian type C proviral genomes.

In order to more precisely identify the conserved regions of the HLM-2 pol gene, the nucleotide sequence of the 3.6 kbp EcoRI fragment (8.0 to 11.6 HLM-2 map units, Figure 1) was determined (unpublished data). A comparison of a portion of this nucleotide sequence (9.5 to 10.0 HLM-2 map units) with those of pol genes from other infectious retroviruses revealed regions of significant homology (51,50,44 and 37%) between HLM-2 and respectively MMTV (type B), SMRV (type D), RSV (avian Rous sarcoma type C virus) and HTLV (human T cell leukemia virus). Similar results were obtained by comparing the translated amino acid sequence of this region (45,38,33, and 27%) respectively. No comparable nucleotide or amino acid sequence homology could be detected between this region of HLM-2 and the MuLV pol gene. These findings show that the HLM-2 pol gene probably arose from the same progenitor that gave rise to the pol genes of the infectious type A,B,D and avian type C retrovirus genera.

In conclusion, we have identified MMTV gag, pol, env and LTR related sequences in human cellular DNA. These sequences do not appear to be organized in a manner expected for a human MMTV related endogenous proviral genome. Instead, the MMTV gag-pol related sequences are found within a new class of human endogenous retroviral genomes which appear to be a mosaic of sequences related to different retroviral genera. This is consistent with the accumulating evidence (summarized in Ref. 30) that genetic interaction between retrovirus genera has played an important role in their evolution. The LTR-like element of this class of human proviral genomes is also found unassociated with viral structural genes and is highly reiterated in cellular DNA. The effect which these "solitary" LTR elements have on the expression of adjacent cellular genes and their potential role in carcinogenesis will provide a provocative new avenue for future research. With respect to MMTV env related sequences in human cellular DNA there is currently no evidence that they are associated with a complete proviral genome. There appears to be several highly diverged copies of these sequences in human cellular DNA. In each of the two recombinant clones which have been analyzed the major region of homology corresponds to the gp52 portion of the MMTV env gene. The significance of this observation remains to be determined, but is consistent with the large body of literature (reviewed in Ref. 1) suggesting that an antigen related to MMTV gp52 is present in many human breast tumors. Although MMTV LTR related sequences have been detected in human cellular DNA, to date no recombinant DNA clones have been detected which contain these sequences. The existence of human recombinant DNA clones containing retroviral related sequences now offers the opportunity to investigate their role in the etiology of human neoplasia.

REFERENCES

1. Sarkar, N. (1980) in The Role of Viruses in Human Cancer, eds. Giraldo, G. and Beth, E. (Elsevier North Holland, New York) pp. 207-235.
2. Morris, V.L., Medeiros, E., Ringold, G.M., Bishop, J.M. & Varmus, H.E. (1977) J. Mol. Biol. 114, 73-91.
3. Schlom J., Drohan, W., Teramoto, Y.A., Hand, P., Colcher, D., Callahan R., Todaro, C., Kufe D., Howard D., Gautsch, J., Lerner R. & Schidlowsky, C; (1978) Origins of Inbred Mice, ed. Morse, C.M. III (Academic Press, New York) pp. 343-368.
4. Drohan, W. & Schlom, J. (1979) J. Natl. Cancer Inst. 62, 1279-1286.
5. Das, M.R., & Mink, M.M. (1979) Cancer Research 29, 5106-5113.
6. Bishop, J.M., Quintrell, N., Medeiros, E., & Varmus, H.E. (1974). Cancer 34, 1421-1426.
7. Axel, R., Schlom, J., & Spiegelman, S. (1972). Nature 235, 32-36.
8. Vaidya, A.B., Black, M.M., Dion, A.S., & Moore, D. (1974) Nature 249, 565-567.

9. Callahan R., Drohan W., Tronick, S. & Schlom, J. (1982) Proc. Natl. Acad. Sci. USA 79, 5503-5507.
10. May, F.E.B., Westley, B.R., Rochefort, H., Buetti, E. & Diggelman, H., 1983 Nucl. Acids. Res. 11, 4127-4139.
11. Lawn, R.M., Fritsch, E.F., Parker, R.C., Blake, G. & Maniatis, T. (1978) Cell 15, 1157-1174.
12. Williams, B. & Blattner, F.R. (1979) J. Virol. 29, 555-575.
13. Wirth, T., Gloggler, K., Baumruke, T., Schmidt, M., & Horak, I. (1983) Proc. Natl. Acad. Sci. USA 80, 3327-3330.
14. Wheeler, D.A., Butel, J.S., Medina, D., Cardiff, R.D., & Hager, G.L. (1983) J. Virol. 46, 42-99.
15. Van Ooyen, A.J.J., Michalides, R.J.A.M., & Nusse, R. (1983) J. Virol. 46, 362-370.
16. Fenner, F. (1976) Virology 71, 371-376.
17. Schidlowsky, G. in Cancer Research: Cell Biology, Molecular Biology and Tumor Virology, Gallo, R. Ed., CRC, Cleveland, Ohio (1977) pp. 189-245.
18. Dalton, A. (1972) J. Natl. Cancer Inst. 49, 323-330.
19. Biczysko, W., Pienkowski, M., Solter, D. & Koprowski, H.J. (1973) J. Natl. Cancer Inst. 51, 1041.
20. Callarco, P.G. & Szollosi (1973) Nature 243, 91-93.
21. Chase, P.G. & Piko, L. (1973) J. Nat. Cancer Inst. 51, 1971-1976.
22. Dalton, A.J., Potter, M. & Merwin, R.M. (1961) J. Natl. Cancer Inst. 26, 1221-1226.
23. Perk, K. & Dahlberg, J.E., (1974) J. Virol. 14, 1304-1309.
24. Callahan, R., Kuff, E.L., Lueders, K.K. & Birkenmeir, E. (1981). J. Virol. 40, 901-908.
25. Herberling, R.L., Barker, S.T., Kalter, S.S., Smith, G.C. & Helmke, R.J. (1977) Science 195, 289-294.
26. Barbacid, M., Long, L.K. & Aaronson, S.A. (1980) Proc. Natl. Acad. Sci. USA 77, 72-76.
27. Stephenson, J.R., Hino, S., Garrett, E.W. & Aaronson, S.A. (1976) Nature 261:609-612.
28. Devare, J.G., Hanson, R.E. & Stephenson, J.R. (1978) J. Virol. 41, 801-808.

29. Cohen, M., Rice, N., Stephens, R. & O'Connell, C. (1982) J. Virol. 41, 801-808.
30. Chiu, I.M., Callahan, R., Tronick, S.R., Schlom, J. & Aaronson, S.A. (1984) Science 223, 364-370.
31 Schlom J. in Molecular Biology of RNA tumor Viruses, Stephenson, J. ed., Academic Press, Inc. New York, 1980, pp. 447-484.
32. Wilson, S.H. & Kuff, E.L. (1972) Proc. Natl. Acad. Sci. USA 69, 1531-1535.
33. Scolnick, E., Rands, E., Aaronson, S.A. & Todaro, G.J. (1970) Proc. Natl. Acad. Sci. USA 67, 1789-1793.

CLOSE STRUCTURAL SIMILARITIES BETWEEN THE LTRs OF BOVINE LEUKEMIA AND HUMAN T-CELL LEUKEMIA VIRUSES

Y. Ikawa, N. Sagata, and T. Yasunaga[1]

Laboratory of Molecular Oncology and [1]. Computation Center, The Institute of Physical and Chemical Research (RIKEN), Wako, Saitama 351-01, Japan

A proviral DNA of bovine leukemia virus (BLV) was cloned in a Charon 4A λ-phage vector (BLV-1) from the leukemic tissue of Japanese cattle. Comparison of its restriction sites with those of other BLV isolates revealed its resemblance to an American isolate but not a to Belgian isolate except the 3' end region. After subcloning into pBR322, both 5' and 3' long terminal repeats (LTRs) were completely sequenced.

The BLV-LTR consisted of 530 bp with a 6 bp inverted repeat at its 5' and 3' ends. A $tRNA^{Pro}$ binding site followed the R' LTR and a polypurine tract of GAGGGGGAG preceded the 3' LTR. The U_3 region possessed putative transcriptional promoters, CAT and TATA boxes. Upstream of these sequences was observed a potential enhancer element which resembled that of an immunoglobulin gene. This may explain why BLV can target B lymphocytes.

Like human T-cell leukemia virus (HTLV)-I LTR, BLV-LTR had an extremely long R region (228 bp) which separated a poly (A) addition signal (AATAAA) from a poly (A) site as far apart as 260 bp. This region appeared to form a large hairpin structure on a nascent RNA chain, making the two signal sequences come closer. About 50% sequence homology was observed in the R regions of HLTV-I and BLV LTRs, indicating their distant evolutionary relationship.

COMMON FEATURES OF BOVINE LEUKEMIA VIRUS AND HUMAN T-CELL LEUKEMIA VIRUS

BLV and HTLV share several biological characteristics such as a totally exogenous nature to the target hosts, natural transmission, geographic peculiality, low incidence (one in several thousands of sero-positive individuals) of induced leukemia, and difficulties in infecting and transfecting cultured cells.

MOLECULAR CLONING OF THE BLV GENOME AND CONSERVATION OF THE pX_{BL} SEQUENCE

We previously investigated existence of the BLV genome in the B cell lymphosarcoma cases of Japanese cattle and reported the clonal nature of the tumor (1). We then made a gene library from the leukemic tissue with a few BLV genomes, and cloned its complete proviral genome into a Charon 4A phage-vector (BLV-1) (2).

Comparison of its restriction cleavage map with those of other BLV isolates revealed that our clone is close to an American isolate, but not so close to a Belgian isolate except for its 3' end region (Figure 1). The 3' region contained several unidentified coding frames (designated pXBL region) and 3' LTR. The conservation of Pb_{BL} in all the BLV isolates suggests that it has a biological function(s).

GENERAL STRUCTURES OF THE BLV-LTR

The LTR plays an important role in retroviral replication, possessing regulatory sequences necessary for transcription (3). Accordingly, we started sequencing of

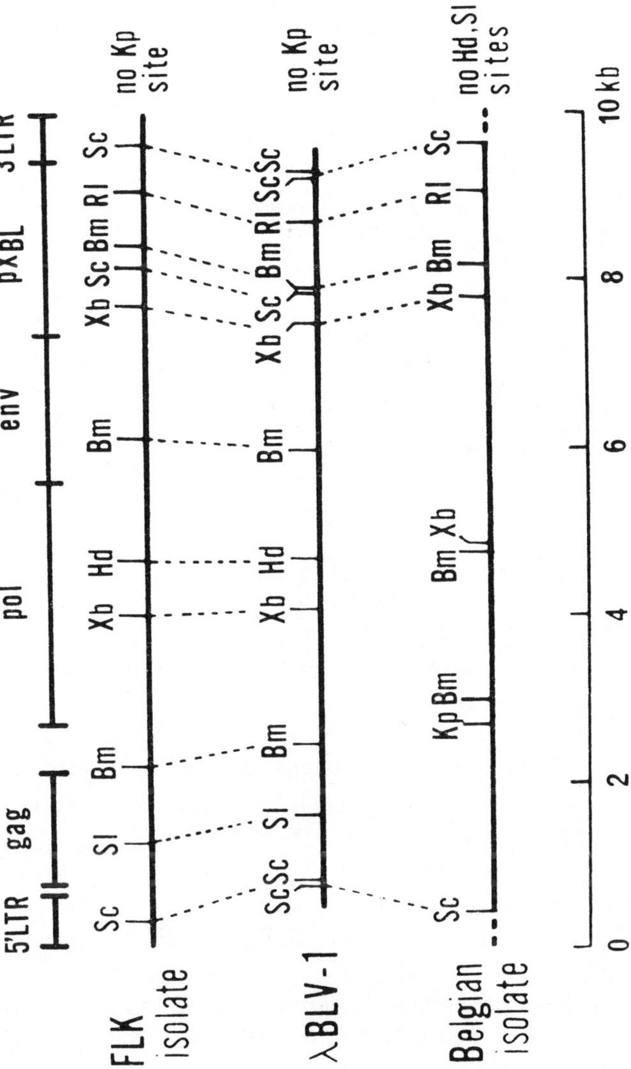

Figure 1. Restriction mapping of three different BLV isolates.

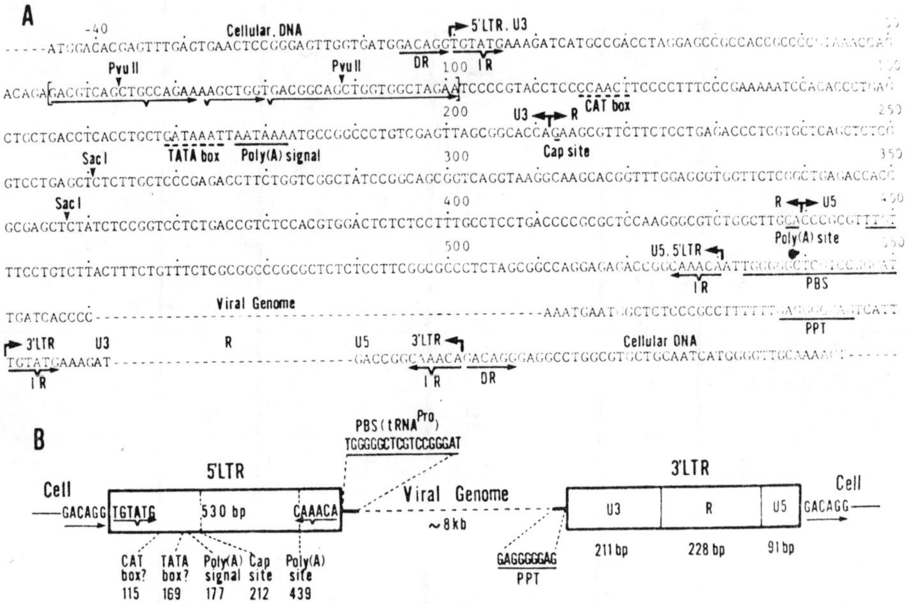

Figure 2. Complete nucleotide sequence of 5' and 3' LTRs of a BLV proviral clone (BLV-1) (A) and their schematic features (B).

both 3' and 5' LTRs of the BLV proviral clone, revealing the structure shown in Figure 2 (4).

To summarize the general structures described in Figure 2, the BLV-LTR consisted of 530 bp with 6 bp inverted repeats at its 5' and 3' ends, flanked by a 6 bp direct repeat of host cell origin. A $tRNA^{Pro}$ binding site for initiation of reverse transcription followed the 5' LTR, and a polypurine tract of GAGGGGGAG for minus-strand DNA synthesis preceded the 3' LTR. The U_3 region contained putative transcriptional promoters with somewhat peculiar sequences CCAACT and GATAAAT as CAT and TATA boxes, respectively.

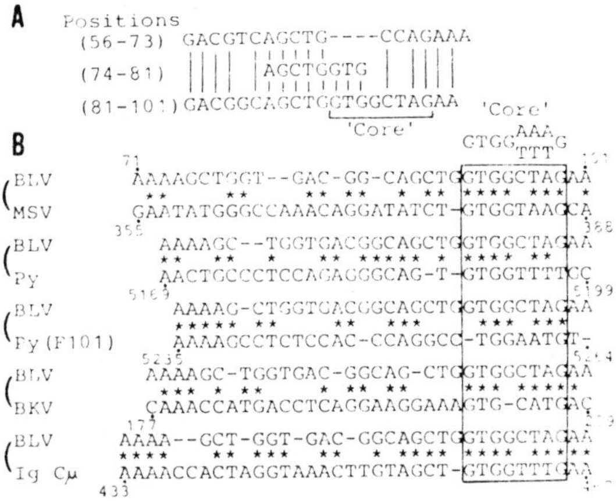

Figure 3. A possible enhancer element of the BLV-LTR and its comparison with viral and cellular enhancers.

UNIQUE STRUCTURE: A POTENTIAL ENHANCER ELEMENT RESEMBLING THAT OF A IMMUNOGLOBULIN GENE

Upstream of the promoter sequences, a potential enhancer element, which was shorter than those of other retroviruses, was observed. Its "core" and surrounding sequences resembled those of other viral and cellular genes (5) (Figure 3), especially of mouse immunoglobulin heavy chain (Cu). This may explain why BLV can target B lymphocytes.

UNIQUE STRUCTURE: LONG R REGION

We attempted to identify the R region, a portion of the LTR unit (U_3-R-U_5) that normally begins with a G residue at the cap site and terminates with a dinucleotide CA at the poly (A) addition site. BLV strong-stop cDNA is 320 bp long (6), which predicts that the G residue at the cap site should precede the $tRNA^{Pro}$ binding site by 320 bp. We found a G residue at exactly the predicted position (position 212 in Figure 2A). This G residue may thus be the cap site or the beginning of the R region. As a possible candidate for the poly (A) site downstream of the putative cap site, on the other hand, 10 CA dinucleotides were found. However, only the CA dinucleotide at positions 438-439 formed a part of 11 bp stretch (TCTGGCTTGCA) which closely matched the transcription termination signal (TTTGCNG(orC)TTGCA) of other retroviruses (7). From these observations, the R region of BLV-LTR was estimated to be 228 bp long, the U_3 region 211 bp long and the U5 region 91 bp long. The R region is thus much longer than those of other retrovirus LTRs but is quite similar to that of HTLV-I LTR (6).

UNIQUE STRUCTURE: POSSIBLE HAIRPIN STRUCTURE BETWEEN POLY(A) SIGNAL AND POLY(A) SITE

The canonical signal sequence (AATAAA) for polyadenylylation is located 10-20 bp upstream from the poly(A) site in most retroviruses. In the BLV LTR, this hexanucleotide was not at the expected position but as far as 260 bp upstream (positions 177-182) from the poly(A) site. We then performed computer-aided construction of a possible secondary structure of the 3' terminus of the BLV RNA transcript, to determine whether the poly(A) signal-like sequence and the poly(A) site could become close together by folding of the RNA transcript. Figure 4 shows the secondary structure formed by nucleotide sequences between positions 170-440. This region formed a large hairpin structure, involving the entire R region and having a high G-C pair content (71%), particularly at the base of the main stem. Consequently, the hexanucleotide AATAAA became located close (as close as 6 bp) to the poly(A) site. If such a secondary structure is formed in vivo, the AATAAA sequence could serve as a "normal" poly(A) addition signal on the RNA transcript. We note that HTLV-I LTR has also a poly(A) signal in an unusual location and can form a similar secondary structure (8).

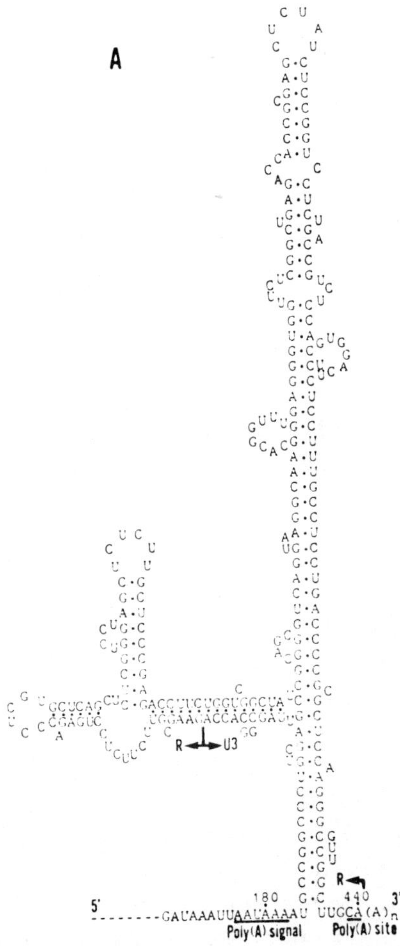

Figure 4. A possible secondary structure formed between the poly(A) signal and poly(A) site.

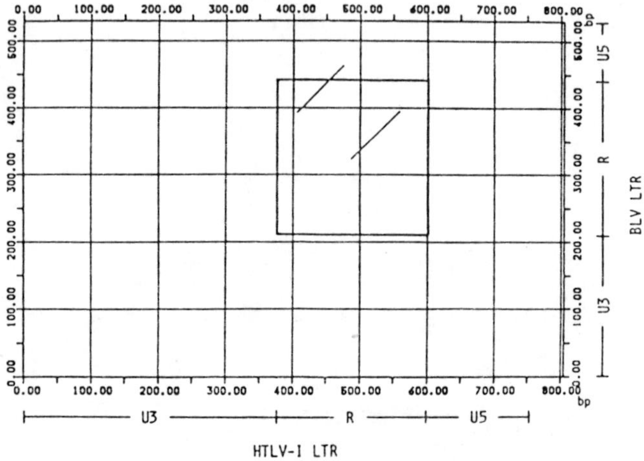

Figure 5. Two-dimensional homology matrix comparison of the LTR sequences of BLV and HTLV-I under conditions detecting more than 50% homology in 70 contiguous nucleotide sequences.

HOMOLOGY BETWEEN HTLV-I LTR AND BLV LTR SEQUENCES

By the computer-assisted two-dimensional homology matrix (9), we compared the LTR sequences of BLV and other retroviruses to find no significant homology between them (under the conditions detecting 20 bp unit sequences with more than 60% homololgy). However, further analysis under less stringent conditions (50% homology detection) revealed a relatively long stretch (about 100 bp) of LBV sequence with homology to only HTLV-I LTR (Figure 5). This stretch was located in the R region (228 bp long in both viruses).

The computer alignment between the R regions of the BLV and HTLV-I LTRs was then made by introducing several gaps to maximize the homology (Fig. 6). Overall homology was 48% (117 matches among 246 nucleotides). In addition, we found a stretch of 91 bp (underlined in Figure 6 and corresponds to a homologous diagonal line in Figure 5) that gave 46% homology without any gaps. The probability of an occurrence of such a homologous stretch in the corresponding regions was calculated to be as low as 4 x 10^{-5}, showing the significance of the homology observed.

In summary, the structural similarity and nucleotide sequence homology between the BLV and HTLV-I LTRs demonstrate that these retroviruses are evolutionarily related.

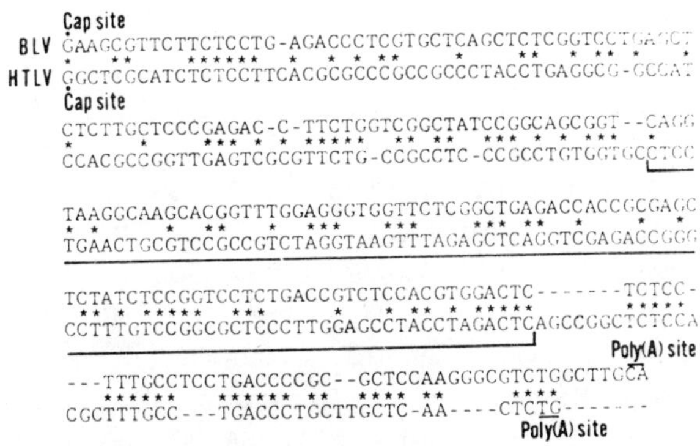

Figure 6. Computer-assisted alignment of the R sequences of BLV and HTLV-I LTRs.

USEFULNESS OF THE BLV SYSTEM TO UNDERSTAND ONCOGENESIS BY HTLV

We have recently determined the complete nucleotide sequence of the BLV genome: the genomic structure has now turned out to be very similar to that of HTLV-I, including the so-called pX region and a newly identified gene coding for a gag precursor protein-cleaving protease, which is located between the gag and pol genes (10,11,12). BLV would thus provide a suitable model for understanding oncogenesis by HTLV.

REFERENCES

1. Onuma, M., Sagata, N., Okada, K., Ogawa, Y., Ikawa, Y. & Oshima, K. (1982) Microbiol. Immunol. 26, 813-820.
2. Sagata, N., Ogawa, Y., Kawamura, J., Onuma, M., Izawa, H. & Ikawa, Y. (1983) Gene 26, 1-10.
3. Temin, Y. (1983) Gene 26, 1-10.
4. Sagata, N., Uasunaga, T., Ogawa, Y., Tsuzuku-Kawamura, J. & Ikawa, Y. (1984) Proc. Natl. Acad. Sci. U.S.A. 81, 4741-4745.
5. Khoury, G. & Gruss, P. (1983) Cell 33, 313-314.
6. Seiki, M., Hattori, S. & Yoshida, M. (1982) Proc. Natl. Acad. Sci. U.S.A. 79, 6899-6902.
7. Bonner, T.I., O'Connell, C. & Cohen, M. (1982). Proc. Natl. Acad. Sci. U.S.A. 79, 4709-4713.
8. Seiki, M., Hattori, S., Hirayama, Y. & Yoshida, M. (1983) Proc. Natl. Acad. Sci. USA 80, 3618-3622.
9. Toh, M.M., Hayashida, H. & Miyaa, T. (1983) Nature (London) 305, 827-829.
10. Sagata, N., Yasunaga, T., & Ikawa, Y. (in press) FEBS Letters.
11. Sagata, N., Yasunaga, T., Ohishi, K., Tsuzuku Kawamura, J., Onuma, M., Ikawa, Y. (in press) EMBO J.
12. Sagata, N., Yasunaga, Y., Ogawa, Y., Tsuzuku-Kawamura, J., Oishi, JhK. & Ikawa, Y. (in press) Proc. Natl. Acad. Sci. U.S.A.

ANALYSIS AND IMMUNOLOGICAL PROPERTIES OF LYMPHADENOPATHY ASSOCIATED VIRUS (LAV) STRUCTURAL PROTEINS

F. Barre-Sinoussi, J.C. Chermann and L. Montagnier

Institut Pasteur, Viral Oncology Unit, 25, rue du Dr. Roux, 75015 Paris, France

LAV or LAV related viruses were isolated from patients with AIDS or with lymphadenopathy. The results presented here indicate that four major components (p45, p25, p18 and p13) are detected in purified virions. The p25 and the p13 are internal proteins of LAV since they cannot be easily iodinated in the virions. The p25 can be purified by phosphocellulose chromatography and the purified protein can be labelled with ^{125}I. The p18 is either a gag gene product or a transmembrane protein. The major core proteins p25 of different viral isolates are antigenically identical but are not related to the major structural proteins of other retroviruses. Antibodies to LAV p25 are predominantly found in the sera of patients with AIDS or with pre-AIDS but in some cases, antibodies to p18 and p13 are also detected. These results confirm that the various LAV isolates represent a new human retroviruses associated with AIDS.

Lymphadenopathy Associated Virus (LAV) was initially isolated from cultured T cels of a patient with lymphadenopathy syndrome (1). Additional isolates of similar viruses were then easily obtained from AIDS patients belonging to all the groups at risk for the disease (2, 3, 4, 5). Epidemiological studies (6) and the selective tropism of LAV for the helper-inducer T lymphocytes (7) strongly support the involvement of this retrovirus in AIDS. Here, we present biochemical and immunological characterization of the structural proteins of LAV.

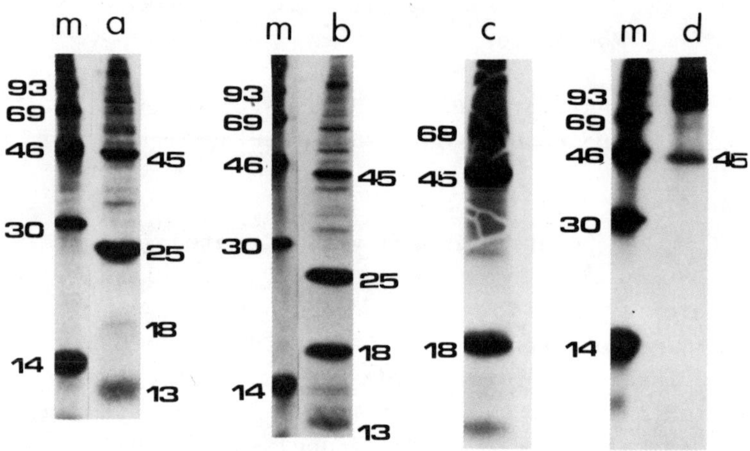

Figure 1. SDS polyacrylamide gel electrophoresis of purified LAV. LAV producing cells were labelled either with ^{35}S methionine (50 uCi/ml) (lane a), ^{14}C amino acids (5 uCi/ml) (lane b) or with ^{14}C glucosamine (lane d) (15 uCi/ml) for 18 hours. Purified labelled viruses were dtergent disrupted (15 minutes at 0-4 ^{o}C) and labelled proteins were analyzed by electrophoresis on 12% polyacrylamide gels (SDS-PAGE). In some experiments (lane c), purified disrupted virus was lebelled with ^{125}I sodium iodine (5 uCi/ug) by iodogen procedure.

LABELLED POLYPEPTIDES OF LAV

Studies on LAV structural proteins were performed using LAV propagated in primary cultures of blood lymphocytes or in human cord blood T cells as previously described (1, 3, 8), and purified by standard sucrose density gradient centrifugation.

Figure 1 shows an analysis by SDS PAGE of LAV proteins labelled either with ^{35}S methionine, ^{14}C amino acids, ^{125}I sodium iodine or with ^{14}C glucosamine.

Four major components with apparent molecular weight of 45,000, 25,000, 18,000 and 13,000 daltons are present in unpurified virions. All these components are labelled with aminoacids whether labelling with ^{35}S methionine indicates that p18 and p13 proteins contain a low amount of this aminoacid. Correspondence of components labelled with aminoacids and glucosamine indicates that the p45 is glycosylated. However, whether this proteins represents the envelope protein or a contamination by a cellular protein could not be determined. A high molecular weight polypeptide (100,000 daltons) is also detected in both cases which may represent either an envelope protein or a precursor of this protein. Localization of constitutitve polypeptides in the virion was also assessed by radioiodination of purified virus. The p25 is not iodinated and the p13 is only slightly labelled. Since purified p25 can be easily iodinated (data not shown) (9), this indicates that these two proteins are internal gag proteins inaccessible to labelling until the virions were sufficiently disrupted. This result is consistent with previously published data considering the p25 as the viral core protein (3, 8, 10). Since the p18 protein is easily iodinated, these experiments do not allow determination of whether this protein is a gag gene product or whether it is a transmembrane protein.

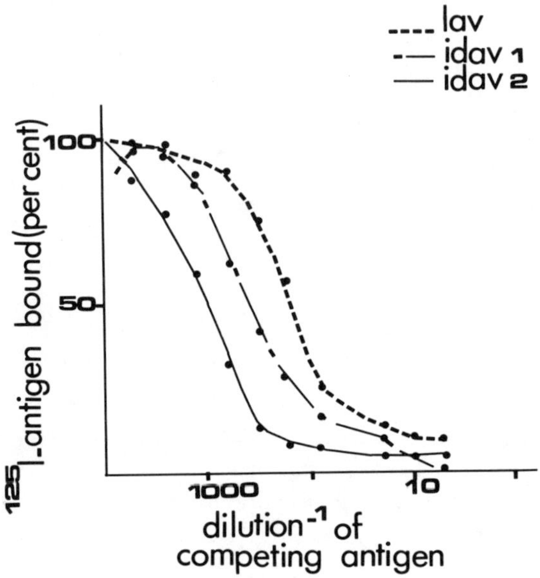

Figure 2. Competition radioimmunoassay for the major structural protein of LAV. Competition radioimmunoassay with our positive reference serum and ^{125}I labelled LAVp25 was carried out as previously published (5, 9). Virus extracts from different isolates were used as competitive antigens.

COMPARISON OF LAVp25 AND MAJOR CORE PROTEINS OF OTHER VIRAL ISOLATES

Purified viruses from two AIDS patients were used as competitive antigens in homologous radioimmunoassays (RIAS) which have been performed by the double antibody method described earlier (9), using as labelled antigen, purified LAVp25 (Figure 2).

The quantitative pattern of the competition observed in this assay indicates that the major core proteins of IDAV1 (isolate from a homosexual with Kaposi's sarcoma) and IDAV2 (isolate from a young B hemophiliac) were identical to LAVp25. This confirmed the similarity previously reported between all the viral isolates obtained from AIDS patients (5, 8, 10).

Similar competition assays have been performed using other human or mammalian retroviruses as competitve antigens (9). None of them, incuding HTLV-I and HTLV-II competes in the homologous LAVp25 assay (data not shown). Such study shows that the major internal protein p25 is a distinct antigen specific for LAV isolates.

ANALYSIS OF SERA FOR ANTIBODIES TO LAV MAJOR PROTEINS

As previously reported (8, 10), LAVp25 is the main protein specifically recognized by patients sera in RIPA using purified ^{35}S labelled virus.

Figure 3 shows an example of the detection of antibodies to this protein in patients sera. Various amounts of antibodies against this protein can be detected in the sera. The major core protein p25 is the only protein labelled with 35S methionine which is recognized by patients sera. No antibodies against an evelope protein can be identified by this assay. Furthermore, these experiments have also shown that all the viral isolates from different AIDS patients are antigenicly related (data not shown).

In order to understand the molecular nature of the antigens recognized by ELISA (Brun-Vézinet et al., this book), selected sera were examined for antibodies to LAV antigens by the sensitive Western Blot technique of Towbin et al. (11). For this study, a lysate of LAV was fractionated by SDS polyacrylamide gel electrophoresis and transferred to a nitrocellulose sheet by the electrophoretic blotting method. The nitrocellulose sheet was cut into 0.5 cm strips and reacted with samples of the human sera. Antigen-antibody complexes formed were detected by immunoenzymatic reaction after incubation of the strips with goat anti-human IgG peroxydase and then diaminabenzidine and H_2O_2.

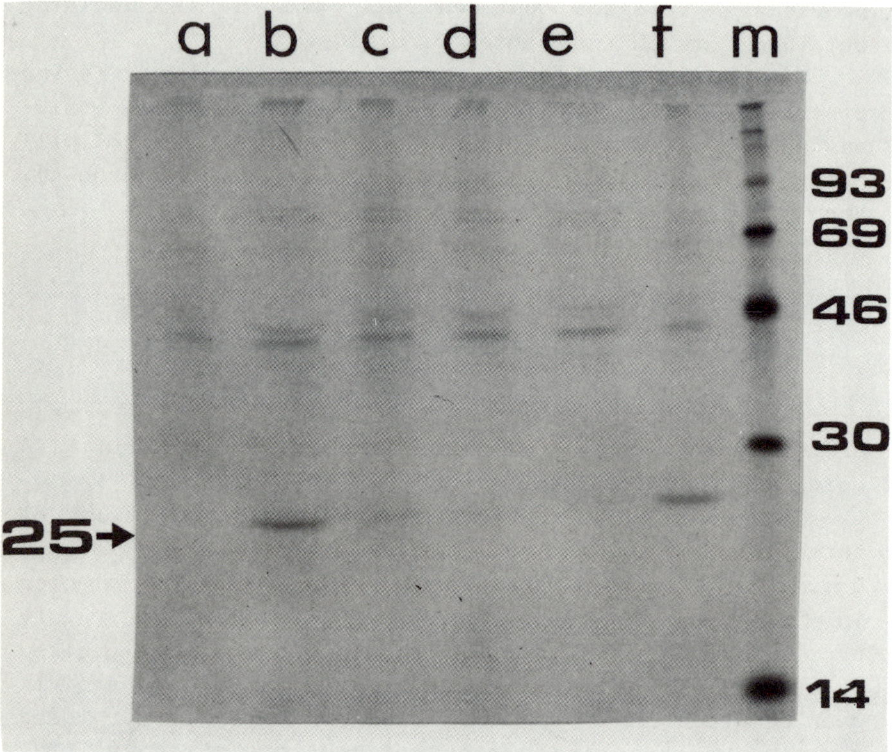

Figure 3. Polyaclylamide gel electrophoresis of immune-complexes between ^{35}S labelled LAV and antibodies in patients sera. Radioimmunoprecipitation experiments were performed as previously described (1, 8). Briefly, ^{35}S methionine labelled virus was concentrated by ultracentrifugation and lysed in RIPA buffer. For immunoprecipitation, aliquots ($2x10^6$ cpm) were incubated with 5 ul of various sera (2 hours at 37 ^oC, 18 hours at 4 ^oC). Immune complexes were isolated by protein A sepharose beads and analysed by electrophoresis on polyacrylamide gels. The sera used for this assay were normal human serum (lane a); our positive reference serum (lane b); sera from patients with AIDS or with pre-AIDS (lane c to f).

Figure 4 shows representative patterns of antibody reactions in the Western Blot assay with selected sera from patients with AIDS or with lymphadenopathy. Although most patients' sera react predominantly with LAVp25, some sera react with the lower molecular weight proteins such as p18 or, in few cases, p13. Therefore, three viral antigens are, at least, specificly recognized by antibodies in the serum of patients with AIDS or pre-AIDS, whereas none of them is detected with a normal human serum. This experiment confirms that p25, p18 and p13 can be considered as virus coded proteins.

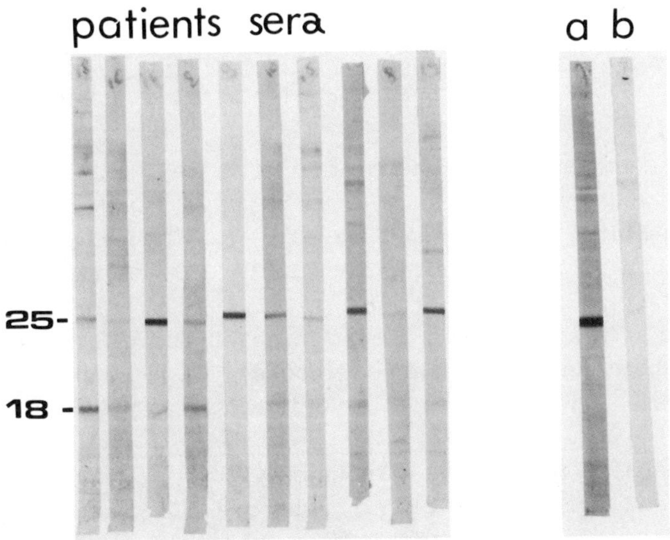

Figure 4. Analysis of sera for antibodies to LAV by Western Blot. This assay was performed according to Towbin et al and is described in more details in the text. On the left, sera from patients with AIDS or with lymphadenopathy. On the right, our positive reference serum (lane a) and a normal human serum (lane b).

CONCLUSIONS

Among the four major components found in LAV, p25, p18, and p13 are the three viral antigens specificly recognized by antibodies in the serum of AIDS or pre-AIDS patients. p25 and p13 are probably gag encoded proteins whereas p18 can be either a gag product or a transmembrane protein. LAVp25 is a highly conserved determinant, as it is for all major core proteins of retroviruses.

The complete nucleotide sequence of LAV genome, recently cloned (M. Alizon et al., submitted) with allow confirmaton of these data and identificaton of the env gene product.

REFERENCES

1. Barre-Sinoussi, G., Chermann, J.C., Rey, F., Nugeyre, M.T., Chamaret, S., Gruest, J., Dauguet, C., Axler-Blin, C., Brun-Vezinet, F., Rouzioux, C., Rozenbaum, W. & Montagnier L. (1983) Science 220, 868-871.
2. Vilmer, E., Rouzioux, C., Vezinet-Brun, F., Fischer, A., Chermann, J.C., Barre-Sinoussi, F., Gazengel, C., Dauguet, C., Manignet, P. & Griscelli, C. 1984. Lancet ii, 753-757.
3. Chermann, J.C., Barre-Sinoussi, F. & Montagnier, L. Acquired immune deficiency syndrome UCLA symposia on molecular and cellular biology; new series; Volume 16 eds. Michael S. Gottlieb and Jerome E. Groopman, Alan R. Liss, Inc., New York 1984, p. 31-46.
4. Ellrodt, A., Barre-Sinoussi, F., Le Bras, Nugeyre, M.T., Palazzo, L., Rey, F., Brun-Vezinet, F., Rouzioux, C., Segond, P., Caquet, R., Montagnier, L. & Chermann, J.C. (1984) Lancet i, 1383-1385.
5. Feorino, M.P., Kalyanaraman, V.S., Haverkos, H.W., Cabradilla, C.D., Warfield, D.T., Jaffe, H.W., Harrison, A.K., Goldringer, D., Gottlieb, M.S., Chermann, J.C., Barre-Sinoussi, F., Spira, T.J.,

McDougal, J.S., Curran, J.W., Montagnier, L., Murphy, F.A. & Francis D.P. (1984) Science 225, 69-72.

6. Brun-Vezinet, F., Rouzioux, C., Barre-Sinoussi, F., Klatzmann, D., Saimaot, A.G., Rozenbaum, W., Montagnier, L. & Chermann J.C. (1984) Lancet i, 1253-1256.
7. Klatzmann, D., Barre-Sinoussi, F., Nugeyre, M.T., Dauguet, Ch., Vilmer, E., Grisceli, C., Brun-Vezinet, F., Rouzioux, C., Gluckman, J.C., Chermann, J.C. & Montagnier L. (1984). Science 225, 59-63.
8. Montagnier, L., Chermann, J.C., Barre-Sinoussi, F., Chamaret, S., Gruest, J., Nugeyre, M.T., Rey, F., Dauguet, C. & Axler-Blin, C. (1984) Cold Spring Harbour Publication Meeting on "Human T-cell leukemia Viruses" 1 vol., 363-379.
9. Kalyanaraman, V.S., Cabradilla, C.D., Getchell, J.P., Narayanan, R., Braff, E.H., Chermann, J.C., Barre-Sinoussi, F., Montagnier, L., Spira, T.J., Kaplan, J., Fishbein, D., Jaffe, H.W., Curran, J.W. & Francis D.P. (1984) Science 225, 321-323.
10. Barre-Sinoussi, F., Chermann, J.C. & Montagnier, F. (1984) Manipulation of Host Defense Mechanisms" ed. Tadao Aoki (Japan), 1 vol.
11. Towbin, H., Staehlin, T. & Gordon J., (1979) Proc. Natl. Acad. Sci. USA 76, 4350-4353.

RNA VIRUSES AND LYMPHOCYTE IMMUNE FUNCTIONS

L. Gazzolo[1], M. Duc Dodon[2], A. Gessain[1], M. Robert-Guroff[3] and G. de-The[1]

1. Laboratoire d'Epidémiologie et d'Immunovirologie des Tumeurs (CNRS), Faculté de Médicine Alexis Carrel, 69372 Lyon Cédex 8, France, 2. Unité de Virologie (INSERM), 69371 Lyon Cédex 8, France, and 3. Laboratory of Tumor Cell Biology, National Cancer Institute, Bethesda, Md., U.S.A.

Among the diverse strategies used by viruses to induce human disease, their ability to cause immune defects has received increasing attention, concurrently with the identification of cells able to mount a large variety of immune responses and secrete numerous factors modulating these responses. In vivo, immunological dysfunctions may result from viral infections and be responsible for acute and/or chronic disorders. In vitro studies have documented the interactions between human lymphocytes and viruses, through which viral infections lead to an aberrant control of immune responses, and to subsequent diseases.

The functions of T and B lymphocyte subsets as well as their dynamic interplay are currently under extensive investigation. Subpopulations of T lymphocytes may amplify (helper cells) or suppress (suppressor cells) the activity of other T lymphocytes or B lymphocytes. Most of the regulatory influences by T lymphocytes are mediated through biologically active molecules called lymphokines. These include T-cell growth factor (TCGF), involved in the proliferation of T lymphocytes activated by lectins or antigens (1), B-cell growth factor (BCGF) and B-cell differentiating factor (BDGF), implicated in the proliferation and differentiaton of B lymphocytes, respectively (2,3). Effector T lymphocytes are responsible for reactions such as delayed cutaneous responses, rejection of foreign tissue grafts or tumours, as well as the elimination of virus-infected cells. Some of these T lymphocytes are cytotoxic, either as natural killer (NK) cells or through antibody-dependent reactions. B lymphocytes synthesize and secrete specific immunoglobulins in response to a broad range of antigens. From this presentation, it is obvious that viral infections of T or B cells may be linked to a variety of disorders characterized by immunodeficiency and autoimmunity. In this brief review, we shall:

1) evaluate the immunological consequences of acute viral infections by orthomyxoviruses (measles virus) or paramyxoviruses (influenza virus).

2) outline the involvement of human retroviruses in immunodeficiencies and in hematologic diseases, using data from the French West Indies.

MYXOVIRUSES, IMMUNODEFICIENCY AND AUTOIMMUNITY

It has been shown that measles viral antigens are expressed in lymphocytes harvested from patients during acute infection (4). Similarly, influenza viral antigens have been found on the surface of lymphocytes in the blood of patients suffering from an acute infection (5). In vitro, both viruses were able to replicate in monocytes, in B and T lymphocytes (6,7). One recent experiment (8) indicated that measles virus blocked the proliferation of infected lymphocyte cultures, but without any cytocidal effects. This silent infection resulted in the abortion of functional properties of T and B lymphocytes: loss of NK activity of the T cells, and shut-off of IgG and IgM synthesis by B cells. Similar observations were made on lymphocyte cultures infected with influenza virus: they failed to synthesize immunoglobulins, but retained their NK activity (8).

The abrogation of the lymphocyte functions by measles and influenza viruses is dependent on infecting these cells before their differentiation into mature T and B cells. Indeed, the infection of IgM-producing lymphoblasts with measles virus did not alter immunoglobulin synthesis and secretion, which persisted during the release of infectious particles. Concerning the influenza-infected lymphoblasts, the synthesis of viral proteins did not affect that of immunoglobulins, which is maintained until the cell lysis. However, we have shown that the action of the viral neuraminidase led to the secretion of immunoglobulins lacking the last terminal sugar, i.e., sialic acid (9). This qualitative alteration is of paramount importance, since such hyposialylated immunoglobulins have been shown to be immunogenic, at the origin of immune complexes (10), to mediate the release of myeloperoxydase from monocytes (11), and to be arthritogenic, inducing the inflammatory and degenerative lesions characteristic of rheumatoid arthritis (12).

In summary, the immunosuppression observed during the course of some acute viral infections results from the direct interactions of these viruses with lymphocytes and from the subsequent impairment of their specific functions. Moreover, viral infections may affect immunoglobulins secreted by mature B lymphocytes. These qualitative alterations somehow outlast the viral cytocidal effects, an argument in favor of the viral etiology of some autoimmune diseases.

HUMAN RETROVIRUSES AND IMMUNOLOGICAL DISORDERS

The discovery of human T-lymphotropic viruses (HTLV) was consecutive to the isolation and characterization of TCGF (1) and to the findings that feline leukemia virus (FeLV) and bovine leukemia virus (BLV) were the causative agents of naturally occurring leukemias and lymphomas in cats and in cattle, respectively (13,14,15). Moreover, the observations that FeLV induced severe immunodepression of pet cats and predisposed them to numerous opportunistic infections, have provided an interesting model in the search for a viral etiology for the acquired immune-deficiency syndrome (AIDS) in humans (14).

Others in this volume will review in detail the pathobiology and molecular biology of viruses belonging to the HTLV family. These viruses display a T-lymphotropism, with an apparent preference for helper T lymphocytes, and share some sequence homology and antigenic determinants. HTLV-I was shown to be associated to adult T-cell leukemia/lymphoma, present in regions where HTLV is endemic (Southwest Japan, and the Caribbean). HTLV-III/LAV has been isolated from patients with lymphoadenopathy and AIDS (16,17). In those patients the quantitative decrease of the helper subset of T cells, and the concomittant reversal of the helper/suppressive ratio are accompanied by numerous T-cell abnormalities. Moreover, B cells are polyclonally activated, which results in an hypergammaglobulinemia. In vitro, these cells do not respond to signals for B cell activation (18,19).

Besides the prominent property of HTLV-1 to immortalize T cells (13), this virus has been shown to be an equally important modulator of the immune functions of these cells. Thus, HTLV-positive leukemic cells appeared to act as suppressors of immunoglobulin synthesis, despite having a helper phenotype (20). Moreover, HTLV-transformed cells secrete a wide array of lymphokines (21). Finally, recent observations indicate that HTLV-I can infect B cells or B cell precursors, which are immortalised, even in the absence of the Epstein Barr virus genome (22,23).

The ability of HTLV-I to interfere with lymphocyte functions should therefore be considered in areas of HTLV-I endemic infection. Thus, on the island of Martinique (French West Indies), a high prevalence of HTLV-I antibodies (Table I) was observed not only in patients with non-Hodgkin's lymphoma (24), but also in those with monoclonal gammopathies (a B cell disease).

Table 1. HTLV antibodies in Martinique

Group Characteristics	No. Tested	HTLV-I positive	HTLV-III positive
Patients:			
non-Hodgkin's lymphoma	24	9(37.5)	0
chronic lymphocytic leukemia	7	0	0
acute lymphoblastic leukemia	8	0	1
Hodgkin's disease	5	0	0
monoclonal gammapathies	6	3(50.0%)	0
Blood donors (age 30-60)	108	4(3.7%)	1(0.9%)
Old people (age 60-90)	114	16(14.0%)	NT
Sickle cell anemia			
homozygotes SS	57	8(14.0%)	1(1.8%)
heterozygotes AS	21	1(4.8%)	0

NOTE: HTLV-I and HTLV-III antibodies were detected by using linked immuno-absorbent assay (ELISA), and confirmed in competition assays for HTLV-I, and by Western blot techniques for HTLV-III. NT = not tested.

In healthy individuals, the antibody prevalence correlated with age. In fact, among blood donors in the age range 30-60 years, approximately 4% were positive, versus 14% positive among old people (over age 60). Whatever the explanations of the correlation between age and antibodies (virus latency or late infection), immunodeficiency associated with HTLV-I might add to the loss of immune competence with age. Such synergism would contribute to an increased susceptibility of HTLV-infected elderly people to infectious and neoplastic diseases.

Repeated blood transfusions are probably at the origin of the prevalence of HTLV-I antibodies observed in sickle cell anemia patients (homozygous SS) (25). Whether antibody-positive patients develop infectious diseases more often than antibody negative-ones is currently being determined.

Finally, a very low prevalence of HTLV-III antibodies was observed. This relative absence of such antibodies brings further evidence that HTLV-I and HTLV-III have different epidemiological patterns.

The seroepidemiological survey in Martinique delineates the implications of HTLV in normal and pathological conditions, and provides guidelines for a broader survey still to be conducted in African populations. Indeed, in Africa, which is most probably the reservoir of HTLV (13,36), the impairment of immune functions by these viruses represents a public health problem, since it may affect the quality of response to vaccination to different antigens and explain the gravity of parasitic and infectious diseases on that continent.

CONCLUSIONS

The unique interactions between immunocompetent cells and RNA viruses provide a better understanding of the pathobiological strategies used by these viruses to impair the immune responses, and to cause immune defects, which might be linked to the etiology of some chronic disorders. Indeed, injury of the immune system by these viruses may result from: a) subtle effects on cell metabolism and function without any structural change; b) immortalization and proliferation of the infected cells, at the origin of the homeostatic imbalance among the different populations, and c) cytocidal effects resulting in a depletion of a subset of immunocompetent cells, both leading to mild or severe immunodeficiencies. Finally, if one takes into account the regulatory influences of T lymphocytes on haematopoiesis (27), HTLV in regions of endemic infection may be implicated in a wide range of haematological diseases.

ACKNOWLEDGEMENTS

We thank Dr. R.C. Gallo for most stimulating discussions, and for permitting L.G. to work in his laboratory, within the framework of an ICRETT fellowship. Technical support of Ms. Andrea Jennings was deeply appreciated. This study was made possible through financial help from CNRS (GIS 410017), INSERM (CRL no 812027), the Virus Cancer Prevention Association of Martinique, and Fondation pour la Recherche Médicale, France.

REFERENCES

1. Robert-Guroff, M., Sarngadharan, M.G. & Gallo, R.C. (1984) In Growth and maturation factors, vol. 2, ed. Guroff, G., (J. Wiley & Sons, New York), pp. 267-308.
2. Melchers, F. & Andersson, J. (1984) Cell 37, 715-720.
3. Smith, K.A. (1984) In Fundamental Immunology, ed. Paul, W.E. (Raven Press, New York), pp. 559-576.
4. Whittle, H.C., Dossetor, J., Oduloju, A., Bryceson, D.M. & Greenwood, B.M. (1978) J. Clin. Invest. 62, 678-687.
5. Wilson, A.B., Planterose, D.N., Nagington, J., Park, J.R., Barry,R.D., & Coombs, R.R.A. (1976) Nature 259, 582-284.
6. Sullivan, J.L., Barry, R.W., Lucas, S.J., & Albrecht, P. (1975) J. Exp. Med. 142, 773-784.
7. Jacobson, S. & McFarland, H. (1982) J. Gen. Virol. 63, 351-357.
8. Casal, P., Rice, G.P.A. & Olstone, M.B.A. (1984) J. Exp. Med. 159, 1322-1337.
9. Duc Dodon, M., Gazzolo, L., Quash, G.A. & Wild, F.W. (1982) J. Gen. Virol. 63, 441-450.
10. Duc Dodon M. & Quash, G.A. (1981) Immunology 42, 401-408.
11. Duc Dodon, M., Gazzolo, L. & Quash, G.A. (1984) Immunology 52, 291-297.

12. Galloway, G., Leung, A.Y.T., Hunneyball, I.M. & Stanworth, D.R. (1983) Immunology 49, 511-519.
13. Gallo, R.C. (1984) Cancer Surveys 3, 114-159.
14. Hardy, W.D., Jr., (1984) In Human T-cell leukemia/lymphoma virus, eds. Gallo, R.C., Essex, M.E. & Gross, L. (Cold Spring Harbor Laboratory) pp. 35-43.
15. Burny, A., Bruck, C., Couez, D. Deschamps, J., Ghysdael, J., Kettman, R., Mammerickx, M., Marbaix, G. & Portetelle, D. (1984) In Human t-cell leukemia/lymphoma virus, eds. Gallo, R.C., Essex, M.E. & Gross, L. (Cold Spring harbor Laboratory) pp. 17-24.
16. Papovic, M., Sarngadharan, M.G., Read, E. & Gallo, R.C. (1984) Science 224, 497-500.
17. Barré-Sinoussi, F., Chermann, J.C., Rey, F., Nugeyre, M.T., Chamaret, S., Gruest, J., Dauguet, C., Axler-Blin, C., Vézinet-Brun, F., Rouzioux, C., Rozenbaum, W. & Montagnier, L. (1984) Science 220, 868-870.
18. Lane, H.C., Masur, H., Edgar, L.C., Whalen, G. & Fauci, A.S. (1983) N. Eng. J. Med. 309, 453-458.
19. Siegal, F.P. (1984) Seminars in Oncology 11, 29-39.
20. Waldmann, T.A., Greene, W.C., Sarin, P.S., Saxinger, C., Blayney, D.W., Blattner, W.A., Goldman, C.K., Bongiovanni, K., Sharrow, S., Depper, J.M., Leonard, W., Uchiyama, T. & Gallo, R.C. (1984) J. Clin. Invest. 73, 1711-1718.
21. Mann, D.L., Clark, J., Clarke, M., Reitz, M., Popovic, M., Fanchini, G., Trainoir, C.D., Strong, D.M., Blattner, W.A., & Gallo, R.C. (1984) J. Clin. Invest. 74, 56-62.
22. Ongo, D.L., Gelmann, E.P., Cossman, J., Young, R.A., Gallo, R.C., O'Brien, S.J. & Matis, L.A. (1984) Nature 310, 505-506.
23. Markham, P.D., Salahuddin S.Z., & Gallo, R.C. (1984) Clinics in Haematology 13, 423-446.
24. Gessain, A., Jouanelle, A., Escarment, P., Calender, A., Schaffar-Deshayes, L. & de-Thé, G. (1984) Lance, i, 1183-1184.
25. Gessain, A., Gazzolo, L., Yoyo, M., Fortier, L.,

Robert-Guroff, M. & de-Thé, G. (1984) Lancet, submitted for publication.

26. Gessain, A., Calender, A., Strobel, M., Lefait-Robin, R. & de-Thé (1984) C.R. Acad. Sci. (Paris), in press.
27. Premier forum d'immunologie (1984) Ann. Immunol. 135C, 261-302.

ANTI HTLV-III AND ANTI T-CELL ANTIBODIES IN AIDS AND ARC PATIENTS

H.L. Ioachim, W.J. Cronin, B.H. Dorsett, D. Triglia, and F.C. Jensen

Departments of Pathology of Lenox Hill Hospital and College of Physicians and Surgeons of Columbia University, New York, N.Y., and Cytotech, San Diego, Ca.

The number of surface immunoglobulins (SIg)-positive lymphocytes was found to increase when normal lymphocytes were incubated with sera of AIDS or ARC patients. These circulating antilymphocyte antibodies were selectively reactive with OKT4- but not with OKT8-staining T-cells. In the present study, AIDS, ARC and control patients were evaluated for antilymphocyte antibodies, anti HTLV-III antibodies and helper/suppressor (h/s) T-cell ratios. In the AIDS group, 23 of 24 patients had circulating HTLV-III antibodies, 24 of 24 showed markedly decreased h/s T-cell ratios and 19 of 21 patients showed marked elevation of anti-lymphocyte antibodies. In contrast, in control patients, none of 14 had HTLV-III antibodies, 13 of 14 had normal h/s T-cell ratios and 3 of 11 showed small increases in antilymphocyte antibodies. In the ARC group, 16 of 16 had circulating anti HTLV-III antibodies. 11 of 15 had decreased h/s T-cell ratios and 6 of 11 showed elevated anti T-cell antibodies. The correlations obtained between these tests and clinical diagnoses indicate their potential usefulness in the detection and monitoring of AIDS and ARC patients.

In the 3 years since first reported in 1981, male homosexuals in major American cities and abroad have been the principal victims of an epidemic of severe opportunistic infections and neoplasias, collectively referred to as acquired immune deficiency syndrome (AIDS). In the same interval and locations, male homosexuals have even more frequently presented with a syndrome of fever of unexplained origin, weight loss and generalized lymphadenopathy, AIDS related complex (ARC), that has often preceded by up to three years the opportunistic infections and neoplasias of AIDS (1). Morphologic studies of the lymph nodes involved, revealed lesions of acute, severe lymphadenitis entirely similar to those observed in the lymphadenitides of infectious mononucleosis, vaccinia, herpes zoster and CMV, thus strongly supporting the hypothesis of a viral infection as the basis of AIDS (2-3). Several viruses including EBV, CMV, and HBV to which AIDS patients have significantly high antibody titers, were each considered as the potential agent inducing the critical immune deficiency (4-6). More recently, strong evidence has been provided for the implication of human lymphotroic retroviruses in the etiology of AIDS. HTLV-III and LAV were repeatedly isolated from peripheral blood and lymph node T-lymphocytes of patients with AIDS (7-8) while antibodies against HTLV-III were detected in 88% of patients with AIDS and in 79% of patients with ARC as compared to less than 1% in normal controls (9). Retroviruses have been known to induce immune deficiency in murine and feline hosts thus suggesting that in AIDS the initial viral infection may cause the immune deficiency by selective annihilation of specific populations of lymphocytes. To explore the mechanisms of lymphopenia and of the reversed helper/suppressor ratios in patients with ARC and AIDS, we examined their sera for the presence of antibodies reactive with normal lymphocytes. The percentage of surface immunoglobulin (SIg)-positive cells (B-cells) present in a preparation of Ficoll-Hypaque-isolated lymphocytes of a normal control were determined. Normal

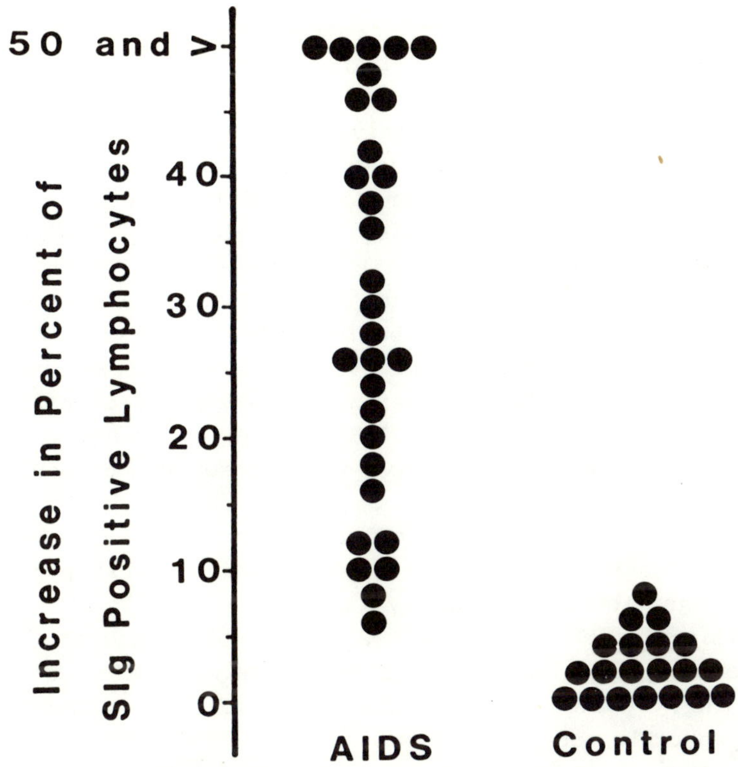

Figure 1. Augmentation of SIg-positive counts after incubation with AIDS and control sera.

lymphocytes from the same source were then incubated with normal sera or sera of AIDS or ARC patients, washed and incubated with FITC-labeled $F(ab')_2$ fragment of goat anti-human immunoglobulin. The presence of anti-lymphocyte antibodies was determined by the increase in the number of SI-positive lymphocytes that occurred as a result of prior incubation with the sera tested. 29 sera of 30 AIDS patients tested, generated increases in SIg-positive cells ranging from 6 to 75 cells per 100. All sera of 20 normal controls produced SIg-positive cell increases of 8% or less (Figure 1). To determine whether the anti-lymphocyte antibodies in AIDS sera were preferentially reactive with helper or suppressor T-cells, double labeling experiments with specific monoclonal antibodies were used.

Normal lymphocytes were sequentially incubated with test sera, monoclonal antibodies OKT4, OHT8, or OKT11 and FITC-labeled antimouse immunoglobulins (non reactive with human immunoglobulins). Patient anti-lymphocyte antibodies were detected with TRITC-labeled anti human immunoglobulins (non reactive with mouse immunoglobulins). The results of these tests on 4 AIDS patients sera and 4 normal controls demonstrated that antibody reactivity was directed against cells that were OKT4 or OKT11 positive. No significant reactivity was detectable with OKT8 positive cells (Figure 2). Normal donors' sera, demonstrating low levels of antilymphocyte antibody binding, showed no apparent specificity toward any T-lymphocyte sub-populations.

Although some variation in the SIg-positive lymphocyte counts with target cells from different donors was noted, the AIDS sera consistently generated significant increases while normal sera did not. Preliminary results using monospecific second antibodies suggest that the anti-lymphocyte activity in AIDS serum is due to IgGs.

In a correlative study, the augmentation in SIg-positive lymphocytes (ASIgL) test was performed in parallel with the determination of anti-HTLV-III antibody titers by an enzyme immuno-assay (ELISA) and with the estimation of T-cell helper/suppressor ratios (Table 1).

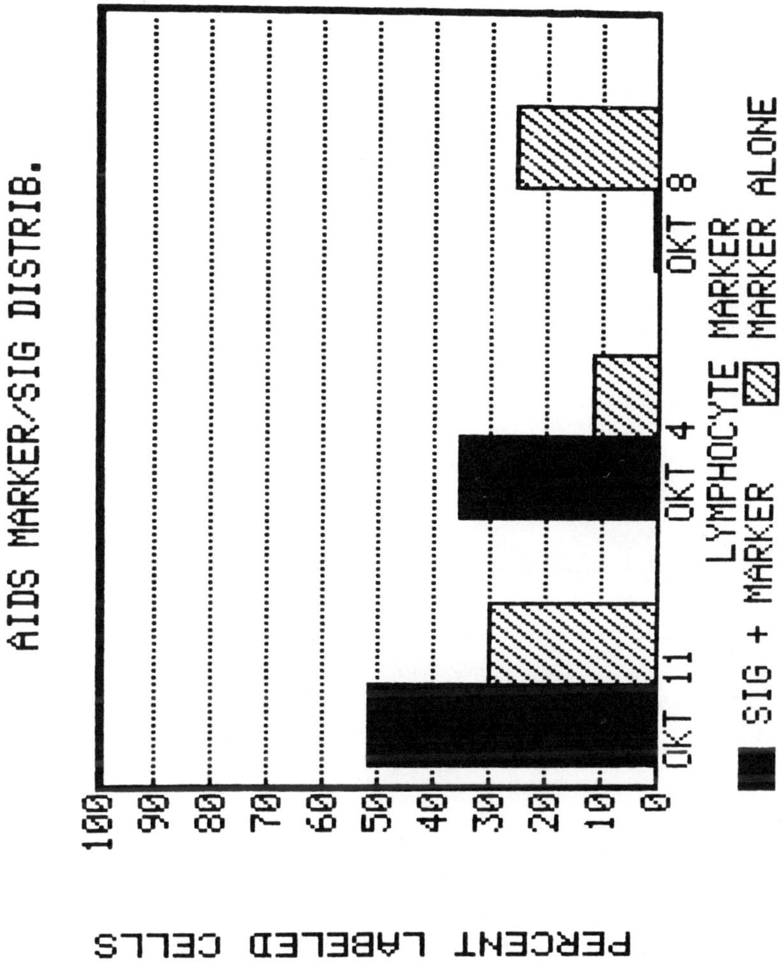

Figure 2. Double labeling of lymphocytes after incubation with serum of AIDS patient and anti T-cells monoclonal antibodies.

Of 24 patients with AIDS, 23 were positive for HTLV-III. In the same group the h/s ratio had a range of .01-.7 and a mean of .28, while the ASIgL test showed a range of 6 to 75 and a mean of 35.3. The two patients who showed no significant increase in the ASIgL test were deeply immunosuppressed with h/s ratios of .05 and 0.1 respectively and have subsequently expired. In the group of ARC patients, 16 of 16 were positive for HTLV-III. The h/s ratio had a range of .1 to 1.4 with a mean of .59 in 15 patients tested. The ASIgL test showed a mean increase of 14.5 with a range of 2 to 43 in 11 patients tested. Finally in the group of non-AIDS controls, all 14 were negative for HTLV-III antibodies. The h/s ratio was within normal limits with a mean of 1.57 ranging well above .8 in all but one 74

Table 1. Anti HTLV-III antibodies, helper/suppressor ratios and anti-lymphocytes antibodies in AIDS, ARC and control patients

Groups	HTLV-III	h/s		ASIgL	
		24/24 -	.8	19/21 -	8%
AIDS	23/24 pos.	mean	.28	mean	35.3
		median	.3	median	36
		range	.01-.7	range	6-75
		11/15 -	.8	6/11 -	8%
ARC	16/16 pos.	mean	.59	mean	14.5
		median	.6	median	9
		range	.1-1.4	range	2-43
		13/14	.8	3/11	8%
Controls	0/14 pos.	mean	1.57	mean	7.6
		median	1.6	median	7
		range	.7-2.4	range	1-16

year-old man with non-AIDS Kaposi's sarcoma whose ratio was .7. The ASIgL test showed a mean increase of 7.6 ranging from 1 to 16. Two of the 3 patients showing slight elevations had non-AIDS Kaposi's sarcoma.

The present results indicate that both AIDS and ARC patients have circulating anti lymphocyte antibodies reactive with an antigen present on helper but not on suppressor T-cells. They also show the presence of anti HTLV-III antibodies in both AIDS and ARC patients with overall higher activity in the latter group. A significant correlation was obtained between the presence of HTLV-III antibody, h/s ratios and ASIgL counts in all three groups of patients tested. The estimation of circulating anti lymphocyte antibodies and of anti HTLV-III antibodies represent valuable tests for the detection and monitoring of the AIDS and ARC patients.

REFERENCES

1. Ioachim, H.L., (1984) Editorial. Acquired Immune Deficiency Disease after Three Years. The Unsolved Riddle. Lab. Invest. 51, 1-6.
2. Ioachim, H.L., Lerner, W.C. & Tapper, M.L. (1983) The Lymphoid Lesions Associated with the acquired immunodeficiency syndrome. Am. J. Surg. Pathol. 7,543.
3. Ioachim, H.L., Lerner, W.C. & Tapper, M.L. (1983) Lymphadenopathies in homosexual men: relationships with the acquired immune deficiency syndrome. JAMA 250, 1306.
4. Sonnabend J., Witkin, S.S. & Purtilo, D.R. (1983) Acquired immunodeficiency syndrome, opportunistic infections, and malignancies in male homosexuals. JAMA 249, 2370.
5. Drew W.L., Miner, R.C., Ziegler, J.L., Gullett, J.H., Abrams, D.I., Conant, M.A., Huang, E.S., Groundwater, J.R., Volberging, P. & Mintz, L. (1982) Cytomegalovirus and Kaposi's sarcoma in young homosexual men. Lancet 1, 125.

6. McDonald, M.I., Hamilton, J.E. & Durack, D.T. (1983) Hepatitis B surface antigen could harbour the infective agent of AIDS. Lancet 1, 882.
7. Gallo, R.C., Salahuddin, S.Z., Papovic, M., et al.(1984) Frequent detection and isolation of cytopathic retroviruses (HTLV-III) from patients with AIDS and at risk for AIDS. Science 224, 500.
8. Barré-Sinoussi, F., Chermann, J.C., Rey, F. et al.(1983) Isolation of a T-lymphotropic retrovirus from a patient at risk for acquired immune deficiency syndrome (AIDS). Science 220, 868.
9. Sarngadharan, M.G., Popovic, M., Bruch, L. et al.(1984) Antibodies reactive with human T-lymphotropic retroviruses (HTLV-III) in the serum of patients with AIDS. Science 224, 506.

SEROEPIDEMIOLOGICAL STUDY OF LYMPHADENOPATHY ASSOCIATED VIRUS, BY ELISA, IN ACQUIRED IMMUNODEFICIENCY SYNDROME

F. Brun-Vezinet and Ch. Rouzioux

Laboratoire Central, Virologie, Hopital Claude Bernard, Paris, France

Lymphadenopathy Associated Virus (LAV) was isolated from T-cultured lymphocytes of a homosexual man with lymphadenopathy syndrome (LAS) in 1983. Since then, it has been repeatedly isolated from AIDS patients belonging to different risk groups: homosexual, haemophiliac, Haitian and Zairian. We present here the results of the detection of IgG antibodies to LAV by ELISA, in patients with AIDS or AIDS related diseases compared to different control groups. First, we show the high seropositivity in both French AIDS patients (75%; 67/90) and French LAS patients (90%; 99/110). Very similar results were obtained from sera of American AIDS or LAS patients. Second, we present the results in 3 groups of haemophiliacs under different treatment. The last part concerns seroepidemiological results in Zairian AIDS patients: 88% LAV-ab-positive (32/36) compared to the control groups. The high prevalence of IgG antibodies to LAV in AIDS patients provides strong evidence for the role played by the virus in AIDS.

In early 1983, a human retrovirus was isolated from T-cultured lymphocytes of a homosexual man showing the lymphadenopathy syndrome (LAS) (1). Since then, this virus named Lymphadenopathy-Associated Virus (LAV) has been repeatedly isolated from different cases of AIDS: homosexual men, haemophiliacs, Haitian and African patients (2) (3) (4). We performed an ELISA in order to investigate the presence of IgG antibodies to LAV in patients with AIDS or AIDS related diseases compared to different control groups.

LAV-ELISA

The method is described in detail elsewhere (5). Briefly, for the antigen preparation, LAV was propagated in T-lymphocytes of a healthy donor or adapted to a B-lymphoblastoid cell line (6). The cell-free supernatant was precipitated by 10% polyethylene-glycol. The virus was purified by banding two or three times on a 20-60% sucrose gradient. After concentration by high speed centrifugation, the virus was disrupted by 1% triton. A lysate of the same uninfected lymphocytes was used as control antigen. For coating, viral and control antigens were used at the same protein concentration (2-2.5 ug/ml). Each serum, prediluted at 1/40, was tested in duplicate on both antigens. Sera were considered as positive when the differential optical density was equal to or higher than 0.30 A negative control serum was included at 1/40 dilution, and the positive reference serum was tested at four dilutions (a standard curve can be used to measure the antibody titers).

RESULTS

In France 75% (67/90) of AIDS patients have IgG antibodies to LAV (5). They belong to different risk groups: 63% are homosexual men, 13% Africans, 9% Haitians, 1% are haemophiliacs and 1% are transfusion associated AIDS cases. In France no cases of AIDS have been reported in drug addicts.

Table 1. Lav serology in French patients.

DONORS/PATIENTS	IgG-LAV POSITIVE	PERCENT POSITIVE
AIDS	67/90	74.4%
LAS, ARC	99/110	90%
French controls		
Contacts of homosexual AIDS cases		
Sexual contacts	16/34	50%
Non sexual contacts	0/10	
Gay control group	14/54	26%
Unselected blood donors	1/300	
Laboratory workers	0/30	
Rheumatoid arthritis	0/30	

In the group of patients with LAS the seropositivity is about 90% (Table 1).

The test of specificity included in this ELISA is very important because it reveals the unspecific binding of sera which contain the Rheumatoid Factor or Immune Complexes or Auto-Immune antibodies. These reactions may occur during AIDS and without the test of specificity AIDS patient's sera would easily give false positive results.

Sequential sera were provided from patients with AIDS: they showed a real decrease of LAV antibody titer during the course of the disease (5). This fact may explain why LAV-ab are not detected in all AIDS cases.

Different control groups were selected for comparison and we show significant differences between those groups. In a control group of 300 unselected blood donors, one serum was IgG LAV positive (a healthy, 19-year-old woman) no positive serum was found among 30 laboratory workers (Table 1). In a gay control group with multiple partners

Table 2. LAV serology in 251 haemophiliacs

Donors	IgG-LAV POSITIVE	%
GROUP I heavily transfused with french and american blood products		
French	79/134	59%
A Haemophiliacs	67/105	68.8%
B Haemophiliacs	12/23	52.2%
Willebrand's disease	0/6	
GROUP II lightly transfused with french and american blood products		
French	6/58	10.3%
A Haemophiliacs	4/49	8.2%
B Haemophiliacs	2/9	22.2%
GROUP III heavily and lightly transfused only with local blood products		
Belgium	2/59	3.4%

Statistical significance (P) : group I vs II < 0.0005, group I vs III < 0.0005, group II vs III $= 0.13$

Table 3. LAV serology in American patients.

PATIENTS	IgG-LAV POSITIVE	PERCENT POSITIVE
AIDS	83/114	72%
LAS, ARC	33/38	87%
Gay population (N.Y.)	29/90	32%

18% (8/44) had antibody to LAV. Among sexual partners of French homosexual AIDS cases, without any clinical symptoms, the seropositivity was 50% (16/34). None of the non-sexual contacts of AIDS patients had antibody to LAV (0/10) (unpublished data).

Similar results were obtained by testing coded sera from American patients (New York and CDC): 72% (83/114) of AIDS patients, 87% (33/38) of LAS and 17% (3/18) of gay control group had IgG antibodies to LAV (Table 3).

Whatever the different manifestations of AIDS, the positivity is not significantly different:

AIDS with Kaposi Sarcoma (KS) alone:	14/24 (58%)
AIDS with Opportunistic Infections (OI):	23/36 (64%)
AIDS with KS + OI:	9/14 (64%)

In these American patients LAV was isolated from two intravenous drug users with AIDS and from one homosexual with LAS (7).

Table 4. IgG-LAV positivity in haemophiliacs according to extent of transfusion during 1983

GROUP	TRANSFUSION U/Kg/Y	IgG-LAV POSITIVE	(%)
GROUP I	800	32/73	44%
	800	47/61	77%
GROUP II	800	4/53	7.5%
	800	2/5	

A significant higher number of patients treated with > 800 U/Kg/Y had LAV antibody in group I, and in group I and II taken together.

Table 5. AIDS in a B Haemophiliac.

PATIENT	LAV ISOLATION	IgG-LAV POSITIVE	
AIDS patient		Feb 82	1:320
		Feb 83	1:80
	+	May 83	1:40
		Dec 83	1:40
His brother			
asymptomatic B haemophiliac		Feb 83	1:160
	+	May 83	1:160
		Dec 83	1:160
His mother	–	May 83	1:40
His father	–	May 83	1:40

Two groups of French haemophiliacs and one of Belgian haemophiliacs, differently treated were tested for IgG-abs to LAV (8, Table 2). The French haemophiliacs were perfused indifferently by French and foreign blood products (coming from paid blood donors of USA); Group I was heavily perfused and group II was very lightly treated. Group III was composed of Belgian haemophiliacs who were treated only with local products (coming from unpaid blood donors). The results show a significant difference ($p < 0.0005$) of seropositivity between the intensively perfused group I: 59% (79/134) and the less transfused group II: 10.3% (6/58). Group III had the lowest seropositivity 3.4% (2/59) significantly different from the other two groups (Table 4).

Moreover, three haemophiliacs (A or B) with AIDS (opportunistic infections) were tested for LAV antibody. All were positive. A sequential sera study of a B haemophiliac showed a real decrease of seropositity during the course of AIDS (Table 5), while LAV was repeatedly isolated from his peripheral blood lymphocytes (3). This

LAV was transmitted via transfusion of blood derived products and resisted the treatments used to prepare factor VIII and IX concentrates and cryoprecipitates. A possibility is that in some patients LAV seropositivity may only represent antibodies to proteins of inactivated virus.

Coded sera from Zairian AIDS patients, collected in 1983, were also screened for antibodies to LAV (9, Table 6). 32/36 (88%) were found to be positive by ELISA. In a control group of 26 patients with infectious diseases (tuberculosis and malaria) 5 (19%) were positive. All had a low T4/T8 ratio with T4 cells 400/mm^3. In 1980, 100 sera were collected from Zairian mothers and 5 were LAV positive. From 100 sera obtained from patients without infectious diseases, in 1983, 7 were LAV positive (Table 6).

Table 6. LAV serology in Zairian patients.

PATIENTS	IgG-LAV POSITIVE	PERCENT POSITIVE
AIDS (1983)	32/36	88%
ARC (1983)	4/4	
Zairian Controls		
Hospitalized patients for infectious diseases 1983	5/26	19%
Hospitalized patients for non infectious diseases 1983	7/100	7%
Mother's sera for hepatitis B studies 1980	5/100	5%

A good correlation was found between the results of LAV serology by ELISA and radioimmunoprecipitation assay (RIPA) (5, 9). This last test, using metabolic labelling of the virus with ^{35}S-methionine, detected mainly antibodies to p25 major core protein. In a few cases, sera were negative by ELISA but highly positive by RIPA indicating a higher sensitivity of this last assay for the detection of antibody to p25. In contrast some positive results were obtained by ELISA and not by RIPA, suggesting that the patients' sera contained antibodies to other viral proteins. This was verified by western blot analysis and radioimmunoprecipitation using ^{125}I viral proteins. With these tests, antibodies to p18 and p13 could also be detected in some patients'sera.

These seroepidemiological studies showed a prevalence of IgG antibodies to LAV in patients with AIDS and AIDS related diseases, compared to control groups. A selective tropism of LAV for helper-inducer T-lymphocytes was demonstrated (10) and LAV was easily isolated from numerous AIDS patients. All these data provide very strong evidence for the role played by LAV in AIDS.

REFERENCES

1. Barre-Sinoussi F., Chermann J.C., Rey F., Nugeyre M.T., Chamaret S., Gruest J., Dauguet C., Axler C., Brun-Vezinet F, Rouzioux Ch., Rozenbaum, W., Montagnier L. (1983) Science 220:868-870.
2. Montagnier L., Barre-Sinoussi F., Rozenbaum W., Brun-Vezinet F., Rouzioux Ch, Klatzmann D., Gluckman J.C. & Chermann J.C.. (1983). Cancer Cell CSH Vol. III
3. Vilmer E., Barre-Sinoussi F, Rouzioux Ch., Gazengel C., Brun-Vezinet F., Dauguet C., Fisher A., Manigne P., Chermann J.C., Grischelli C., Montagnier L. (1984). Lancet 753-757.
4. Ellrodt A., Barre-Sinoussi F., Lebras Ph., Nugeyre M.T., Palazzo L., Rey F., Brun-Vezinet F., Rouzioux Ch., Segond P., Caquet R., Montagnier L., Chermann

J.C. (1984) Lancet 1383-1385.

5. Brun-Vezinet F., Rouzioux Ch., Barre-Sinoussi F., Klatzmann D., Saimot A.G., Rozenbaum W., Christol D., Gluckman J.C., Montagnier L., Chermann J.C. (1984) Lancet 1253-1256.
6. Montagnier L., Gruest J., Chamaret S., Dauguet C., Axler C., Guetard D., Nugeyre M.T., Barre-Sinoussi F., Chermann J.C., Brunet J.B., Klatzmann D., Gluckman J.C. (1984) Science 225:63-66.
7. Barre-Sinoussi F., Usha-Mathur-Wagh, Rey F., Brun-Vezinet F., Rouzioux Ch., Yancovitz S., Montagnier L., Mildvan D., Chermann J.C. (1984) Annals of Internal Medicine (in press).
8. Rouzioux Ch., Brun-Vezinet F., Courrouce A.M., Gazengel C., Vergoz D., Desmyter J., Vermylen J., Vermylen C., Klatzmann D., Geroldi D., Barreau C., Barre-Sinoussi F., Chermann J.C., Christol D., Montagnier L. (1984) Submitted.
9. Brun-Vezinet F., Rouzioux Ch., Montagnier, L., Chamaret S., Gruest J., Barre-Sinoussi F., Geroldi D., Chermann J.C., McCormick J., Mitchell S., Piot P., Taelman H., Bila K., Wobin O., Mbendi N., Mazebo P., Kayembe K., Bridts C., Desmyter J., Feinsod F.M., Quinn T.C. (1984) Science (in press).
10 Klatzmann D., Barre-Sinoussi F., Nugeyre M.T., Dauguet C., Vilmer E., Griscelli C., Brun-Vezinet F., Rouzioux Ch. Gluckman J.C., Chermann J.C., Montagnier L. (1984) Science 225:59-63.

IgG ANTIBODIES TO SAIDS-D VIRUS ASSOCIATED ANTIGENS IN PATIENTS WITH AIDS AND AT RISK FOR AIDS

J. Goudsmit, M. Gravell, F.W. van der Walls, J.L. Sever, C.J. Gibbs Jr. and D.C. Gajdusek

Virology Department of the University of Amsterdam, the Netherlands, and NINCDS (LCNSS & IDB), National Institutes of Health, Bethesda, Md., U.S.A.

A new type D retrovirus (SAIDS-DV) has been identified as the cause of simian AIDS. Because of the similarity between simian and human AIDS the rates of exposure to SAIDS-DV in patients with AIDS and at risk for AIDS relative to the normal population were determined. One of 6 AIDS patients and 5 of 15 pre-AIDS patients had antibodies to SAIDS-DV compared to 20 of 78 healthy homosexuals, 20 of 53 hemophiliacs and 17 of 52 normal controls. No cross-reactivity with HTLV-I and LAV(HTLV-III), but some cross-reactivity with Mason-Pfizer monkey virus (MPMV) was observed.

A new type D retrovirus related to but distinct from Mason-Pfizer monkey virus (MPMV) has recently been identified as the cause of simian acquired immune deficiency syndrome (SAIDS) (1). Monkeys of the genus *Macaca* housed in three regional primate centres in the USA have acquired SAIDS by natural means. Highly purified virus isolated from a monkey with SAIDS transmitted the disease to previously healthy monkeys 2 to 4 weeks after intravenous inoculation (2). SAIDS-D virus (SAIDS-DV) shared gag-related antigens with MPMV, but not with type C retroviruses of monkeys or the human retroviruses HTLV-I (3) or LAV(HTLV-III).

SAIDS resembles human AIDS and is characterized by immunosuppression opportunistic infections and tumors and chronic wasting. Because of these similarities we decided to determine if patients with AIDS and at risk for AIDS had increased rates of exposure to SAIDS-DV relative to the normal population.

Serum samples were obtained from six patients with AIDS, 15 patients with Lymphadenopathy syndrome (LAS) or Gay Bowel syndrome (GBS), 78 unmatched healthy homosexual men, 53 healthy hemophiliacs and 52 healthy blood donors not belonging to any risk-group for AIDS. These samples were tested under blind conditions for antibodies to SAIDS-DV by ELISA using purified virus(IDB-2) as antigen. The virus used as antigen was grown in rhesus monkey cells and purified by discontinuous and continuous density gradient centrifugation in neutral sucrose and had an isopyknic density of 1.15 g/ml. Peak absorbance of 254 nm and reverse transcriptase activity coincided in the pooled fractions used as antigen. In the ELISA the absorbances of the test samples were determined at 490 nm and sera were regarded as positive when the optical density of the test sample exceeded a negative control serum three times at a dilution of 1:40. Control positive sera at four dilutions and a control negative serum were tested in each test.

To test for cross-reactivity with MPMV, HTLV-I and HTLV-III both ELISA and indirect immunofluorescence tests were used.

One of 6 AIDS patients and 5 of 15 LAS/GBS patients had antibodies to SAIDS-DV. These proportions did not differ significantly from those observed in healthy homosexual men (20/78), hemophiliacs (20/53) or normal controls (17/52) (Table 1). Cross-reactivity of neutral antibodies to SAIDS-DV with the human type C and D retroviruses HTLV-I and LAV(HTLV-III) was not observed, confirming the previously reported antigenic

Table 1. Antibodies to the type D retrovirus SAIDS-DV and MPMV in patients with AIDS and at risk for AIDS

Subject	Number tested	Anti-SAIDS-DV (%)	Anti-MPMV (%)
patients with AIDS	6	1(-)	1(-)
patients with LAS/GBS	15	5(30)	2(13)
Homosexual men	78	20(26)	5(6)
Hemophiliacs	53	20(38)	7(13)
Normal controls	52	17(33)	15(29)

distinction between these viruses (3). Limited cross-reactivity, however, was observed between antibodies to SAIDS-DV and MPMV in accord with the reported antigenic relatedness of SAIDS-DV and MPMV (4). Conflicting reports have appeared on the presence of antibodies to MPMV associated antigens in human sera (5,6). We find that only a very small proportion of the human population tested had antibodies to MPMV without antibodies to SAIDS-DV, indicating that in most cases these antibodies reflect cross-reactivity with SAIDS-DV associated antigens. No cross-reactivity with the human retrovirus LAV(HTLV-III), strongly associated with AIDS in humans, and no association between the presence of antibodies to SAIDS-DV and frank AIDS or pre-AIDS could be established. Although cross-reactivity with cellular antigens copurifying with SAIDS-DV and MPMV cannot be excluded, our data suggest that antibodies to SAIDS-DV associated antigens in human sera reflect the circulation of viruses antigenically related to SAIDS-DV in the human population.

ACKNOWLEDGEMENTS

We thank Drs. R.A. Coutinho, C. Breederveld, and K.W. Slaterus for providing serum samples and clinical information and Drs. R.C. Gallo and M. Popovic for providing HTLV-I(MT-2) and HTLV-III(H9-HTLV-III).

REFERENCES

1. Daniel, M.D. et al. Science 223, 602 (1984).
2. Gravell M. et al. Lancet i, 334 (1984)
3. Marx, P.A. et al. Science 223, 1083 (1984)
4. Stromberg K. et al. Science 224, 289 (1984)
5. Charmann H.P. et al. Int. J. Canc. 19, 498 (1977)
6. Thiry, L. et al. J. gen. Virol. 41, 587 (1978)

IS A RETROVIRUS-LIKE PARTICLE EXPRESSED AT A SPECIFIC STAGE DURING HUMAN OOCYTE MATURATION ?

E. Larsson[1], I. Suni[2], A. Vaheri[2], P. Sundstrom[3] and O. Nilsson[4]

1. Department of Pathology, Div. Tumorbiology., University of Uppsala, Box 553, S-751 85 Uppsala, Sweden, 2. Department of Virology, University of Helsinki, Finland, 3. Department of Obstetrics and Gynecology, Allmanna Sjukhuset, S-214 10, Malmo, and 4. Department of Human Anatomy, Biomedical Centre, Box 571, S-751 23 Uppsala, Sweden

We have previously shown that human oocytes sometimes express particles with striking resemblance to C-type retroviruses and that corresponding follicular fluids, derived mainly from preovulatory follicles, were analyzed for their contents of RD114 p30 related antigen. Taken together, 70% of the fluids contained detectable levels of such antigen. Attempts were made to correlate the amount of p30-like antigen to the follicle maturation. This was done by calculating a maturation index based on the pattern of follicular steroids and correlating the levels of virus like antigen to that index. However, no positive correlation could be found between the degree of follicular maturation and levels of retroviral related antigen. Some of the fluids also contained RT-like activity.

Endogenous retroviruses are present in the genome of most, if not all, vertebrates. These proviruses are often reinterated in their host's genome, and consist both of defective and nondefective genomes (4,5). A complete replication competent human endogenous retrovirus has, however, never been isolated, yet recently three independent laboratories have reported the detection of apparently different proviral-like sequences from human recombinant DNA libraries (1,2,10,13,14,15). It is, however, not clear if any of those retroviral related sequences code for a complete viral particle. In humans the indications of the expression of presumed endogenous retroviruses repeatedly have been seen in organs involved in fertilization and early embryo genesis (6,8,11,17,19). This has lead to the speculation that such sequences or particles might influence the differentiation process. So far there are no experimental data supporting such a theory. We have recently reported the detection of C-type virus like particles (VLP) in some human oocytes, reverse transcriptase (RT) like activity and a retrovirus related protein (RD 114 p30) in the surrounding follicular fluid (9,12). These findings together with the other above mentioned reports encouraged us to investigate more follicular fluids and oocytes for the presence of VLP and virus related proteins. We also wanted to see if the VLP are expressed at a certain stage during the oocyte maturation.

The follicular fluids were recovered from women who were laparascopied to recover oocytes for in vitro fertilization and embryo transfer. The women were infertile mainly due to Fallopian tube damage. Before laparascopy they were treated with the ovulation-inducing drugs Clomiphenecitrate (Clomivid^{R}) and human chorion gonadotropic hormone (HCG) according to a special schedule. The details have been described earlier (20). The hormones (estradiol and progesterone) were assayed by radioimmunoassays as described earlier (20).

Purified RD 114 p30 was iodinated by the Iodogen procedure (IODO-GEN^{TM}, Pierce, Rockford, IL) for homologous radioimmunoassay.The anti-RD114 p30 goat hyperimmune serum (gift from S. Oroszlan, National Cancer Institute, Frederick, MD) diluted in PTA buffer (phosphate-buffered saline, pH 7.4 containing 0.05% Tween 20 and 0.05% NaN_3), supplemented with 1% heat treated (+56°C, 30 min) goat serum, was used as the primary antiserum and rabbit anti-goat IgG (Miles Yeda, Rehovot, Israel) as the secondary antiserum. For the assay the follicular fluid samples were diluted 1:2 or 1:5 in PTA buffer. The precipitation of immune complexes was enhanced with a final concentration of 8% w/vol polyethylene glycol (PEG; Fluka, Buchs, Switzerland) at pH 8.0. Purified RD114 p30 was used as standard and the protein contents were determined by the Lowry method.

The oocytes were fixed and prepared for transmission electron microscopy as described before (9).

Assays for reverse transcriptase (RT) were done according to standard methods (16) and as described before from follicular fluids (9).

With electron microscopy, virus-like particles (VLP) could be demonstrated in more than 50% of the investigated oocytes. Free lying particles have a maximal diameter of 80-90 nM, which is slightly smaller than classical C-type particles (Fig. 1). Analysis of corresponding follicular fluids for RD 114 p30 related antigens and RT-like activity were made. All together 246 follicular fluids were included in this study and in 70% antigens could be demonstrated by competitive radioimmunoprecipitation (RIA). The sensitivity of the RIA was 5 ng/mg protein. 34 (14%) fluids contained 40 ng/mg RD114 p30 related antigen, 70 (27%) contained 10-40 ng/mg, and the rest 39%, 5-10 ng/mg. RT-like activity was detected in 8/10 fluids with high amounts of p-30 related antigen, ($>$ 40 ng/mg), but only in 2/10 fluids with low amounts of antigens (5-10 ng/mg).

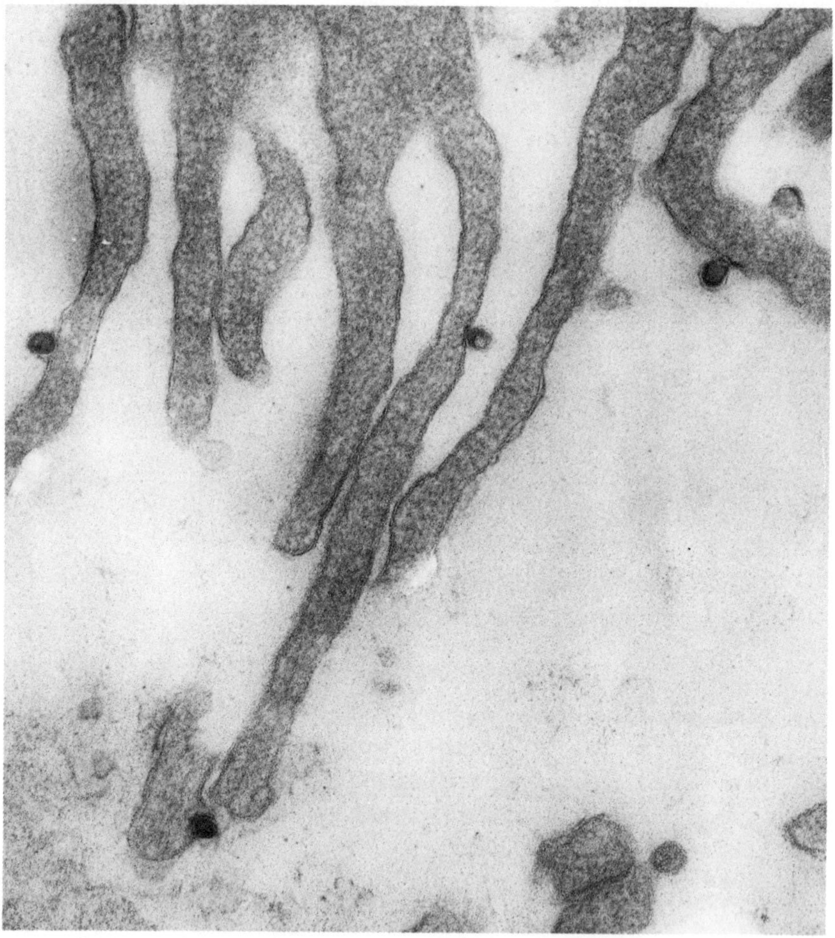

Figure 1A. Human oocyte surface microvilli with budding virus like particles (x 50,000).

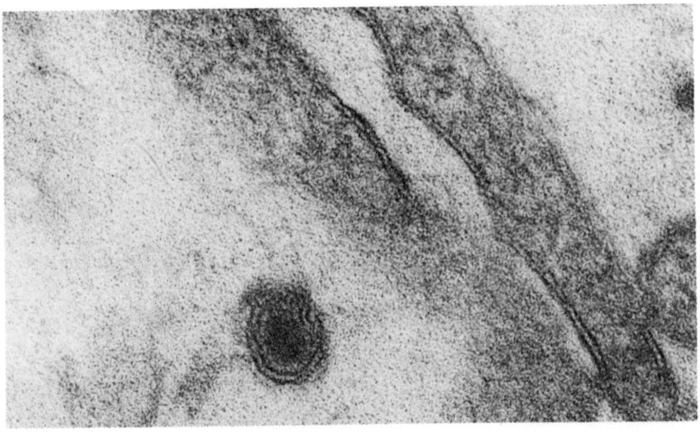

Figure 1B. Free lying particle (x 200,000).

To find out if the VLP and virus-related protein are expressed at a specific stage during the oocyte maturation, the follicle steroid hormone values were first plotted in various ways in an attempt to find a pattern which would be consistent with the general view that progesterone and estrogen first are increasing towards ovulation and that estrogen then decreases preovulatory. We found that using progesterone as the parameter (X-axis) will take into account that progesterone increases with maturation and taking the quotient progesterone/estrogen (Y-axis) will reflect the change in the relationship between these two hormones, that is, an increase of the quotient close to ovulation. A plot based on these parameters resulted in a pattern with concomitantly increasing values which could be expected. A maturation index was then obtained for each sample of follicular fluid by calculating the rectangular area of each coordinate (progesterone x progesterone/estrogen). This index was then displayed on the abscissa, and the virus related protein p30 on the ordinate. The distribution of p30 among the maturation stages is given in Fig.2 . The

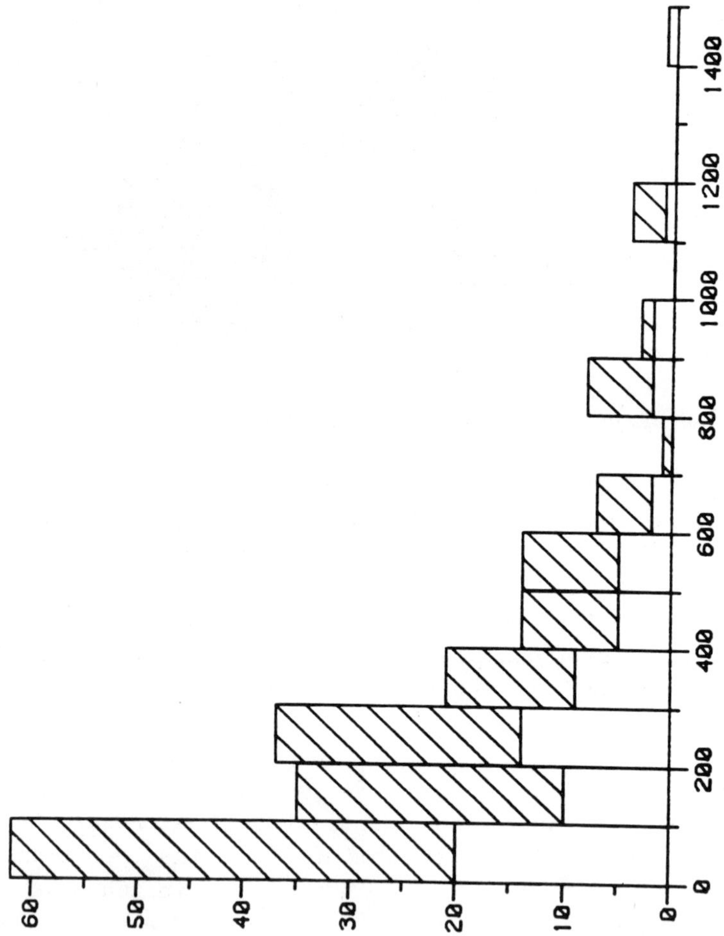

Figure 2. Number (Y-axis) of follicular fluids with p30 related antigen (shaded bars) and fluids without detectable amounts of such antigen (empty bars) in relation to the maturation index (X-axis).

proportion of follicles containing virus related protein in arbitrary chosen parts of maturation was rather similar, varying between 60 and 80%.

We consider that our data clearly indicate the presence of at least one retrovirus related protein (possibly the translation product from one of the endogenous retroviral like sequences). The attempts to correlate retroviral like expression to a specific stage have so far failed. However, our working hypothesis is still that VLP expression is not random, but reflects a specific stage of maturation. Our failure to find a specific stage could depend on several reasons. The final maturation of a human follicle to create a mature, fertilizable oocyte includes several rapid changes in the oocyte itself (structural, functional and genetic) and in its environment (the follicle wall, granulosa cells) and the follicular fluids (for a review see 7, 18). The parameters we use to establish the degree of maturation are morphology and hormone levels, but because the women have been treated with hormones we are studying a somewhat artifical situation.

Our main hypothesis is that in vivo the retroviral like sequences are activated by changes in the hormone levels. An endogenous retrovirus could activate genes important for maturation either through transposition following transcription and reverse transcription into C-DNA, or by simple chromosome rearrangement which could bring the retroviral related sequences close to genes important for maturation. Such a process would not need the production of a complete particle. Relocation of an endogenous intracisternal A-particle genome has been found to be responsible for activation of the C-mos oncogene in a mouse plasmacytoma (3). It is possible that under physiological conditions no particle is produced, but only after artifical hormone stimulation. To study this an ideal model would be to follow the oocyte maturation process in vitro and try to detect retroviral production at different maturation stages.

ACKNOWLEDGEMENTS

This work was supported by grants from the Swedish cancer society, project number 2037-B85-01X.

REFERENCES

1. Bonner T.I., O'Connell C., and Cohen M. (1982) Proc. Natl. Acad. Sci. USA 79, 4709-4713.
2. Callahan R., Drohan W., Tronick S., and Schlom J. (1982).Proc. Natl. Acad. Sci. USA 79, 5503-5507.
3. Canaani E., Dreagen O., Klar A., Rechavi G., Ram D., Cohen J.B. and Givol D. (1983) Proc. Natl. Acad. Sci. USA 80, 7118-7122.
4. Coffin J. (1982) Endogenous virus. In "RNA Tumor Viruses" (R. Weiss et al) Cold Spring Harbour Monograph Series, New York, 1109-1204.
5. Cohen M., Rein A., Stephens R.M., O'Connell C., Gilden R.V., Shure M;, Nicolson M.O., McAllister R.M. Davidson N. (1981) Proc. Natl. Acad. Sci. USA 78, 5207-5211.
6. Harzman R., Lower J., Lower R., Bichler K., Kurth R. (1982) The Journal of Urology, vol. 128, 1055-1060.
7. Jones R. (ed.) The vertebrate ovary. Comparative Biology and Evolution. Plenum Press, New York 1978.
8. Kalter, S.S., Helmke, R.J., and Heberling, R.C. (1973). J. Nat. Cancer Inst. 50, 1081-1084.
9. Larsson, E., Nilsson, O., Sundstrom, P., and Widehn, S..(1981) Int. J. Cancer 28, 551-557.
10. Martin, M., Bryan, T., Rastad, J. and Kahn A.S. (1981) Proc. Natl. Acad. Sci. USA 78, 4892-4896.
11. Mondahl, H., and Hofschneider, H. (1982). Int. J. cancer. 30, 281-287.
12. Nilsson, O., Larsson E., Sundstrom, P., and Widehn S. (1981) Ups. J. Med. Sci. 86, 225-232.
13. O'Brien, S.J., Bonner, T.I., Cohen, M., O'Connell, C., Nash, W.G. (1983). Nature (London) 393, 74-77.
14. Rabson, A., Steele, P., Garon, C., Martin, M. (1983)

Nature 306, 604-606.

15. Repaske, R., O'Neill, R.R., Steele, P.E. and Martin, M.A. (1983) Proc. Natl. Acad. Sci. USA 80, 678-682.
16. Sarngadharan M.G., Sarin P.S., Relts M.S. and Gallo R.C. (1972) Nature New. Biol. 240, 67-70.
17. Suni, J., Wahlstrom, T. and Vaheri, A. (1981). Int. J. Cancer 28, 559-566.
18. Terranova, Greenwald (1983) Factors regulating ovarian function. Raven Press, New York.
19. Vernon , M.L. McMahon, I.M., and Hackett I.I. (1974) J. Nat. Cancer. Inst. 52, 982-992.
20. Wramsby, H., Kullander S., Liedholm, P., Rannevik, G., Sundstrom, P., and Thorell, J. (1981) Fertil Steril. 448-454.

PSORIASIS -- A RETROVIRUS DISEASE?

O.-J. Iversen and A.B. Dalen

Department of Microbiology, Faculty of Medicine, University of Trondheim, Trondheim, Norway

Virus-like particles have been demonstrated in psoriatic lesions and in the serum and the urine from psoriatic patients. The particles have a morphology resembling that of a C-type retrovirus, banding in sucrose gradients at densities of 1.15-1.18 g/cc and being composed of an outer glycoprotein (gp70), a major internal protein (p27) and two minor internal proteins (p15 and p12). Neither RNA-directed DNA polymerase nor polyadenylated 70S RNA have been detected in the particles. Psoriatics express the p27 antigen on B and T lymphocytes and NK-cells (frequencies 0.1-1%). Small quantities of antibodies against p27 were detected in the serum from psoriatic patients while large amounts of IgG and IgA with specificity for p27 could be extracted from psoriatic scales.

Psoriasis is a disease with an abnormally high turn-over of epidermal cells both in clinically affected and unaffected skin. An altered immune activity including a depressed cellular immune response to mitogens and antigens (1,7,8) has been recognized in this disease. We have observed virus-like particles in psoriatic plaques, in the urine from psoriatic patients and in the growth medium of cultivated cells from psoriatic lesions (2,4).

Immunological cross-reactivity has been demonstrated between the particles released from cultivated cells and those obtained from the urine (4). The particles have a retrovirus-like morphology and band at densities between 1.15 and 1.18 g/cc in sucrose gradients. The particles from urine isolated by sucrose gradient centrifugation, could be further purified by Con A Sepharose fractionation and immuno-sorbent chromatography with antibodies against virus-like particles from cultivated psoriatic cells. A component of molecular weight 70,000 (gp 70) bound to Con A, while three other components, p27, p15, and p12 did not bind to Con A. The urine particles could be adsorbed to immunobeads with antibodies against gp70. Differential radiolabelling of the absorbed material demonstrated that the glycoprotein was externally located on the particle, while the three other proteins, p27, p15, and p12 were labelled only after detergent disruption of the particles. This showed that the four proteins were located in the particle with gp70 as the surface protein and p27, p15, and P12 as internal proteins (3). The separation of the internal proteins of the particles using SDS-PAGE is shown in Figure 1. The internal proteins were separated by a final gel filtration on Sephacryl S-300 in 6 M guanidine hydrochloride (4). Estimates of molecular weights made by this method differed slightly from those obtained by SDS-PAGE (27,000, 15,000, 12,000 versus 30,000, 18,000, 15,000). The composition of the particles thus resembled that of murine retroviruses, with an external glycoprotein (gp70), a major internal protein (p27) and two minor proteins.

p27 isolated by gel chromatography (Figure 1) and which appeared homogenous by SDS-PAGE, was used for immunization of rabbits. The antiserum obtained reacted in high dilution in an ELISA test using purified p27 as antigen, indicating a hyperimmune serum against p27.

Virus-like particles have been observed in blood from psoriatic patients (2), and the anti-p27 serum was used in an attempt to demonstrate antigen expression in blood cells from psoriatic patients. Lymphocytes were isolated by the one step Lymphoprep (Nyegaard et Co., Oslo) procedure, and the cells were adsorbed to polylysine coated coverslips and fixed in methanol. The cells were incubated with anti-p27 serum (1:50) and fluorescein conjugated anti-rabbit antibodies. About 0.5% of the cells obtained from psoriatic patients showed a positive reaction with a cytoplasmatic and a more intense outer membrane fluorescence (Figure 2a).

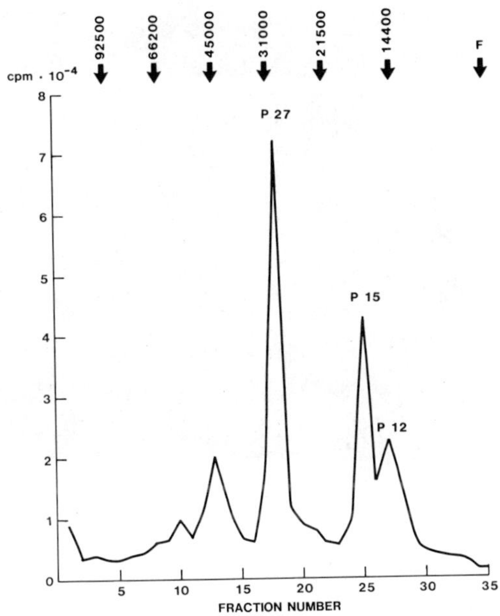

Figure 1. SDS-PAGE of internal proteins of virus-like particles isolated from the urine of a psoriatic patient. The particles were collected by ultracentrifugation, banded at 1.17 g/cc in a sucrose gradient, purified by immunosorbent chromatography and passed through Con A Sepharose. Labelling was performed using the Bolton Hunter reagent.

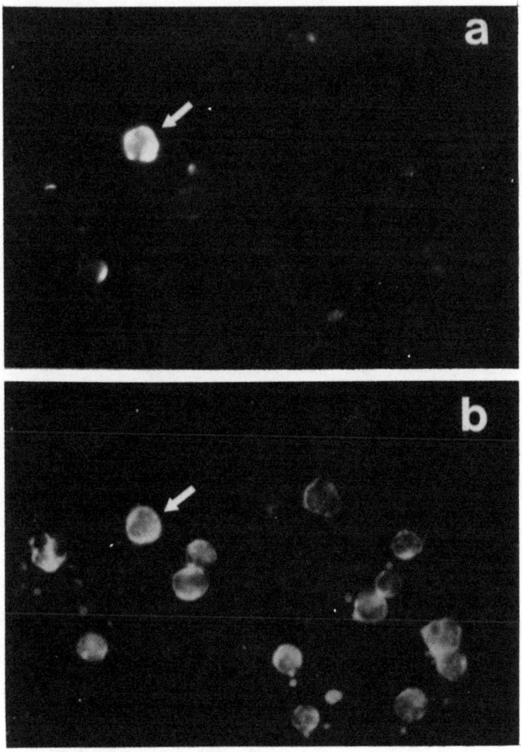

Figure 2. Indirect immunfluorescence of lymphocytes from a psoriatic patient. a) Lymphocytes stained with anti-p27 antibodies and fluorescein marked anti-rabbit immunoglobulins showing a positive p27 cell (arrow). b) The same field stained with monoclonal mouse anti-T lymphocyte antibodies (leu 4) and Texas Red conjugated anti-mouse immunoglobulin.

A double blind study was peformed including six

patients with moderate to extensive psoriasis and six healthy controls without known cases of psoriasis in their families. p27 positive cells were detected in all preparations from the patients (frequency between 1 and 0.1%) while no p27 positive cells were seen in the preparations from the controls (frequency $<$ 0.01%).

Among the p27 positive cells were lymphoctes with markers for B cells, T cells as well as NK cells. These cells were identified by monoclonal antibodies, BMA 0120 (Behringwerke AG), anti-leu 4 and anti-leu 11 (Becton Dickenson), and Texas Red conjugated anti-mouse immunoglobulin as second antibody.

Serum antibodies against purified p27 in psoriatic patients were demonstrated by the ELISA method. The analysis was performed with serum from 12 psoriatics with moderate to extensive psoriasis and 12 healthy controls without known cases of psoriasis in their families. Only small quantities of free antibodies against p27 were demonstrated in sera from the patients as well as controls. Psoriatic scales, which are known to contain large amount of IgG and IgA antibodies (6), were extracted with 1 M proprionic acid. Anti-p27 reactivity of both IgG and IgA from scale extracts was demonstrated. The activity exceeded that of serum by a factor of 1000 and a positive reaction was obtained with 1 ng of both IgG and IgA.

The virus-like particles associated with psoriasis have morphological resemblance to retroviruses and composition similar to murine retroviruses. Neither RNA-directed DNA polymerase activity nor polyadenylated 70 S RNA have been detected in the particles (5). These studies have been done on material from patients with a disease of long standing. Analysis of patients in an early phase of the disease and studies of cultured lymphocytes have not yet been done. The particles are expressed in a number of cells including epidermal and urogenital cells and lymphocytes. The expression in lymphocytes seems to be of particular interest in view of the altered immune response observed in psoriatics. We also believe that the humoral response with large amounts of anti-p27 antibodies located in psoriatic scales further indicates a pathogenic role of the particle in the disorder. The depletion of anti-p27 antibodies in serum from psoriatics might be due to antigen expression in psoriatic lesions, and might contribute to the inflammatory reaction seen in psoriatic skin.

REFERENCES

1. Clot, J., Dardenne, M., Brochier, J., Andary, M. & Guilhou, J.J. (1978) Clin. Immunol. Immunopathol. 9, 389.
2. Dalen, A.B., Hellgren, L., Iversen, O.-J. & Vincent, J. (1983). Acta Path. Microbiol. Immunol. Scand. Sect. B, 91, 221-229.
3. Iversen, O.-J., (1983) Acta Path. Microbiol. Immunol. Scand. Sect. B, 91, 407-412.
4. Iversen, O.-J., & Dalen, A.B. (1983). Acta Path. Microbiol. Immunol. Scand. Sect. B, 91, 343-349.
5. Iversen, O.-J., Nissen-Meyer, J., & Dalen, A.B. (1983) Acta Path. Microbiol. Immunol. Scand. Sect. B, 91,413-417.
6. Krogh, H.K. & Tonder, O. (1973) Scand. J. Immunol. 2, 45-51.
7. Krueger, G.G., Hill, H.R. & Jederberg, W.W. (1978) J. Invest. Dermatol. 71, 189.
8. Krueger, G.G., Jederberg, W.W., Ogden, B.E. & Reese, D.L. (1978) J. Invest. Dermatol. 71, 195.

PURIFICATION AND CHARACTERIZATION OF A HIGH MOLECULAR WEIGHT HUMAN MILK RIBONUCLEASE: ITS POTENTIAL USE FOR DIAGNOSIS AND PROGNOSIS OF HUMAN MAMMARY NEOPLASIA

Hemavathj R., and Das M.R.

Centre for Cellular & Molecular Biology, Hyderabad 500007, India

A high molecular weight ribonuclease (MW 80,000 daltons) from human milk (HMRNase) has been isolated and purified to homogeneity. Antiserum raised against this enzyme does not cross react with any of the human serum proteins, suggesting that the enzyme is synthesized in the mammary cells and secreted into the milk. The anti HMRNase antibody is expected to be a useful reagent for diagnostic and prognostic studies of human mammary neoplasia in view of the reverse correlation of the amount of ribonuclease present in human milk and mammary tumour incidence implicated in earlier studies (1).

We have reported earlier the presence of a ribonuclease activity in human mik plasma, capable of breaking down genomes of known RNA tumour viruses. It was also demonstrated that the level of RNAse present in milk samples from donors of the Parsi community is much lower compared to the level of the enzyme present in samples from donors belonging to other communities (1). In Parsi women, breast cancer accounts for 49% of all malignant diseases and the age-adjusted incidence is about thrice as high as that of the entire population of greater Bombay (2,3). In order to study possible specificity of the human milk RNAse in terms of RNA substrates of viral or proto-oncogenic origin we have undertaken to purify and characterize the ribonuclease or antibodies raised against the purified enzyme as reagents for diagnostic or prognostic studies of human mammary neoplasia.

CHARACTERIZATION OF THE HUMAN MILK RIBONUCLEASE

In order to identify the ribonuclease present in the human milk plasma prior to purification, activity staining of milk plasma samples was carried out. Following electrophoresis on SDS polyacrylamide gels, the ribonuclease activity was detected in two bands of ribonuclease activity corresponding to the molecular weights of 80,000 and 14,000 daltons.

The purified high molecular weight ribonuclease (80 kd) shows an activity band identical to that in plasma. The enzyme appears to be a single polypeptide (Figure 1) as judged by the absence of any change in its electrophoretic mobility in the presence of beta-mercapto ethanol. We have also shown using periodic acid Schiff's staining that the enzyme is a glycoprotein. It binds irreversibly to Con A Sepharose and cannot be eluted with either 1 M alfa-methylmannoside or buffers containing NaCl upto a concentration of 4 M. The enzyme binds to DNA cellulose and can be eluted with 9.5 M NaCl. The purified enzyme is devoid of any contaminating DNAse, alkaline phosphatase, phosphodiesterase or esterase activities.

The enzyme has a broad pH optimum between pH values 7.5 and 8 and is likely to be a secretory ribonuclease unlike the nonsecretory RNase having acidic pH optima around 6.5 (4).

The effect of cations on the activity of the enzyme is presented in Table 1. It can be seen that several divalent cations are inhibitory, including Ca^{2+}. In this respect it distinctly differs from the ribonuclease

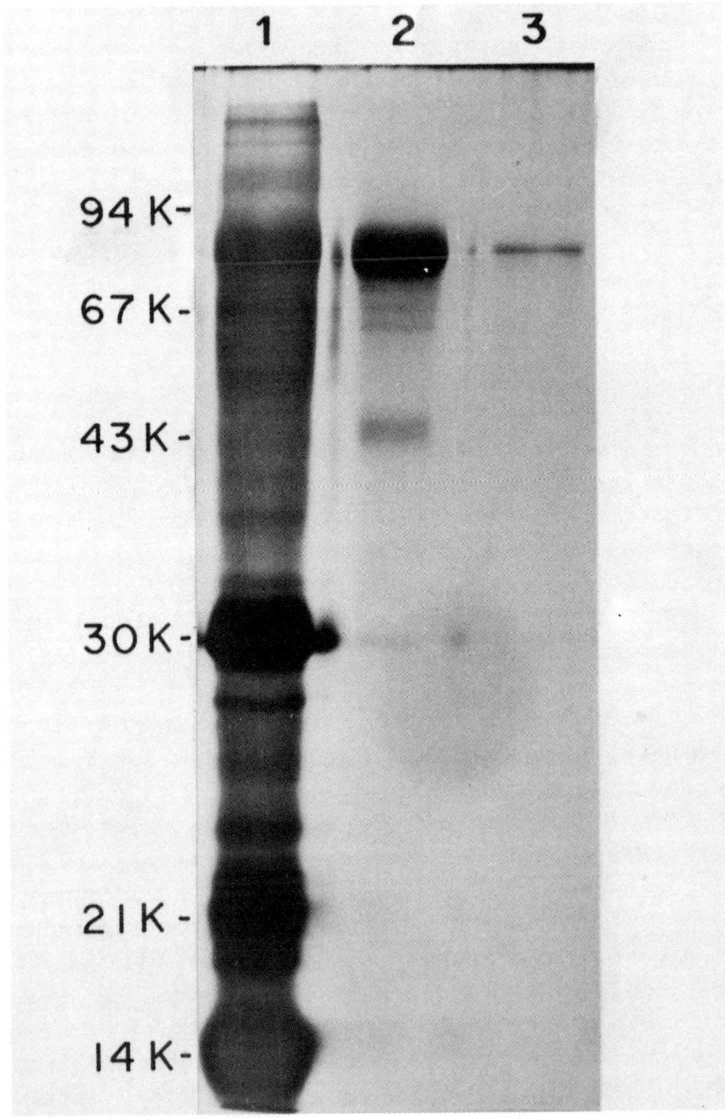

Figure 1. SDS-PAGE (9) profile of the purified high molecular weight ribonuclease from human milk plasma, and crude plasma samples at different stages of purification. The dialysed plasma were subjected to phosphocellulose column chromatography and eluted using 0.2-1.5M linear

Figure 1 (continued).
sodium chloride gradient. The peak eluting between 0.7-0.9M NaCl contained the major ribonuclease activity. This was further purified by gelfiltration chromatography. Fractions containing the enzyme activity were pooled and concentrated by dialysis against saturated sucrose in Tris-HCl 10mM pH 7.5. After SDS-PAGE, the gel was stained by silver staining technique (10). Lane 1: Milk plasma, Lane 2: Phosphocellulose eluate, Lane 3: sephadex G-150 eluate.

---

present in rat milk reported by Liu and Owens (5). The strategy suggested by the above workers in distinguishing ribonucleases of mammary origin, making use of the stimulation of the enzyme activity by Ca^{2+} is clearly inapplicable in the case of the HMRNase.

A striking feature of the 80-kd ribonuclease is that it is somewhat unstable compared to other ribonuclease activities so far reported. On keeping at 4°C it initially breaks down to different molecular species corresponding to molecular weights of 65, 50, 40, 20 and 14 K daltons. These products do show ribonuclease activity but if kept longer than 72 hours at 4°C the enzyme gradually loses its activity. However, the enzyme can be preserved for longer periods at -20°C. Addition of DTT did not have any influence on the stability of the enzyme, but the presence of 10% glycerol moderately increased the stability.

The purified 80-kd ribonuclease appears to have the highest molecular weight compared to all other ribonucleases so far reported from body fluids of Vertebrate animals. An earlier report by Dalaly et al. (6) describes the purification of a 14 kd enzyme from human milk. This corresponds to the lower molecular weight band which could have arisen from the breakdown products of the 80 kd protein.

Table 1. Effect of different cations on the activity of human milk rebonuclease

Ion	Concentration (mM)	% Activity
Na^{+}	50	114
	200	90
	800	0
K^{+}	50	123
	200	93
	800	0
Mg^{+2}	2	95
	5	50
	10	0
Mn^{+2}	2	2.6
Ca^{+2}	2	2.0
Fe^{+3}	1	60.3
Fe^{+2}	1	0
Cu^{+2}	1	0
Zn^{+2}	1	0
Co^{+2}	1	59.9

Enzyme activity was measured in 10 mM Tris pH 7.6. Cations were tested in reaction mixtures containing 50 mM NaCl in Tris (10 mM, pH 7.6). The reactions were carried out in 50 ul assay mixtures containing 40 ug E. coli RNA Tritium labelled with uridine-5-T and 500 units of the enzyme at 37°C for 15 min. An aliquot of 25 ul reaction mix was spotted on a 2x10 cm Whatman No. 3 paper strip over a streak of glacial acetic acid and chromatographed in a solvent system containing equal volumes of 1 M Ammonium acetate and 95% ethanol (7). The origin of the chromatographed strip was cut, dried and counted in a toluene based scintillation fluid. Enzyme unit = the amount of the enzyme that degrades 1 ug of E. coli RNA in 15 mins at 37°C (Tris 10 mM, pH 7.6, 50 mM NaCl).

Table 2. Degradation of natural substrates by human milk ribonuclease

Enzyme Concentration Units/ml	% degradation		
	mRNA	rRNA	tRNA
100	50.4	36.1	20.5
200	74.9	64.7	56.5
400	81.1	71.0	77.3
600	91.2	78.5	87.1
800	94.6	90.7	97.2

The assays were carried out in 50 ul reaction mixtures containing 5 ugs of the substrate (tritiated RNA with specific activity of 1500 cpm per ug of RNA) in a buffer containing 10 mM tris HCl pH 7.5 and 50 mM NaCl and aliquots of enzyme as shown above. After incubation of the reaction mixture at 37°C for 15 minutes; the RNase activity was determined by chromatography as described in Table 1. The RNA samples were isolated from the livers of rats injected intraperetoneally with 1 mci tritiated oroticacid T (G) 24 hours prior to sacrificing the animal.

SUBSTRATE SPECIFICITIES

The action of the HMRNase on different kinds of naturally occurring RNAs from rat liver are shown in Table 2. In Table 3 we present the results of degradation of synthetic ribohomopolymers by the enzyme. The enzyme acts readily on AMV viral RNA and also poly A containing mRNAs. The ability of the enzyme to degrade RNAs decreases in the order mRNA rRNA tRNA at low concentrations of the enzyme. It may also be noticed that the purine homopolymers are resistant to the action of the human milk ribonuclease whereas pyrimidine homopolymers are readily degradable. Conformational features of the substrates as well as the presence of purine or pyrimidine stretches in them are likely to influence the degradation pattern of the natural substrates by the enzyme.

IMMUNOLOGICAL SPECIFICITY AND IMPLICATIONS

Antibodies raised against the enzyme show distinct cross reactivity with the milk plasma as detected by Ouchterlony double diffusion technique. On the other hand, these antisera do not show any cross reactivity with human

Table 3. Degradation of synthetic homopolymer substrates by human milk ribonuclease

Substrate	% degradation
Poly rC	73.5
Poly rU	74.6
Poly rA	5.3
Poly rG	1.45
Poly rA:Poly rU	72.1

All the reactions were carried out in 500 ul reaction. mixtures containing 200 units of the enzyme, 100 ugs of unlabelled substrates 10mM Tris H-Cl, pH 7.5, and 50 mM NaCl. After incubation at 37°C for 30' the undegraded polymer was precipitated by the addition of an equal volume of 0.5% uranyl acetate and 16% Perchlonic acid mixture. The contents were chilled in ice bath; centrifuged at 10,000 rpm for 15 mins. The optical density (260 nm) of the clear supernatant was measured; with appropriate blanks to determine the concentration of the degraded material (8).

serum proteins. This observation along with the distinct characteristics of the human milk ribonuclease described above would suggest that the enzyme is synthesized in the mammary cells and secreted into the milk. In the light of the reverse correlation of the amount of ribonuclease present in human milk and mammary tumour incidence as implicated in our earlier observations (1), it is reasonable to test the reactivity of the antibody raised against the enzyme with mammary tumour tissues and other control tissues to check the potential use of the reagent for diagnostic and probably prognostic purposes. These experiments are in progress.

REFERENCES

1. Das, M.R., Padhy, L.C., Koshy, R., Sirsat, S.M. & Rich, M.A. (1976) Nature (London) 262, 802-805.
2. Jussawalla, D.J., Deshpande, V.A. & Haenszel, W. (1970) Brit. J.Cancer 24, 56-66.
3. Paymaster, J.C. & Gangadharan P. (1970) Int. J. Cancer 5, 426-431.
4. Sierakowska, H. & Shugar D. (1977) in Prog. Nucleic. Acid. Res. Mol. Biol. 20, 59-130.
5. Liu, D.K. & Owens G.F. (1983) Int. J. Biochem. 15, 1273-1277.
6. Dalaly, B.L., Eitenmiller, R.R., Friend, B.A. & Shahani, K.M. (1980) Biochem. Biophys. Acta 615, 381-389.
7. Scheit, K.H., Reddy, E.S.P.& Bhargava, P.M. (1979) Nature (London) 279, 728-731.
8. Kalnitsky, G., Hummel, J.P. & Dierks, C. (1959) J. Biol. Chem. 234, 1512-1516.
9. Laemmli, U.K. (1970) Nature 227, 680-685.
10. Oakley, B.R., Kirsch, D.R. & Morris, N.R. (1980) Anal. Biochem. 105, 361-363.

THE ROLE OF RETROVIRUSES IN AIDS AND SLOW INFECTIONS

R.W. Smith

Institute for Postgraduate Interdisciplinary Studies, P.O. Box 60846, Palo Alto, Calif.

Evidence of several (possibly identical) lymphotrophic retroviruses has been identified in blood and sera from many persons with the acquired immunodeficiency syndrome (AIDS). Although various investigators have postulated that these retroviruses may be the cause of AIDS, definitive and convincing proof of these claims remains elusive. Moreover, evidence of high titers of several herpesviruses can be found in all reported cases of AIDS-like diseases in man and other animals. The apparent ubiquity of these herpesviruses has led many investigators to conclude that they cannot play an etiologic role in this apparently new disease. This report therefore examines necessary conditions for distinguishing causation from opportunity in AIDS. Even if the lymphotrophic retroviruses are associated with substantial morbidity or mortality in AIDS, available evidence now suggests that they may be opportunistic in AIDS with underlying immune modification being caused largely by the titer and dilution of Epstein-Barr viruses (EBV) and their secondary products. A careful analysis of the possible roles of EBV in AIDS also reveals a novel model of slow infectivity possibly providing clues to the slow and progressive features of AIDS and other slow progressive diseases (SPD), and to the structure and function of retroviruses in AIDS and other slow infections.

Epidemics of AIDS-like diseases recently have been described in humans (1,2) and non-human primates (3,4). An earlier epidemic of an AIDS-like disease in sheep can be inferred (5) from reports by Sigurdsson (6-8) describing three unusual slow infections which arose following the importation into Iceland of 20 karakul breed sheep from Halle, Germany in 1933. The latter inference is made without the benefit of direct measurements of the ratio of helper T cells (Th) to suppressor T-cells (Ts) which could not be measured at the time of Sigurdsson's reports. Nevertheless, it now is apparent that outbreaks of maedi, Johne's disease, rida and possibly jaagziekte in the Icelandic sheep may have been largely opportunistic, with the underlying cause of the immune deficiency still remaining a mystery. An interesting finding in each of these epidemics is the occasional reports of retroviruses associated with disease. A lymphadenopathy-associated retrovirus (LAV) (9) and several variants of other T-cell lymphotrophic retroviruses (HTLV) (10-13) have been associated with AIDS in humans. Of these retroviruses, LAV and HTLV-III have been shown to have the highest correlation with AIDS or its possibly prodromal lymphadenopathy syndromes. A variant of a type D Mason-Pfizer monkey retrovirus (MPV) has been associated with simian AIDS (14). Maedi/visna retroviruses (MVV) are associated with ovine AIDS (6). Although complete characterization of the agent causing jaagziekte remains unclear, reverse transcriptase (RT) activity has been associated with this disease and, by inference, in ovine AIDS described by Sigurdsson (6-8). Interestingly, MVV and another lentivirus designated the "caprine arthritis-encephalitis retrovirus" (CAEV) share many structural and functional characteristics of LAV and HTLV-III despite their having slightly different (though progressive) effects on immune dysfunction. The presence of retroviruses in epidemics of AIDS-like diseases therefore raises important questions about the possible roles they play in AIDS. Are they the cause of disease? Are they opportunistic? Why are the retroviruses implicated in

AIDS-like diseases relatively rare pathogens -- at least in comparison to other infectious agents in the environment surrounding the host? In view of the link between AIDS and slow infections by their apparent long "incubation" periods and progressive infectious courses (8), are retroviral mechanisms directly or indirectly implicated in the mechanisms of slowness and persistency in AIDS? What molecular mechanisms associated with host or retroviral function are implicated if these associations are not merely coincidental? Is RT fundamentally consistent with AIDS-like sequelae? Are specific subcategories of retroviruses implicated in AIDS and, if so, upon what basis can those subcategories be described?

The recent attention on the phenomenology of AIDS poses an even more enigmatic situation if one recognizes that there is evidence of profound infections by several herpesviruses in all persons with AIDS. These data often are not appreciated because of the apparent ubiquity of herpesviruses and because of the infrequency or inappropriateness of clinical or other investigations of these agents. Significantly, attention often is also directed to associations between herpesvirus and retrovirus infections (15-18). Is there a substantive basis for these associations and, if so, how is one to distinguish primary events from secondary events?

Undoubtedly, having answers to the above questions would advance our understanding of AIDS and other SPD. This report summarizes relevant results of a three year investigation of AIDS, other SPD and autoimmune diseases providing possible answers to several of these questions. A model now can be formulated accounting for all reported features of AIDS and the other SPD under investigation. This novel model of slow infectivity suggests that all retroviruses are likely to be opportunistic (but not causative) in AIDS-like diseases -- even if those retroviruses are lymphotrophic and cause substantial morbidity or mortality. Recognition of specific retroviruses in AIDS-like diseases depends on the relative rareness of those retroviruses in the environment. Causes of AIDS-like diseases may be attributable to agents interfering with host RNA translational and post-translational processing (especially in B lymphocytes) with the "immune deficiency" being largely abnormal tolerance. On the other hand, available evidence suggests that retroviruses may interfere with RNA translation, however, there may be some contribution to AIDS directly. Results of this research also suggest reasons why proponents of LAV and HTLV-III as causes of AIDS are less likely to discover underlying reasons for EBV and EBV secondary products being principal determinants of underlying immune modification and progressive immune dysfunction.

REFERENCES

1. Centers for Disease Control (1981) MMWR 30(21), 250-252.
2. Centers for Disease Control (1984) MMWR 32(52), 688-691.
3. Hendrickson, R.V., Osborn K.G., Madden, D.L., Anderson, J.H., Maul, D.H., Sever, J.L., Ellingsworth, L.R., Lowenstine, L.J. & Gardner, M.B.,(1983) Lancet i, 388-390.
4. Letvin, N.L. Eaton, K.A., Aldrich, W.R, Sehgal, P.K., Blake, B.J., Schlossman, S.F., King, N.W. & Hunt, R.D. (1983) Proc. Natl. Acad. Sci. USA (1983) 80, 2718-2722.
5. Smith, R.W. (1984) Ann. N.Y. Sci., in press.
6. Sigurdsson, B. (1954) Brit. Vet. J. 110, 255-270.
7. Sigurdsson, B. (1954) Brit. Vet. J. 110, 307-322.
8. Sigurdsson, B. (1954) Brit. Vet. J. 110, 341-354.
9. Barre-Sinoussi, F., Chermann, J.C., Rey, F., Nugeyre, M.T., Chamaret, S., Gruest, J., Daugnet, C., Axler-Blin, C., Vezinet-Bun, F., Rouzioux, C., Rozenblum, W. & Montagnier, L.(1983) Science 220, 868-871.
10. Gallo, R.C. Sarin, P.S., Gelmann, E.P., Robert-Guroff,

M., Richardson, E., Kalyanaraman, V.S., Mann, D., Sidhu, G.D., Stahl, R.E., Zolla-Pazner, S., Leibowittch, J. & Popovic, M. (1983) Science 220, 865-867.
11. Popovic, M., sarngadharan, M.G., Read, E. & gallo R.C. (1984) Science 224, 497-500.
12. Gallo, R.C., Salahuddin, S.Z., Popovic, M., Shearer, G.M., Kaplan, M., Haynes, B.F., Palker, T.J., Redfield, R., Oleske, J., Safai, B., White, G., Foster, P. & Markham, P.D. (1984) Science 224, 500-503.
13. Brun-Vezinet, F., barre-Sinoussi, F., Saimot, A.G., Christol, D., Montagnier, L., Rouzioux, C., Klatzmann, D., Rozenbaum, W., Gluckmann, J.C. & Chermann, J.C. (1984) Lancet i, 1253-126h56.
14. Marx, P.A., Maul, D.H., Osborn, K.G., Lerche, N.W., Moody, P., Lowenstine, L.J., Hendrickson, R.V., Arthur, L.O., Gilden, R.V., Gravell, M., London, W.T., Sever, J.L., Levy, J.A., Munn, R.J. & Gardner, M.B. (1984) Science 223, 1086-1089.
15. Martin, W.B., Scott, F.M.M., Sharp, J.M, Angus, K.W. & Norval, M. (1976) Nature 264, 183-184.
16. Hampar, B., Aaronson, S.A., Derge, J.G., Chakrabarty, M., Showalter, S.D. & Dunn, C.Y. (1976) Proc. Natl. Acad. Sci. USA 73, 64-650.
17. Iakovleva, L.S., Plakhov, I.V., Voronov, A.V., et al. (1982) Eksp. Onkol. 4, 18-21.
18. Rosadio, R.H. (1983) Master's Thesis, Washngton State University, Pullman, Wa.

4. Retroviruses and Oncogenes

RETROVIRUSES WITH TWO ONCOGENES

D. Stehelin and P. Martin

Inserm U 186, Institut Pasteur 15 Rue C. Guerin - 59019 Lille - FRANCE

Less than a decade ago the first retroviral oncogene was discovered (1) and shown to be derived from a normal cellular gene (2). Today over twenty different retroviral oncogenes have been found, all derived from cellular counterparts. How a single oncogene can cause cancer is still not fully understood. Natural cancers are known to involve multi-step molecular changes, raising a paradox as compared to cancers induced by retroviral oncogenes. To turn a cellular gene into an active retroviral oncogene, an overexpression due to the very potent retroviral promotor may suffice in a few cases, whereas in most cases several modifications are probably required. These modifications might involve enhanced transcription, truncation of the gene, specific mutations, deletions or insertions (Fig. 1) as well as the viral route of transmission. In this respect a retroviral oncogene may then be regarded as a single gene having accumulated stepwise, through many replication cycles and selections by researchers (these viruses do not exist in nature) several modifications in order to become a potent cancer gene. Such a process represents a somewhat artificial situation never to be challenged for statistical reasons by a cellular oncogene during the life-time of the host-cells. Nevertheless, cellular oncogenes that were identified through retroviruses seem to be involved in some natural cancers, where they are for example de-regulated through chromosomal translocation (c-myc) or mutations (13) (c-ras). Although they appear much "wheaker" transforming genes than their viral counterparts, they legitimate the use of retrovirus as tools. It follows that natural cancers are more likely to involve probably single alterations on several distinct genes that cooperate in the tumorigenic process. Recently a first example of cooperation was demonstrated by in vitro studies showing that the activated ras and myc oncogenes could transform rat embryo fibroblast in a way that neither gene could achieve alone (3) and some human tumor cell-lines were found to contain the cellular ras and myc oncogenes both altered. How can we identify more such cooperative genes? Among a few other methods retroviruses may again represent useful tools. In 1979, studying acute avian leukemia retroviruses, we raised the possibility (4) that some retroviruses undergoing modifications could have, among those, transduced not one, but two distinct cellular genes that could cooperate in the viral-proned transformation processes. There are now three examples of such retroviruses (Fig. 2) that we would like to review briefly.

AVIAN ERYTHROBLASTOSIS VIRUS (AEV).

The genome of AEV contains the two oncogenes erbA and erbB (5). Deletion mutants in one or the other oncogene have shown that in adult bone marrow the erbB product transforms erythroblasts which subsequently cannot mature properly anymore. The erbA product alone does not modify erythroid cells in a detectable way (6). In contrast, wild type AEV blocks tightly erythroid cells at an immature stage (erythroid colony forming units or CFUe) (7). Thus erbA potentiates the transforming activity of the erbB gene product. The nucleotide sequencing of the erbA gene appears unrelated to any of the oncogenes characterized so far and related to carbonic anhydrases, enzymes known to play a major role in red blood cells, the progenitors of which are precisely the target cells for AEV (see C.

Henry, this volume). Other studies performed on embryonic tissue of the primitive streak indicate that AEV affects also target cells that appear to preceed the BFUe stage (see Moscovici et al. this volume).

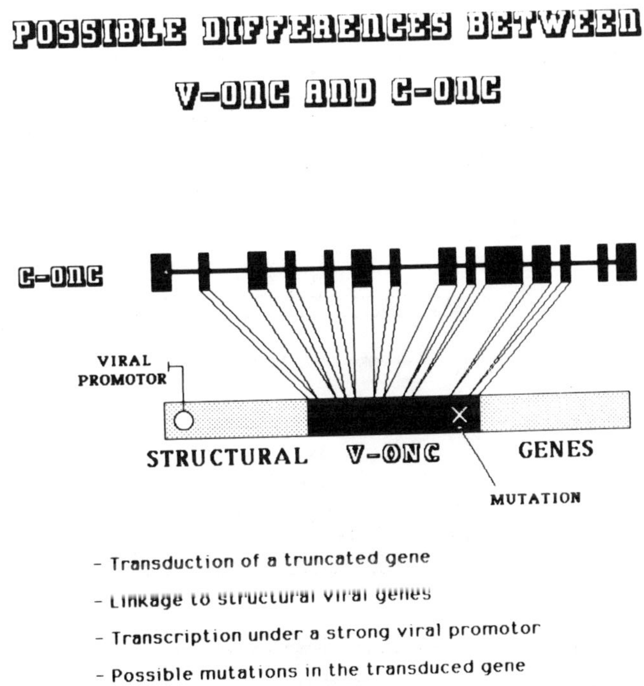

Figure 1. Possible differences between v-onc and c-onc.

AVIAN ERYTHROBLASTOSIS VIRUS E26.

The genome of E26 virus contains the two oncogenes myb and ets (8), expressed in infected cells as a triple fusion proteins $P130^{gag-myb-ets}$ (5). E26 appears able to transform uncommitted erythroid-myeloid hemopoietic cells as well as cells committed in the erythroid and myeloid lineages (see Moscovici et al., this volume). How the two oncogenes myb and ets are involved in the transforming properties of E26 virus awaits the construction of mutants deleted in one or the other of the genes. We recently obtained a molecular clone of E26 provirus that is biologically active (D. Leprince et al., in preparation) and that should facilitate the construction of such mutants.

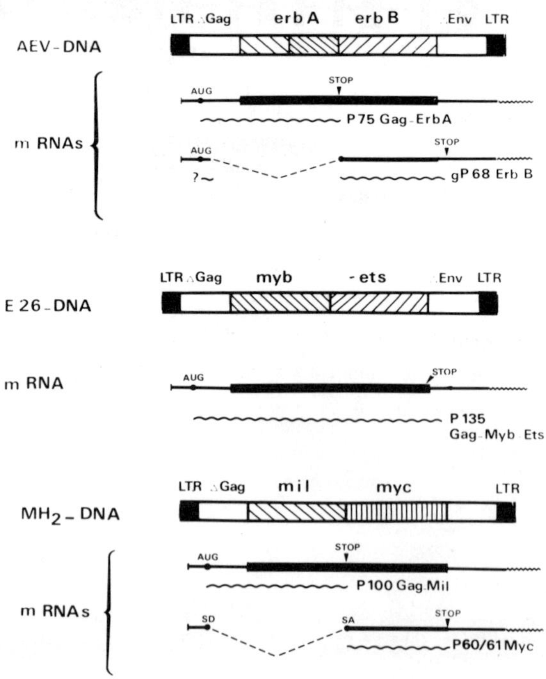

Figure 2. Retroviruses with double oncogenes.

MILL-HILL-2 RETROVIRUS (MH2)

The avian retrovirus Mill-Hill-2 (MH2) is a replication defective retrovirus that causes, like other avian myc containing retroviruses (MC29, CMII, OK10), mainly liver and kidney carcinomas in the chicken, and transforms chicken fibroblasts and macrophages in culture (5). MH2 appears more aggressive that the other myc-containing viruses in its tumorigenic potential and its genome contains a second oncogene, mil (9), yielding in infected cells the two onc-proteins $P100^{gag-mil}$ and $p57^{myc}$ (10). In order to examine the respective roles of the two proteins in the transformation process, we attempted the isolation of spontaneous or constructed mutant expressing properly only the mil or only the myc oncogene product. Two classes of spontaneous mutants were isolated with the group of G. Calothy (Institut du Radium, Orsay, France) using fibroblasts and neuroretinal (NR) cells prepared from 7 day old chick embryos. The choice of this latter cell system was bount to the observation that MH2 wild type virus was shown to stimulated the growth and to transform NR cells that remain usually quiescent in culture (11, and Table 1). Such an effect was not detected with retroviruses like MC29 (Table 1) that contain only the myc oncogene (11) and transform readily chicken fibroblasts (5). Class I mutants (Table 1) were selected on the basis of their inability to induce NR cell proliferation, whereas they still transformed fibroblasts. MH2 C116 exhibited such properties and was shown to suffer an extensive deletion in the mil gene. A mutant (MH2-OB) with similar biological properties was constructed by inducing a frameshift in the v-mil gene in a molecularly cloned MH2 provirus, resulting in a premature termination of the v-mil translation product.

The class II mutant (i.e. MH2 PA 200) was selected on the ground that it induced NR cells to proliferate with the same efficiency as wt-MH2, but failed to transform fibroblasts (Table 1). This mutant also failed to morphologically transform NR cells and showed upon

Table 1. Characterization of MH2 mutants.

Virus	Fbl*	NR*		Apparent functional oncogene	
	T*	M*	T*		
MC29	+	–	–	myc	
wt* MH2	+	+	+	myc + mil	
MH2 Cl 16	+	–	–	myc	(class I)
MH2 OB	+	–	–	myc	
MH2 PA 200	–	+	–	mil	(class II)
MH2 LI 200	–	+	–	mil	

* Fbl = Fibroblasts; NR = neuroretinal cells; T = transformed; ,M = mitogenized; wt = wild type.

analysis that it was extensively deleted in the myc gene. A mutant (MH2 LI 200) with similar biological properties (Table 1) was constructed by inducing a frameshift in the v-myc gene of molecularly cloned MH2 provirus that resulted in a premature termination of the v-myc translation product.

The results presented here indicate that the ability to induce sustained proliferation and transformation of NR-cells from 7 day-old chicken embryos is a remarkable property distinguishing MH2 among other myc-containing retroviruses, and requireing the coordinate expression of both mil and myc oncogenes. Class I mutants lacking a functional mil gene (MH2 Cl 16, MH2 OB) do not induce NR cell-proliferation nor transformation, although they still transform fibroblasts (and macrophages: T.Graf, pers. comm.). Conversely, mutants expressing only the mil oncogene (MH2 PA 200, MH2 LI 200) induce NR cell proliferation without morphological transformation.

So far, the viral myc oncogene (or the large T of Polyoma virus) was shown to cooperate with the EJ bladder carcinoma activated ras oncogene (or middle T of Polyoma virus) for rat embryo fibroblasts transformation (3). We show now that the myc oncogene can also cooperate with the mil oncogene (the latter being structurally related to the src-gene family, 12) for the transformation of NR cells. Thus the myc oncogene may cooperate with two distinct types of oncogenes depending on the cell-types considered. Whether myc plays a key role in two distinct pathways leading to transformation, or whether the three types of oncogenes (myc-, ras- and mil-like) belong to a single pathway leading to cell-growth stimulation, where transformation can occur when some of them become deregulated whereas others might be perhaps constitutively expressed at specific stages of cell-maturation or in specific cell-types, remains to be examined. Earlier work on Polyoma migh be recalled in this respect. Although the oncogenes of this virus were not shown to have cellular counterparts, the large T and middle T Polyoma genes were shown to cooperate for fibroblast transformation as do the activated myc and ras genes, respectively (13). in addition, the middle T was shown (14) to bind specifically in the transformed fibroblast the cellular protein pp60 src that was shown activated in the complex.

In conclusion research begins slowly to unwrap the cooperation of genes in normal and pathological cell-growth stimulation, and retroviruses with double oncogenes represent convenient tools in such investigations. They have allowed to discover three new oncogenes (erbA, ets and mil) that potentiate previously described oncogenes (erbB, myb and myc, respectively) in their transforming activity or allow these viruses to transform new target cells. Whether the corresponding couples of cellular oncogenes participate in the formation of natural human cancers is under investigation.

Note: the results presented here for MH2 correspond to a collaborative investigation between our laboratory (P. Martin, J. Coll, F. Denhez, S. Saule, J. Ghysdael and D. Stehelin) and two groups in Paris (C. Bechade and G. Calothy, Institut Curie, and B. Pessac, Hopital Broussais).

REFERENCES

1. Stehelin, D., Guntaka, R.V., Varmus, H.E. and Bishop, J.M. (1976) J. Mol. Biol. 101:349-356.
2. Stehelin, D., Varmus, H.E., Bishop, J.M. and Vogt, P.K. (1976) Nature 260:170-173.
3. Land, H., Parada, L.F., and Weinberg, R.A. (1983) Nature 304:596-602.
4. Roussel, M. et al. (1979) Nature 281:452-455.
5. Graf, T. and Stehelin D. (1982) Biophys Biochim. Acta 651:245-271.
6. Frykberg, L. et al. (1983) Cell 32:227-238.
7. Samarut, J., and Gazzolo, L. (1982) Cell 28:921-929.
8. Leprince, D. et al. (1983). Nature 306:395-397.
9. Coll, J. et al. (1983) Embo J. 2:2189-2194.
10. Pachl, C., Biegalke, B. and Linial, M. (1983) J. Virol. 45:133+139.
11. Calothy, G. et al. (1979) Cold Spring Harbor Symp. Quant. Biol. 44:983-990.
12. Galibert, F. et al. (1984) EMBO J. 3:1333-1338.
13. Cuzin, F. (1984) Biophys. Biochim. Acta 781:193-204.
14. Courtneidge, S.A., and Smith, A.E. (1983) Nature 303:435-439.

MOLECULAR ASSAYS FOR DETECTION OF ras ONCOGENES IN HUMAN AND ANIMAL TUMORS

H. Zarbl, S. Sukumar, D. Martin-Zanca, E. Santos, and M. Barbacid.

Developmental Oncology Section, NCI-Frederick Cancer Research Facility, P.O. Box B, Frederick, Maryland 21701.

The recent discovery of oncogenes in human and animal tumors has made it possible to investigate the molecular basis of neoplastic transformation. Oncogenes are altered versions of normal cellular genes, generically known as proto-oncogenes (25, 67). Although the role of these proto-oncogenes is for the most part unknown, it is generally believed that they code for proteins functional in the regulation of cell differentiation and/or proliferation. Recent findings demonstrating a high degree of similarity between certain oncogenes and growth factors or growth factor receptors corroborate this general hypothesis. Whereas the sis oncogene has been found to be one of the polypeptide chains of the platelet-derived growth factor, the erb-B oncogene appears to be a truncated form of the epidermal growth factor receptor (18,19,75). Activation of such growth regulatory proteins by mutations, overexpression, or expression in inappropriate cells would be expected to result in uncontrolled growth, the hallmark of transformed cells.

Oncogenes are known to acquire their malignant properties by a variety of different mechanisms. v-onc, the oncogenes to acute transforming retroviruses arose by complex recombinational events between replication competent nontransforming retroviruses and cellular proto-oncogenes (25, 67). Some retroviruses are known to carry more than one oncogene implicating that several recombination events between distant cellular loci took place (28, 34). Integration of retrovirus regulatory elements in the vicinity of cellular proto-oncogenes such as the myc and mos loci leading to increased expression of their respective gene products is involved in the development of bursal lymphomas of chickens and mouse plasmacytomas, respectively (32, 49). Chromosomal translocations such as the 8:14 translocation, characteristic of Burkitt's lymphoma, involve translocation of the myc proto-oncogene from its normal location in chromosome 8 to the immunoglobulin loci of chromosome 14 (1,14,57,66,74). As a consequence the myc locus becomes constitutively expressed in these tumor cells under the influence of immunoglobulin regulatory elements (3). Other well-characterized translocations such as Philadelphia chromosome are also responsible for activation of cellular oncogenes. In this case the abl gene acquires its malignant properties as a consequence of its translocation from chromosome 9 to chromosome 22 (33). Gene amplification has also been implicated in oncogene activation. For instance, the myc locus is amplified and over-expressed in human leukemia cells and small cell lung carcinomas (10,13,36). More recently an association between N-myc amplification and the late stages of neuroblastoma development has been reported (6). Integration of mouse mammary tumor virus genomes within a cellular locus, designated int-1, has been implicated in the development of mammary carcinomas induced by this virus (42). It is postulated that integration of this viral genome disrupts the normal functions of the putative int-1 proto-oncogene. Finally, point mutations, such as those responsible for the malignant activation of ras oncogenes, have been found in a significant fraction of human as well as animal tumors (51, 68, 70) and will be the central subject of this review.

Proto-oncogenes were initially detected by nucleotide sequence homology with the transforming regions of retroviral genomes (25,67). The advent of gene transfer techniques, however, provided the first direct assay for proto-oncogene activation (58). Gene transfer experiments have been used to demonstrate the presence of oncogenes in human cancers as well as in chemically induced animal tumors. To date, a significant fraction (15-20%) of human tumors have oncogenes capable of inducing the malignant transformation of cell lines of rodent origin (12). Most of these oncogenes have been identified as members of the ras gene family (16,44,53,63) originally identified as the transforming principle of a number of strains of murine sarcoma virus (2,21,48). Interestingly, there is no apparent correlation between activation of a given ras oncogene and the pathological characteristics of the tumor (47). In contrast, carcinogen-induced animal model tumor systems exhibit a good correlation (70-90%) between oncogene activation and tumor development (4,5,29,68,69). Moreover, the same oncogene appears to be specifically activated in each tumor system. Balmain et al. (4,5) have shown the specific activation of the H-ras oncogene in 5 of 6 DMBA-induced mouse skin carcinomas. Similarly, Guerrero and co-workers (29) have shown the reproducible activation of K-ras and N-ras in mouse thymomas induced by X-rays and NMU, respectively. In our laboratory we have demonstrated the presence of a transforming H-ras oncogene in each of nine NMU-induced mammary tumors of Buf/N and in four of six guinea pig cell lines induced by in vivo or in vitro treatment with different chemical carcinogens (68,69). The discrepancy between the frequency and specificity of oncogene activation in human and carcinogen-induced animal tumors suggests that the presence of a particular ras oncogene in a tumor may be more related to its etiology and the genetic background of the host than to its pathological properties. This may not be the case, however, for the oncogenes. Activation of myc and abl oncogenes is specifically associated with the chromosomal translocations responsible for the development of Burkitt's lymphomas and chronic myelogenous leukemia, respectively (35,52). In this review, we will describe the latest results regarding the activation of ras oncogenes in human neoplasmas as well as in carcinogen-induced animal tumors.

TRANSFORMING ras GENES IN HUMAN TUMORS

Oncogenes have been detected in about 15% of human tumors including the most common forms of cancer such as carcinomas of the lung, breast and colon, as well as in several types of sarcomas and leukemias (12). Most of the transforming genes detected by gene transfer assays are members of the ras gene family which, so far, includes three loci, H-ras (26,46,59), K-ras (8,39,41,61), and N-ras (31,62). H-ras and K-ras are the cellular homologs of the oncogenes carried by the prototype Harvey and Kirsten strains of murine sarcoma virus, respectively (16,44,53). The N-ras gene is distantly related to the other ras genes and has no known retroviral homology (63).

The molecular structure of the three known human ras oncogenes has been recently established (7,8,26,39,44,50, 59,61,62,73). They exhibit a large variability in genetic complexity ranging from 4.5 kilobase pairs (kbp) for H-ras to 40-50 kbp for K-ras (Figure 1). However, ras genes contain similar coding sequences whose splice junctions are precisely conserved, suggesting a common ancestral gene with a minimum of four exons. The K-ras gene has an alternative fourth exon, conferring the potential to encode an additional protein (39,61). All three ras genes encode highly conserved proteins of 189 amino acid residues, designated p21 (60). Each of the p21 proteins can be divided into three structural domains (61,73). The first domain is composed of the first 80 amino-terminal residues. Within this region, there is virtually no variation in amino acid sequence among the different p21 proteins. The second structural domain encompasses the next 80 amino acid residues, where extensive homology

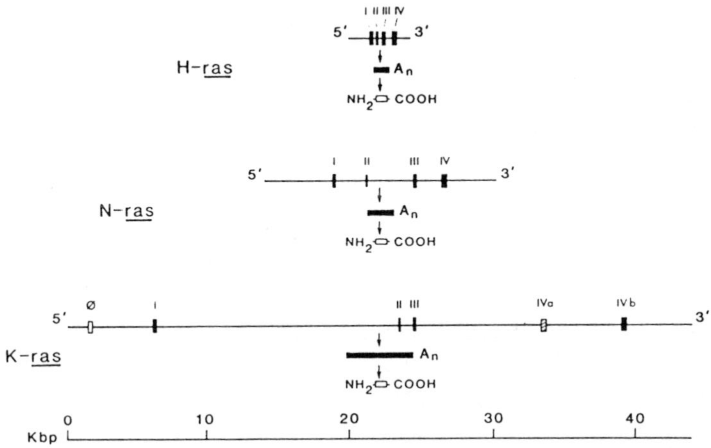

Figure 1. Molecular structure of the human H-ras, N-ras and K-ras genes. Exons are represented by the vertical boxes. The K-ras gene contains two alternate fourth exons (labeled IVa and IVb) as well as an untranslated exon (labeled Ø) which is located upstream of the initiation codon. Their major mRNA transcripts (sizes 1.2, 2.2 and 5.5 kbp for H-ras, N-ras and K-ras, respectively) and their p21 gene products are also represented.

(85%) is maintained between any pair of ras genes. The carboxy-terminal region defines a region of amino acid sequence divergence among the ras genes, and it has been speculated that it may confer physiological specificity to each member of the ras gene family.

ras genes have been highly conserved during evolution. The variation in amino acid sequences among p21 proteins of human and rat origin is less than 5% (68). Recently, ras genes have been detected in yeast by virtue of their nucleotide sequence homology with mammalian ras genes

(15,17,43,45). Although yeast ras genes encode proteins of higher molecular weight (42,000 daltons), they also conform to the three-domain structures defined in the mammalian p21 proteins. Furthermore, a homology of more than 90% of significant amino acids is observed between the amino-terminal domains of the yeast and mammalian ras gene products. Such evolutionary conservation lends further credence to the notion that ras genes encode functions essential to the proliferation of eukaryotic cells.

Comparative nucleotide sequence analysis of ras oncogenes with their normal alleles has allowed the identification of the critical change that confers on the ras oncogenes their transforming properties. In all cases, a single point mutation leading to a single amino acid substitution in the p21 protein product is responsible for the malignant activation of ras oncogenes (51,70,72). Two "hot spots" for activation have been detected so far: codon 12, which is located in the first exon (51, 70, 72), and codon 61, which is located in the second exon (40, 73, 76). Table 1 summarizes the different point mutations which have been detected so far in ras oncogenes of human tumors.

Recently, Fasano et al. (24) used random in vitro mutagenesis of the cloned H-ras gene to test the effect of other point mutations on the ability of the H-ras gene to transform NIH/3T3 cells. When the mutant H-ras genes with transforming activity were subjected to nucleotide sequencing, it was determined that there were three additional targets for activation. Mutations leading to changes in amino acids 13, 59, and 63 were found to confer transforming activity to the H-ras gene. Although mutations at codon 59 are present in the two viral ras proteins, it is not clear why they have not yet been detected in tumor cells. One possible explanation is that mutations capable of transforming NIH/3T3 cells may not be equally capable of inducing neoplastic alterations in other cell types.

Some of the mutations responsible for the malignant

Table 1. Mutations responsible for malignant activation of human ras genes.

Codon	Human Cells	Sequence	Amino Acid	Reference
H-ras:				
12	Normal	GGC	Glycine	51,70
	T24	GTC	Valine	51,70,72
	134-51§	GAC	Aspartic Acid	54
61	Normal	CAG	Glutamine	7,50
	Hs242	CTG	Leucine	76
N-ras:				
12	Normal	GGT	Glycine	73
	PA1	GAT	Aspartic Acid	71
61	Normal	CAA	Glutamine	73
	Sk-N-SH	AAA	Lysine	73
	SW-1271	CGA	Arginine	77
K-ras:				
12	Normal	GGT	Glycine	39,55
	Calu 1	TGT	Cysteine	61
	SW480	GTT	Valine	8
	PR371	TGT	Cysteine	41
	A2182	CGT	Arginine	55
	A1698	CGT*	Arginine	55
	LC-10	CGT*	Arginine	55
61	Normal	CAA	Glutamine	39
	PR310	CAT	Histidine	40

§NIH/3T3 cells transformed by a spontaneously activated human H-ras oncogene. * Determined by Sac I polymorphism.

activation of ras oncogenes introduce restriction enzyme fragment length polymorphisms (RFLP). By utilizing appropriate DNA probes, the resulting RFLPs can be utilized as molecular markers to identify transforming ras genes in human DNAs. Some of the predicted polymorphisms are listed in Table 1. In collaboration with Drs. M. Pierotti and G. Della Porta (Istituto Tumori, Milan), we have successfully utilized the Sac I RFLP created by a G → C mutation in nucleotide 34 of the first coding exon of the human K-ras locus to detect K-ras oncogenes in human tumors (55). The first exon of the normal K-ras locus is located in a 14 kbp Sac I DNA fragment. As a consequence of the $G^{34} \rightarrow C$ mutation, two new Sac I fragments of 5.8 kpb and 8.2 kbp are created which can be easily identified by Southern blot analysis (Figure 2). Of a total of sixty tumors analyzed, a squamous cell lung carcinoma was found to possess the diagnostic Sac I polymorphism (Figure 3) (55). This is the expected frequency considering that K-ras oncogenes are present in about 5-8% of human solid tumors and that at least 14 different point mutations can confer malignant properties to the human K-ras locus. Transfection studies showed that DNA isolated from the squamous cell lung carcinoma had transforming activity. All tested NIH/3T3 transformants derived from this tumor DNA contained the expected 8.2-kbp and 5.8-kbp Sac I DNA fragments characteristic of the activating G → C mutation (Figure 3).

Examination of DNAs isolated from normal tissue of the same patient, including blood lymphocytes as well as bronchial and parenchymal cells, showed that none of them contained the activating G → C mutation present in tumor tissue (Figure 3). Moreover, DNA extracted from these normal tissues did not show transforming activity in NIH/3T3 transfection assays. These results indicate that the mutational event responsible for the malignant activation of the K-ras gene in a squamous cell lung carcinoma is specifically associated with tumor development. Moreover, these findings unequivocally establish the somatic nature of the activating point mutation, implying that external agents were responsible for the malignant activation of the K-ras locus in this patient.

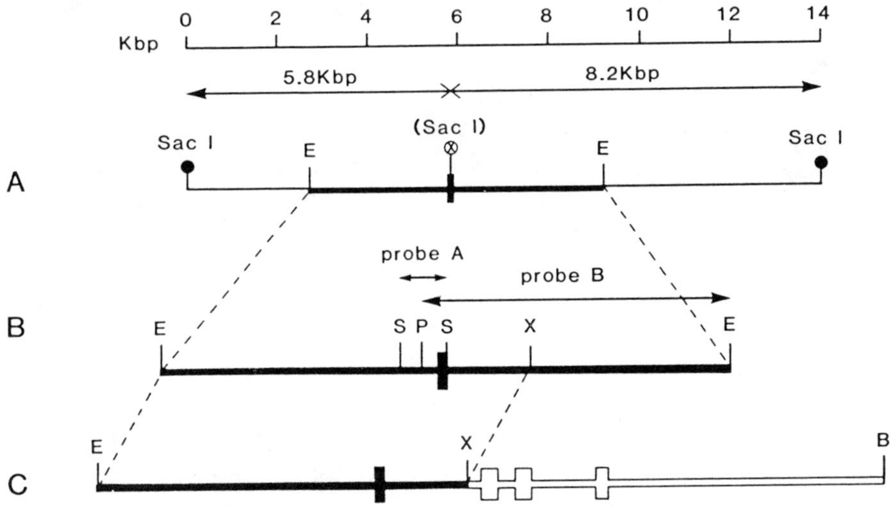

Figure 2. (A) sac I polymorphism created by a G→C mutation in codon 12 of the first exon (▮) of the human K-ras gene. Wildtype (●) and polymorphic (⊗) Sac I cleavage sites. (B). DNA probes utilized to identify this Sac I polymorphism in human DNA: Probe A contains 374 basepairs (bp) of upstream sequences and 96 bp of the first exon. Probe B contains 176 bp of upstream sequences, the entire exon and 3.1 kbp of downstream intron sequences. (C) Chimeric ras oncogene containing the first exon (black box) of the A2182 K-ras oncogene and the second, third and fourth exons (open boxes) of the normal human H-ras gene (54). E, Eco RI; P, PstI; S, Sau 3AI and X, Xba I. Only those restriction endonuclease sites needed to define the probes are indicated.

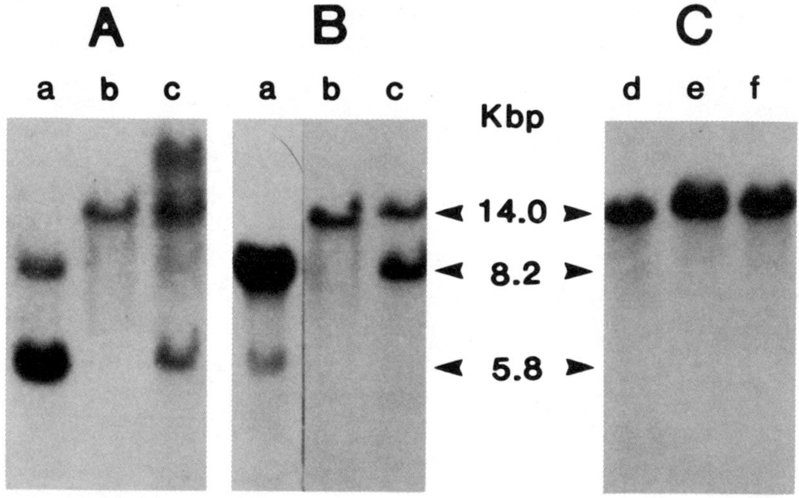

Figure 3. Somatic point mutation responsible for the malignant activation of the K-ras locus in tumor but not in normal tissue of a patient with squamous cell lung carcinoma (LC-10). DNAs digested with Sac I were hybridized to probe A (panel A), probe B (panel B) or probes A & B (panel C). (a) NIH/3T3 cell transformed by LC-10 tumor DNA, (b) normal human foreskin, (c) squamous cell lung carcinoma LC-10, (d) normal bronchia, (e) normal parenchyma and (f) blood lymphocytes of the same patient.

Increased expression of non-mutant ras genes can also lead to malignant transformation. Placing the human H-ras proto-oncogene under the control of retroviral enhancer elements confers this proto-oncogene with transforming properties in the NIH/3T3 transfection assay (9) and makes it capable of "immortalizing" primary embryo fibroblasts (65). Amplification of the K-ras locus has been reported in a mouse adrenocortical tumor cell line (56) and in a human lung carcinoma biopsy (unpublished results). Whereas it is tempting to implicate increased expression of ras genes in the development of naturally occurring malignancies, we must remember that incresed H-ras expression has been detected in normal physiological processes such as regeneration of rat liver (27). Thus, assesment of the role of normal (non-mutated) ras proto-oncogenes in malignancies must await careful and detailed investigation of the crucial threshold of p21 ras protein expression that separates normal from neoplastic growth.

TRANSFORMING ras GENES IN ANIMAL TUMOR SYSTEMS

To establish an unequivocal link between ras oncogene activation and tumorigenesis it is necessary to understand the role that these transforming genes play in well-defined tumor models. During the last two years, we have searched for the presence of ras oncogenes in several model systems in which malignant transformation (in vitro studies) or tumor formation (in vivo studies) was induced by chemical carcinogenes.

A) <u>In vitro studies: ras oncogenes in tumorigenic guinea pig cell lines</u>.

Guinea pig fetal cells exposed to chemical carcinogens are known to proceed through several well-defined preneoplastic stages before becoming tumorigenic (23). Morphological transformation as evidenced by loss of cellular orientation is the earliest change and is usually followed by the ability of these carcinogen-treated cells to form colonies in semisolid medium. These multiple changes appear to be necessary for the acquisition of the complete neoplastic phenotype. These features made this in vitro model system suitable for studying the role of oncogene activation in the multistep process of carcinogenesis.

Guinea pig cell lines, transformed by in vitro treatment with 3-methylcholanthrene (3-MCS), benzo(a)pyrene B(a)P or N-methyl-N-nitro-N' nitrosoguanidine (MNNG), as well as cell lines derived from fetuses, which received a single transplacental injection of MNNG or diethylnitrosamine (DEN) 48 hours prior to its removal (23), were used as a source of DNA in gene transfer assays. A nontreated guinea pig fetal cell culture GP84, and several guinea pig fetal cell pools were used as controls. Foci of morphologically transformed NIH/3T3 cells were induced by DNA from each of the above tumorigenic guinea pig cell lines, but not by DNA from GP84 or from six different cell pools derived from untreated guinea pig embryos (Table 2) (69). Representative transformants derived from each of the five guinea pig cell lines were submitted to Southern blot analysis utilizing ras-specific probes. An 11-kpb Eco RI DNA fragment of guinea pig origin was specifically detected in each of the NIH/3T3 transformants tested, but not in control NIH/3T3 cells (69). This DNA fragment hybridized preferentially to probes derived from human N-ras and H-ras oncogenes and less intensively with a probe specific for the human K-ras locus (69). These results clearly demonstrate that the above tumorigenic guinea pig cell lines contain the same ras oncogene. However, the precise ras locus that became activated in these cells remains to be determined. Frequent detection of ras oncogenes in this well-defined in vitro model system should make it possible to investigate the role of ras gene activation in the multiple stages that carcinogen treated guinea pig cells require to acquire their full malignant phenotype.

B) <u>In vivo studies: carcinogen-induced mammary carcinomas of rats.</u>

Injection of a single dose of nitrose-metyl-urea (NMU) to Buf/N female rats during their sexual development leads to the reproducible induction of mammary carcinomas (30, 38). Initial experiments in our laboratory demonstrated that DNAs extracted from nine excised NMU-induced mammary tumors were positive in transfection assays using NIH/3T3 cells as recipients (68). In contrast, DNAs from normal

Table 2 DNAs isolated from Guinea pig cells treated with chemical carcinogen transformed NIH/3T3 mouse cells.

Source	Carcinogen treatment	Cell line	Transforming activity (foci per ug DNA)
32-day fetuses	None		0.00
48-day fetus	3-MCA	74-C3	0.10
43-day fetus	B(a)P	104-C1	0.15
43-day fetus	MNNG	107-C3	0.10
38-day fetus	DEN	HM2-C1	0.08
49-day fetus	MNNG	HM4-C1	0.09

breast tissues were consistently negative. Molecular characterization of the resulting NIH/3T3 transformants indicated that in each case, the oncogene responsible for their malignant phenotype was the H-ras-1 gene. Molecular cloning and DNA sequence analysis of this transforming gene revealed that its malignant activation was due to the same mutational mechanism previously identified in transforming ras genes present in human tumors (68). Substitution of the second deoxyguanosine of the twelfth codon of the H-ras gene by a deoxyadenosine led to the replacement of glycine by glutamic acid as the twelfth amino acid residue of the transforming p21 protein.

Several RFLPs created by point mutations in codons 12 and 61 of the rat H-ras-1 locus could be utilized to detect transforming H-ras genes (Table 3). For instance, the deoxyguanosine mutated in the cloned NMU-H-ras-1 oncogene is part of the sequence GAGG, which is specifically recognized by the restriction endonuclease Mnl I (68). Mutations in this particular nucleotide (residue +35) or in either of the two deoxyguanosines responsible for the codon properties of codon 13 (residues +37 and +38) will eliminate this cleavage site (Figure 4).

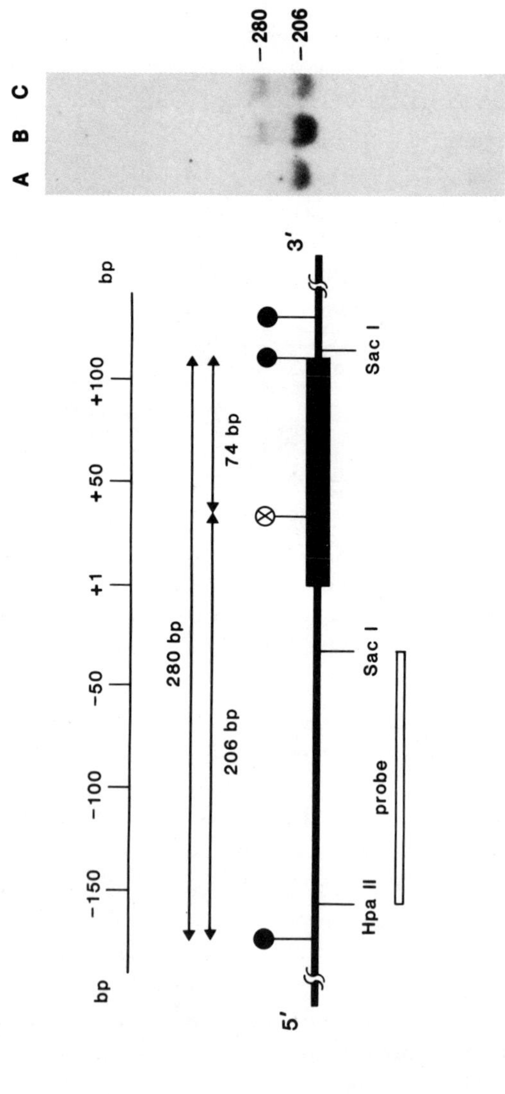
A
B
C
280
206
bp
−150
−100
−50
+1
+50
+100
bp
280 bp
206 bp
74 bp
5′
3′
Hpa II
probe
Sac I
Sac I

Table 3. Restriction enzyme polymorphisms created by point mutations in codons 12 and 61 of the rat H-ras-1 locus.

Codon	Mutation	Polymorphism
12	G^{34} C	New Taq I, Ava I, Xho I sites
	G^{35} N	Lost Mnl I site
	G^{35} C	New Bbv I,Fnu 4HI,Pst I sites
	A^{36} N	Lost MNl I site
61	C^{181} G	New Hph I site
	A^{182} T	New Hba I site
	A^{182} C	New Ava II, Sau 961 sites
	A^{182} G	New Taq I site
	A^{183} T	New Nla III site

Figure 4. Detection of H-ras oncogenes in NMU-induced mammary carcinomas of Buf/N rats by molecular polymorphisms. Wildtype (●) and polymorphic (⊗) Mnl I cleavage sites either within or in the vicinity of the first exon (▬, nucleotides +1 to +111) of the Buf/N rat H-ras-1 locus are indicated. Southern blot analysis of Mnl I cleaved normal rat DNA yields a fragment of 206 bp that can be identified with the indicated 120 bp Hpa II-Sac I ^{32}P-labeled DNA probe. DNAs containing mutations within nucleotides +35 to +38 (GAGG) exhibit a 280 bp DNA fragment because of the elimination of the polymorphic MNl I cleavage site. DNAs tested include those isolated from (A) a normal Buf/N breast and (B,C) representative NMU-induced BuF/N mammary carcinomas.

As a consequence, a RFLP indicative of the malignant activation of the H-ras-1 locus will be created by point mutations in any of these three deoxyguanosines (substitution of the deoxyadenosine residue will not have any biological significance, as it will not alter the codon specificity). We have now tested fifty-eight NMU-induced mammary tumors in three different strains of rats including Buf/N, Sprague-Dawley, and Fischer 344. We have found that more than 80% of the NMU-induced tumors have activated H-ras-1 oncogenes, as determined by the presence of the polymorphic Mnl I cleavage site. In contrast, normal breast tissues or other tissues from the same tumor-bearing rats did not exhibit such polymorphism. This polymorphism, however, could not be detected in DNAs isolated from DMBA-induced mammary carcinomas in spite of the fact that some of them also contain transforming ras genes as determined in gene transfer experiments. These observations suggested that the specific activation of H-ras-1 oncogenes in NMU-induced tumors by mutations located in a region spanning no more than four nucleotides may be due to the direct interaction of NMU with this domain of the H-ras-1 locus.

NMU is known to methylate the N^7 and O^6 positions of deoxyguanosine residues (64). Whereas N^7 methylations elicit a repair response, O^6MeG efficiently directs the incorporation of thymidine residues in the complementary DNA strand. As a consequence, the preferential mutagenic effect of NMU is a G → A transition (20,37). As indicated above, this type of mutation was found to be responsible for the malignant activation of the cloned NMU-H-ras-1 oncogene, Thus, we decided to explore whether the observed Mnl I RFLPs in NMU-induced tumors were in fact due to $G^{35} \rightarrow A^{35}$ mutations. Recently, Conner et al. (11) have demonstrated the ability of synthetic oligonucleotide probes to detect point mutations in specific loci of genomic DNA. Thus, we synthesized nonadecamers corresponding to residues 26 to 44 of the first coding exon of the H-ras-1 locus. These oligonucleotides differ only in a single residue, that corresponding to position

+35 of the H-ras-1 gene. Figure 5 illustrates how these oligonucleotide probes specifically detect the normal and mutated alleles of the H-ras-1 locus under appropriate conditions of stringency. These synthetic oligonucleotide probes were subsequently utilized to examine the sequence status of the twelfth codon of each of the activated H-ras-1 oncogenes present in NMU-induced mammary tumors.

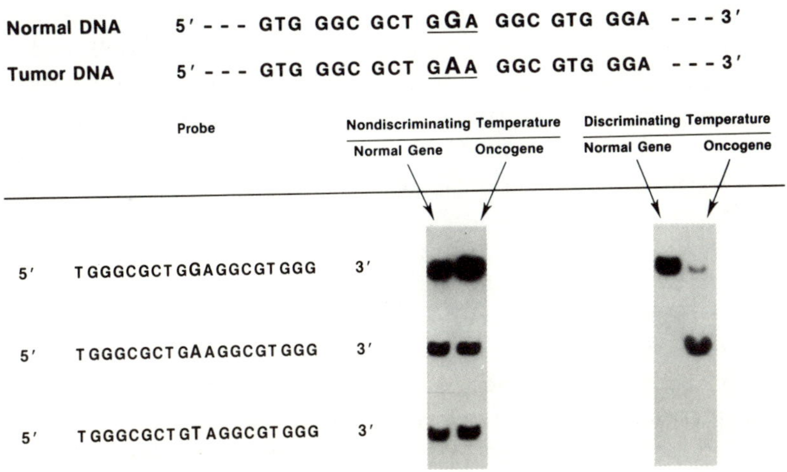

Figure 5. Synthetic nonadecamer probes corresponding to the nucleotide residues 26 to 44 in the first exon of the normal H-ras-1 locus as well as those for $G^{35} \rightarrow A$ and $G^{35} \rightarrow T$ mutations were synthesized. Probes were labeled at the 5' termini with polynucleotide kinase and hybridized to Hind III digested DNA from plasmids containing the normal and transforming alleles of the rat H-ras-1 locus. Nondiscriminating temperature was 42 C; the discriminating temperature was 65 C.

In all cases tested to date (fifteen), the same $G^{35} \rightarrow A^{35}$ point mutation was detected. In contrast each of the DMBA-induced H-ras-1 oncogenes exhibited a normal 12th codon (unpublished observations). These findings strongly suggest that NMU is the direct mutagen responsible for the G→A transitions that activate H-ras-1 oncogenes in NMU-induced tumors.

Several tentative, yet fundamental conclusions can be derived from these findings. First, malignant activation of ras genes cannot be a consequence of the genetic disarray characteristic of neoplastic cells, but instead it must play an important role in tumor development. Furthermore, the extremely short half-life of NMU and the fact that tumors result from a single carcinogenic insult indicates that oncogenic activation of the H-ras gene must be a very early event in tumor development. In agreement with these observations, Balmain and co-workers have identified transforming H-ras genes in premalignant papillomas, also suggesting an early and fundamental role of ras activation in tumorigenesis (4).

The reproducible activation of specific ras oncogenes in other animal tumor systems adds further support to the concept that these oncogenes play a fundamental role in the development of tumorigenesis (4,5,22,29). Furthermore, the similarity between the mechanisms of activation of human and animal ras oncogenes (68) suggests that at least some human cancers may proceed to malignancy through the same pathways delineated by carcinogen-induced animal tumors. The use of these model systems is therefore proving to be an invaluable tool in elucidating the molecular events leading to the initiation and development of human neoplasia

ACKNOWLEDGMENTS

Research is sponsored by the National Cancer Institute, DHHS, under contract No1-CO-23909 with Litton Bionetics, Inc. The contents of this publication do not necessarily reflect the views or policies of the Department of Health and Human Services, nor does mention of trade names, commercial products, or organizations imply endorsement by the U.S. Government. H. Zarbl is the recipient of a Postdoctoral Fellowship from Fonds de la Recherche en Sante du Quebec, Quebec, Canada.

REFERENCES

1. Adams, J.M., Gerondakis, E., Corcoran, L.M., and Gary, S.(1983). Proc. Natl. Acad. Sci. U.S.A., 80:1982.
2. Anderson, P.R., Devare, S.G., Tronick, S.R., Ellis, R.W., Aaronson, S.A., and Scolnick, E.M. (1981): Cell, 26:129.
3. Ar-Rushdi, A., Nishikura, K., Erickson, J., Watt, R., Rovera, G. and Croce, C.M. (1983): Science, 222:390.
4. Balmain, A., and Pragnell, I.B. (1983). Nature, 303:72..
5. Balmain, A., Ramsden, M., Bowden, G.T., and Smith, J. (1984): Nature, 307:658.
6. Brodeur, G.M., Seeger, R.C., Schwab, M., Varmus, H.E., and Bishop, J.M. (1984) Science, 224:1121.
7. Copon, D.J., Chen E.Y., Levinson, A.D., Seeburg, P.H. and Goeddel, D.V. (1983). Nature, 302:33.
8. Capon, D.J., Seeurg, P.H., McGrath, J.P., Hayflick, J.S., Edman, U. , Levinson, A.D., and Goeddel, D.V. (1983): Nature, 304:507.
9. Chang, E.H., Furth, M.E., Scolnick, E.M. and Lowy, D.R. (1982): Nature, 297:479.
10. Collins, S., and Groudine, M. (1982): Nature, 298:679.
11. Conner, B.J., Reyes, A.A., Morin, C., Itakua, K., Teplitz, R.L., and Wallace, R.B. (1983): Proc. Natl. Acad. Sci. USA, 80:278.
12. Cooper, G.M. (1982): Science, 217:801.
13. Dalla Favera, R., Wong-Staal, F., and Gallo, R.C. (1982): Nature, 299:61.
14. Dalla Favera, R., Bregin, M., Erickson, J., Patterson, D., Gallo, R.C., and Croce, C.M. (1982): Proc. Natl.

Acad. Sci. U.S.A., 79:7824.

15. DeFeo-Jones, D., Scolnick, E.M., Koller, R., and Dhar, R. (1983). Nature, 306:707.
16. Der, C.J., Krontiris, T.G., and Cooper, G.M. (1982): Proc. Natl. Acad. Sci. USA, 79:3637.
17. Dhar, R., Nieto, A., Koller, R., DeFeo-Jones, D., and Scolnick, E.M. (1984): Nucleic Acids Res., 12:3611.
18. Doolittle, R.F., Hunkapiller, M.W., Hood, L.E., Devare S.G., Robbins, K.C., Aaronson, S.A., and Antoniades, H.N. (1983): Science, 221:275.
19. Downward, J., Yarden, Y., Mayes, E., Scrace, G., Totty, N., Stockwell, P., Ullrick, A., Schlessinger, J., and Waterfield, M.D. (1984). Nature, 307:521.
20. Eadie, J.S., Conrad, M., Toorchen, D., and Topal, M.D. (1984): Nature, 308:201.
21. Ellis, R.W., DeFeo, D., Shih, T.Y., Gonda, M.A., Young, H.A., Tsuchida, N., Lowy, D.R., and Scolnick, E.M. (1981): Nature, 292:506.
22. Eva, A., and Aaronson, S.A. (1983): Science, 220:506.
23. Evans, C.H., and DiPaolo, J.A. (1975): Cancer Res., 35:1035-1044.
24. Fasano, O., Aldrich, T., Tamanoi, F., Taparowsky, E., Furth, M., and Wigler, M. (1984): Proc. Natl. Acad. Sci. USA, 81:4008.
25. Frankel, A.E., and Fischinger, P.J., (1976): Proc. Natl. Acad. Sci. USA, 73:3705.
26. Goldfarb, M., Shimizu, K., Perucho, M., and Wigler, M. (1982) Nature, 296:404.
27. Goyette, M., Petropoulos, C.J., Shank, P.R., and Fausto, N. (1983): Science, 219:510.
28. Graf, T., and Beug, H. (1983): Cell, 34:7.
29. Guerrero, I., Calzada, P., Mayer, A., and Pellicer, A. (1984): Proc. Natl. Acad. Sci. USA, 81:202.
30. Gullino, P.M., Pettigrew, H.M., and Grantham, F.H. (1975): J. Natl. Cancer Inst., 54:401.
31. Hall, A., Marshall, C.J., Spurr, N.K., and Weiss,.R.A. (1983) Nature, 303:396.
32. Hayward, W.S., Heel, B.G., and Astrin S.M. (1981): Nature, 290:475.

33. Heisterkamp, N., Stephenson, J.R., Groffen J., Hansen, P.F., deKlein, A., Barbam, C.R., and Grosveld, G. (1983): Nature, 306:239.
34. Jansen, H.W., Ruchert, B., Luzz, R., and Bister, K. (1983) EMBO J., 2:1969.
35. Klein, G. (1981): Nature, 294:313.
36. Little, C.D., Nan, M.M., Canery, D.N., Gazdar, A.F., and Minna, J.D. (1983): Nature, 306:194-196.
37. Loveless, A. (1969): Nature, 223:206.
38. McCormick, D.L., Adamowski, C.B., Fiks, A., and Moon, R.C. (1981): Cancer Res., 41:1690.
39. McGrath, J.P., Capon, D.J., Smith, D.H.,Chen, E.Y., Seeburg, P.H., Goeddel, D.V., and Levinson, A.D. (1983): Nature, 304:501.
40. Nakano, H., Neville, C., Yamamoto, F., Garcia, J.L., Fogh, J., and Perucho, M. (1984): In:Cold Spring Harbor Conference on Cell Proliferation and Cancer: The Cancer Cell, vol. 11, pp. 447-454. Cold Spring Harbor Laboratory, Cold Spring Harbor, New York.
41. Nakano, H., Yamamoto, F., Neville, C., Evans, D., Mizuno, T., and Perucho, M. (1984): Proc. Natl. Acad. Sci. USA 81:71.
42. Nusse, R., van Odyen, A., Cox, D., Fung, Y.K.T., and Varmus, H. (1984): Nature, 307:131.
43. Papageorge, A.G., DeFeo-Jones, D., Robinson, P., Temeles, G., and Scolnick, E.M. (1984): Mol. Cell. Biol. 4:23.
44. Parada, L.F., Tabin, C.J., Shih, .C, and Weinberg, R.A. (1982). Nature, 297:474.
45. Powers, S., Kataoka, T., Fasano, O., Goldfarb, M., Strathern, J., Broach, J., and Wigler, M. (1984): Cell, 36:607.
46. Pulciani, S., Santos, E., Lauver, A.V., Long, L.K., Robbins, K.C., and Barbacid, M. (1982): Proc. Natl. Acad. Sci. USA 79:2845.
47. Pulciani, S., Santos, E., Lauver, A.V., Long, L.K., Aaronson, S.A., and Barbacid, M. (1982): Nature, 300:539.
48. Rasheed, S., Norman, G.L., and Heidecker, G. (1983):

Science, 221:155.

49. Rechavi, A., Givol, D., and Canaani, E. (1982): Nature, 300:607-611.
50. Reddy, E.P., (1983): Science, 220:1061.
51. Reddy, E.P., Reynolds, R.K., Santos, E., and Barbacid, M. (1982): Nature, 300:149.
52. Rowely, J.D. (1983): Nature, 301:290.
53. Santos, E., Tronick, S.R., Aaronson, S.A., Pulciani, S., and Barbacid, M. (1982): Nature, 298:343.
54. Santos, E., Reddy, E.P., Pulciani, S., Feldmann, R.J., and Barbacid, M. (1983): Proc. Natl. Acad. Sci. U.S.A., 80, 4679.
55. Santos, E., Martin-Zanca, D., Reddy, E.P., Pierotti, M.A., Della Porta, G., and Barbacid, M. (1984): Science, 223:661.
56. Schwab, M., Alitalo, K., Varmus, H.E., Bishop, J.M., and George, D. (1983): Nature, 303:497.
57. Shen-Ong, G.L.C., Keath, E.J., Piccoli, S.P., and Cole, M.D. (1982): Cell, 31:443.
58. Shih, C., Shilo, B.-Z., Goldfarb, M., Dannenberg, A., and Weinberg, R.A. (1979): Proc. Natl. Acad. Sci. USA, 76:5714.
59. Shih, C., and Weinberg, R.A. (1982). Cell, 29:161.
60. Shih, T.Y., Weeks, M.O., Young, H.A., Scolnick, E.M. (1979): Virology, 96:64.
61. Shimizu, K., Birnbaum, D., Ruley, M.A., Fasano, O., Suard, Y., Edlund, L., Taparowsky, E., Goldfarb, M., and Wigler, M. (1983). Nature, 304:497.
62. Shimizu, K., Goldfarb, M., Perucho, M., and Wigler, M. (1983): Proc. Natl. Acad. Sci. USA, 80:383.
63. Shimizu, K.,Goldfarb, M., Suard, Y., Perucho, M., Li, Y., Kamata, T., Feramisco, J., Stavnezer, E., Fogh, J., and Wigler, M.H., (1983): Proc. Natl. Acad. Sci. USA, 80:2112.
64. Singer, B. (1975): Prog. Nucleic Acids Res. Mol. Biol., 15:219.
65. Spandidos, D.A., and Wilkie, N.M. (1984): Nature, 310:469.
66. Stanton, L.W., Watt, R., and Marcu, K.B. (1983):

Nature, 303:401.

67. Stehelin, D., Varmus, H.E., Bishop, J.M., and Vogt, P.K. (1976): Nature, 260:170.
68. Sukumar, S., Notario, V., Martin-Zanca, D., and Barbacid, M. (1983): Nature, 306:658.
69. Sukumar, S., Pulciani, S., Doniger J., DiPaolo, J.A.,Evans, C.H., Zbar, B., Barbacid, M. (1984): Science, 223:1197-1199.
70. Tabin, C.J., Bradley, S.M., Bargmann, C.I., Weinberg, R.A., Papageorge, A.G., Scolnick, E.M., Dhar, R., Lowy, D.R., and Chang, E.H. (1982): Nature, 300:143.
71. Tainsky, M.A., Cooper, C.S., Giovanella, B.C., and Vande Woude, G.F. (1984): Science, 225:643.
72. Taparowsky, E., Suard, Y., Fasano, O., Shimizu, K., Goldfarb, M., and Wigler, M. (1982): Nature, 300:762.
73. Taparowsky, E., Shimizu, K., Goldfarb, M., and Wigler, M. (1983): Cell, 34:581.
74. Taub, R., Kirsch, I., Morton, C., Lenoir, G., Swan, D., Tronick, S., Aaronson, S.A., and Leder, P. (1982): Proc. Natl. Acad. Sci. U.S.A., 79:7837.
75. Waterfield, M.D., Scrace, T.G., Whittle, N., Stroobant, P., Johnsson, A., Wasteson, A., Westermark, B., Heldin, C.-H., Huang, J.S., and Deuel, T.F. (1983): Nature, 304:35.
76. Yuasa, Y, Srivastava, S.K., Dunn, C.Y., Rhim, J.S., Reddy, E.P., and Aaronson, S.A. (1983): Nature, 303:775.
77. Yuasa, Y., Gol, R.A., Chang, A., Chiu, I.-M., Reddy, E.P., Tronick, S.R., and Aaronson, S.A. (1984): Proc. Natl. Acad. Sci. U.S.A., 81:3670.

THE raf ONCOGENE

U.R. Rapp[1], T.I. Bonner[2], and J.L. Cleveland[1]

1. Laboratory of Viral Carcinogenesis, National Cancer Institute, Frederick, Md. 21701, and 2. Laboratory of Cell Biology, National Institute of Mental Health, Bethesda, Md. 20205

v-raf is the oncogene of 3611 MSV and was isolated from mouse cells by transduction with murine leukemia virus (MuLV). v-raf is a new member of the src family of oncogenes and has associated ser/thr specific protein kinase activity. The active cellular homolog, c-raf-1, maps on chromosome 6 in the mouse and on chromosome 3p25 in man. There is a second gene in man, c-raf-2, which is an inactive pseudogene. the v-raf as well as the c-raf coded proteins are located predominantly in the cytoplasm. The active human gene, c-raf-1, has a complex structure with 15 exons, 9 of which are homologous to v-raf. An avian carcinoma virus, MH2, transduces the avian homologue of v-raf, v-mil, in addition to a second oncogene, v-myc. v-mil shares sequences with 11 exons of c-raf-1. A 3' portion of c-raf-1 containing six of the seven amino acid differences relative to v-raf can substitute for 3' portion of v-raf in a transformation assay. Sequence homologies between c-raf-1 and Moloney leukemia virus at both ends of v-raf indicate that the viral gene was acquired by homologous recombination, probably at the DNA level.

The v-raf oncogene acts synergistically with v-myc in transformation of fibroblastic and hemopoietic cells in vitro and induction of lymphomas in vivo. The basis for this synergism may be the combination of genes coding for "competence" (for cell division) inducing (v-myc) and "progression" inducing (v-raf) factors. Consistent with the hypothesis that v-myc may serve as a proximal effector for several distinct (competence inducing) growth factors, we find that infection with v-myc transducing MuLV abrogates the growth factor requirement of IL-2 and IL-3 dependent cultures.

ISOLATION AND STRUCTURE OF THE v-raf TRANSDUCING RETROVIRUS 3611 MSV

The viral oncogene v-raf was originally isolated from mouse cells by retrovirus transduction. The isolation of retroviral oncogenes has in the past been sporadic and limited mainly to isolations from spontaneous tumors. More recently we and others have designed experiments to generate acutely transforming retroviruses by growth of type C viruses in chemically or phenotypically transformed cells (1-5), followed by selection for tumor induction in vivo (1-3). In the course of these experiments, we have isolated several new transforming viruses, including 3611-murine sarcoma virus (MSV) (6). 3611-MSV transforms embryo fibroblasts and epithelial cells in culture and induces fibrosarcomas in vivo. 3611-MSV is replication defective, requiring a type C helper virus for propagation both in vitro and in vivo. By using endpoint transmission of 3611-MSV to MMCE C17 mouse and FRE 3A rat cells, several nonproductively transformed clonal cell lines have been derived. Pseudotype virus stocks obtained from such clones transform cells in vitro, are highly oncogenic in vivo, and exhibit host range and serological properties that are characteristic of their helper virus component. Analysis of viral antigen expression in 3611-MSV transformed cells has led to the demonstration of a 75,000-molecular-weight (M_r) polyprotein and a 90,000-M_r glycosylated form of this protein, both containing the amino-terminal murine leukemia virus gag gene proteins p15 and p12. In contrast to gene products of many previously described mammalian transforming viruses, 3611-MSV-encoded polyproteins lack detectable tyrosine specific protein kinase activity, and 3611-MSV-transformed cells resemble chemically transformed cell line C3H/MCA-5, from which 3611-MuLV was originally derived, in that they do not exibit elevated levels of phosphotyrosine (6).

We have molecularly cloned the unique acute transforming replication-defective mouse type C virus (3611-MSV) and characterized its acquired oncogene (7). The viral genome closely resembles Moloney (M) murine leukemia virus (MuLV), except for a substitution in M-MuLV in the middle of p30 and the middle of the polymerase gene (pol). Heteroduplex analysis revealed that 2.4 kilobases of M-MuLV DNA were replaced by 1.2 kilobases of cellular DNA. The junctions between viral and cellular sequences were determined by DNA sequence analysis to be 517 nucleotides into the p30 sequence and 1,920 nucleotides into the polymerase sequence. Comparison of the transforming gene from 3611-MSV, designated v-raf, with previously isolated retrovirus oncogenes either by direct hybridization or by comparison of restriction fragments of their cellular homologs showed it to be unique. Transfection of NIH 3T3 cells with cloned 3611-MSV proviral DNA lead to highly efficient transformation and the recovered virus elicited tumors in mice typical of the 3611-MSV virus. Transfected NIH 3T3 cells express two 3611-MSV-specific polyproteins (P75 and P90), both of which contain NH2-terminal gag gene-encoded components linked to the acquired sequence (v-raf) translational product. The cellular homolog, c-raf, is present in one or two copies per haploid genome in mouse and human DNA.

PRIMARY STRUCTURE OF v-raf, A NEW MEMBER OF THE src FAMILY OF ONCOGENES

To assess the possibility of a distant relationship

between the v-raf oncogene gene and other oncogenes, we determined the nucleic acid sequence of v-raf (8). A 1514-base-pair (bp) long DNA fragment of 3611-MSV encompassing v-raf and adjacent viral gag (p30) and polymerase gene domains was sequenced. Examination revealed no sequences characteristic of promoter or splice acceptor regions, nor a polyadenylation signal. This is consistent with the expression of v-raf as a gag-x polyprotein that depends on the virus for transcriptional and translational controls. The single open reading frame translating the gag-raf gene is terminated by an amber codon approximately 180 nucleotides from the presumed 3' end of the inserted cellular sequences. By analogy to the synthesis and posttranslational modification of Moloney murine leukemia virus (MuLV) $Pr65^{gag}$, two raf-containing polypeptides would be expected in transformed cells. The smaller one would be initiated at the AUG (A, adenine; U, uracil; G, guanine) from which the translation of $Pr65^{gag}$ begins. This gag-raf polyprotein which contains gag-specific amino acids and 329 raf-speficic amino acids, has a predicted molecular size of 79,000 daltons. The larger polyprotein, representing the initiation product characteristic of $gPr80^{gag}$, the glycosylated form of $Pr65^{gag}$, should migrate as if it has a molecular size of 94,000 daltons. These predictions agree well with the 90,000 and 75,000-dalton gag-fusion polypeptides observed in 3611-MSV transformed cells (6). The glycosylation of P90 may involve sites on gag as well as a potential site near the carboxyl terminal end of v-raf (8). In further analogy with the gag precursor proteins, we find that only the nonglycosylated form, P75, is phosphorylated at a serine residue and myristilated at the NH2 terminal (9).

The predicted amino acid sequence of v-raf was compared by two-dimensional dot matrix analysis with the predicted amino acid sequences of other oncogenes. Comparison with the proposed sequences for v-src, v-yes, v-abl, v-fps, v-fes, v-mos, and the ovine adenosine 3', 5'-monophosphate-dependent protein kinase revealed regions of significant homology throughout the v-raf sequence.

This suggests that the v-raf oncogene is a member of the evolutionarily related "src family" of transforming proteins. No significant homologies were observed in comparisons of v-raf with the oncogene sequences of myc, fos, rel, sis, Blym, ras, ski, or myb.

Examination of the v-raf amino acid sequence shows that it aligns exclusively with the kinase half of the src family progenitor. The homology begins within a region corresponding to exon 7 of c-src and terminates near the location of v-src c-src sequence divergence. From this analysis v-raf appears to be as closely related to v-src as are v-fps, v-fes, or v-abl. This is surprising since the oncogene proteins of v-fps, v-fes, and v-abl have readily detectable tyrosine-specific kinase activity, whereas we have been unable to detect a similar actity for v-raf. We find that v-mos, another tyrosine kinase-negative src family oncogene, is distantly related to v-raf although extensive regions of homology were prominent at the termini of each sequence. The amino acid sequence relatedness between v-raf and the src family oncogenes varied from 26 percent for v-mos to 29 percent and 25 percent for v-fes and v-src, respectively. By comparison, the corresponding regions of v-src and v-fes show a 39 percent amino acid homology.

Near the amino end of the v-raf sequence lies one of the several regions of greater than 57 percent homology detected in the dot matrix comparisons. This domain is predicted to fold into a beta-sheet-alfa-helix-beta-sheet configuration analogous to that exhibited by lactate dehydrogenase and by the ras family of oncogenes (10). This amino acid sequence is thought to be responsible for a nucleotide binding activity. Such a binding activity has been demonstrated for the ras p21 protein and for $p60^{src}$.

The most distinctive feature in the remainder of the v-raf oncogene sequence lies in the region corresponding to exons 10 and 11 of c-src. Contrally located in this region is the tyrosine acceptor site of the tyrosine kinase-positive oncogenes. In v-raf, there are two regions of more than 60 percent homology separated by 32 amino acids of unique sequence. The proteins coded for by the five oncogenes capable of phosphorylating tyrosine show identical or conservatively altered amino acid sequences (matches occur in 20 of 20 amino acids) throughout this acceptor site region and identical predicted secondary structures. The oncogene v-mos and v-raf, both of which lack a tyrosine acceptor, and also v-erb B, exhibit variations from the consensus sequence (matches in 6 of 20, 8 of 20, and 13 of 20 amino acids, respectively) as well as alterations in the predicted secondary structures. When these differences, which are multifocal, are arranged in a gradient of severity relative to the tyrosine acceptor genotype, a time table for their emergence in evolution is suggested (see below). Although all of the members of this family have unique carboxyl terminal sequences, they all contain positively charged amino acids within a predicted alfa-helical domain. Deletion of these sequences in v-raf removes its transforming activity (M. Goldsborough et al., in preparation).

Using the computer programs ALIGN and MATTOP we compared src family members according to the relatedness of their amino acid sequences. The phylogenetic tree built from these comparisons suggests that the src family of oncogenes evolved from a common ancestor. This phylogenetic arrangement predicts that genetic loci related to v-raf and v-erb B sequences should be present in Drosophila melanogaster and separate from the loci determined for the v-abl v-src, and v-fps sequences. We have found this to be the case for v-raf. We hypothesize that the v-mos sequence represents to oldest known derivative of the ancestral gene, marking a time in evolution at which introns were not present within the family progenitor. The next sequences for which we have a record of diverging would be those of v-raf and v-erb B. It is only after this point in evolution that tyrosine-specific kinase activity is a characteristic of the src family members. Consistent with this evolutionary pattern is the absence of detectable phosphotyrosine in yeast proteins. The possibility, however, exists that the dominant tyrosine-specific kinase demonstrable in the most recent evolutionary members of this family represents a broadening of substrate specificity.

ASSOCIATION OF A ser/thr-SPECIFIC PROTEIN KINASE WITH PURIFIED gag-raf PROTEIN IN VITRO

While we had been unable to detect tyrosine specific protein kinase of gag-raf polyproteins under standard assay conditions, an autophosphorylating activity with specificity for ser/thr was recently demonstrated for purified gag-raf protein (11). For this determination, assay conditions were modified to include Mn^{2+} as divalent ions and gag-raf proteins attached to immunobeads after immunoaffinity chromatograhy with anti-MuLV P30 antibody. A preliminary search for cellular target proteins has not yielded information about protein substrates. It will be important in the future to test certain oncogene proteins such as myc, which is phosphorylated in ser/thr and which acts synergistically with v-raf in transformation, as acceptor molecules for the v-raf-associated protein kinase. The finding of v-raf-associated protein kinase activity is consistent with the last possibility mentioned above for the evolution of src family kinases which suggests emergence of specificity for tyrosine as the result of a broadening of substrate specificity.

STRUCTURE AND BIOLOGICAL ACTIVITY OF THE HUMAN HOMOLOGUES OF THE raf ONCOGENE

We have shown that there are two human genes homologous to the raf oncogene, c-raf-1 and c-raf-2 (12). One of these two genes, c-raf-2, is a processed pseudogene which appears to have been formed early in the evolution of primates. Since c-raf-2 contains numerous insertions and deletions relative to c-raf-1 as well as numerous termination codons in all reading frames, it is unlikely to be functional. The human genomic DNA clones that we have isolated contain all the sequences which are homologous to the viral transforming gene v-raf, and contain the 3' end of the gene as defined by the poly (A) position of cDNA clones from placental and liver mRNAs (Bonner, T.I., Opperman, H., Seeburg, P., and Rapp, U.R., in preparation). However, the sequence of the c-raf-2 gene suggests that it may have been produced from an alternately spliced message in which exon 11 was replaced by another exon(s). If such an exon exists, it is not located in the present clones and must be at least 5.5 kb 3' of the end of the present exon 11.

The exon sequences of the present clones account for 2.2 kb of the 3.1 kb message that we detect in human lymphocytes, and thus, there must be more of the gene to be identified beyond the 5' end of the present clones. Analysis of cDNA clones indicates that only 0.6 kb of the additional 0.9 kb in mRNA is actually coding sequence. Preliminary analysis of clones from the 5' end of c-raf-1 indicates that these additional coding sequences are distributed over another 15 kb. Thus, the entire gene spans more than 36 kb. Given the large sizes of the c-raf-1 gene, it is unlikely to be transferred intact in transfection experiments using human DNA from normal or tumor cells. Thus, one means of assessing what changes in the gene are necessary to activate its tumorigenic potential does not appear to be useful. As a first step toward this goal, we have shown that the c-raf-1 gene can be substituted for the 3' two-thirds of v-raf without impairing its transformation capability in transfecting assays. This eliminates all but one of the seven amino acid changes between v-raf and c-raf-1 as being essential for transformation. Since transformation of mouse NIH 3T3 cells by promoter mediated activation of the cellular mouse gene has been achieved (13), it is unlikely that isolated amino acid changes are necessary to activate the raf gene. Thus, it appears that the raf genes cause transformation by an inappropriately high level of expression of the normal gene product or by expression of a truncated gene product which does not function normally.

THE MECHANISM OF TRANSDUCTION OF v-raf

The transforming retroviruses are generally considered to have arisen from a recombination event between a nontransforming retrovirus and a normal cellular gene. In the case of the 3611-MSV virus, this recombination event would have involved a murine retrovirus which is closely related to the Moloney Leukemia Virus (MoLV) and the mouse gene which is homologous to the human c-raf-1. In comparing the sequences of c-raf-1, v-raf, and MoLV to determine the precise points at which this recombination would have occurred, we find that there is a stretch of 8-16 nucleotides at each end of the v-raf sequence in which the c-raf-1, v-raf and MoLV sequences are nearly identical (Figure 1). Thus, the beginning of v-raf homology occurs in exon 3 of c-raf-1 within the sequence CTGGGACCCAGG which is identical in c-raf-1 and v-raf and differs from the corresponding MoLV sequence only by an extra A in the MoLV sequence. Based on a comparison of only the v-raf and MoLV sequences, we had previously identified (7) the beginning of the raf-specific sequence in v-raf as occurring immediately after this 12 nucleotide sequence. Furthermore, we supposed that the A which is present in MoLV but absent in v-raf was deleted after the recombination event in order to place the v-raf sequence in the proper reading frame. However, since this A is missing in the human c-raf-1 sequence, it is likely that it is also missing in the murine homologue. Thus, it appears that the point of recombination is within the CTG (underlined above) which is common to the three sequences. Similarly, the end of v-raf homology occurs within the 3' untranslated sequence of exon 11 within the sequence AAGGAAGC, which is nearly (7/8 nucleotides) identical to the corresponding sequence, ATGGAAGC, of v-raf and MoLV. The single nucleotide difference presumably reflects evolutionary divergence between the human and mouse genes.

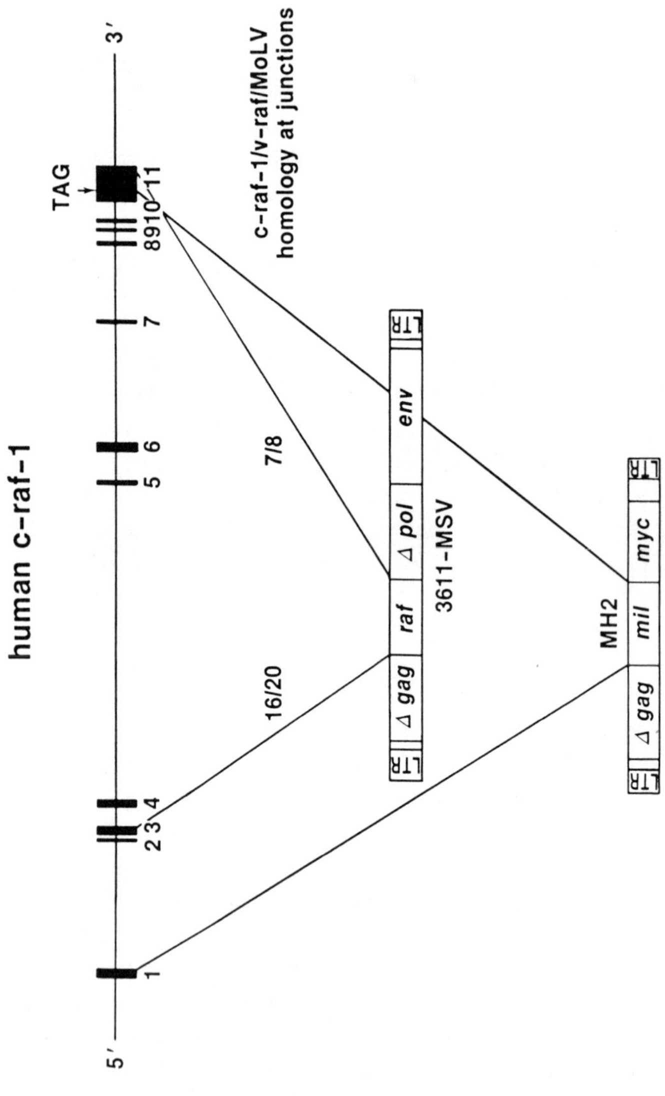

Figure 1. Relationship of v-raf and v-mil to c-raf-1. Exons of c-raf-1 are indicated by black boxes, introns as horizontal lines. Viral genes in 3611 MSV and MH2 are gag = internal structural proteins, pol = reverse transcriptase, env = envelope glycoproteins, = deleted version of gene.

These sequence homologies imply that the point of recombination cannot be assigned to a specific nucleotide at either end of the v-raf sequence. More importantly, the sequence homologies provide clear evidence that the tranduction occurred via homologous recombination (Figure 1). Although short stretches of homology between viral and cellular sequences have been observed in other transforming retroviruses, only in the case of FBJ virus, which contains the fos oncogene, has such homology been observed at both ends of the acquired sequence (14). In most cases, homology is seen at the 5' junction but not the 3' junction. Since the 3' junction is often in the 3' untranslated region, the preservation of these sequences is not required for transforming activity of the virus and may be lost with repeated passage of the virus. If one were to assume that all the viral oncogenes are transduced by a common mechanism, then it should be by homologous recombination at the DNA level since at least two viral oncogenes, v-myb (15) and the v-myc gene in the MH2 virus (16), contain intron sequences. These findings raise as a formal possibility the model for retrovirus transduction outlined in Figure 2. They are also compatible with a modification of previously proposed two-step models which require retrovirus integration next to an oncogene before transduction can begin.

ROLE OF THE raf ONCOGENE IN NATURAL TUMORS

3611-MSV induces fibrosarcomas and hyperplasia of hemopoietic tissues upon inoculation of newborn NFS/N mice. The in vivo infected hemopoietic cells cannot be grown in culture unless a growth factor, such as Interleukin 3 (17) is added to the culture medium (U.R. Rapp and J. Ihle, in preparation). In cell culture 3611-MSV transforms established lines of fibroblastic and epithelial cells (6), primary mouse fibroblast cells, and human fibroblastic and epithelial cell strains (U.R. Rapp, unpublished data).

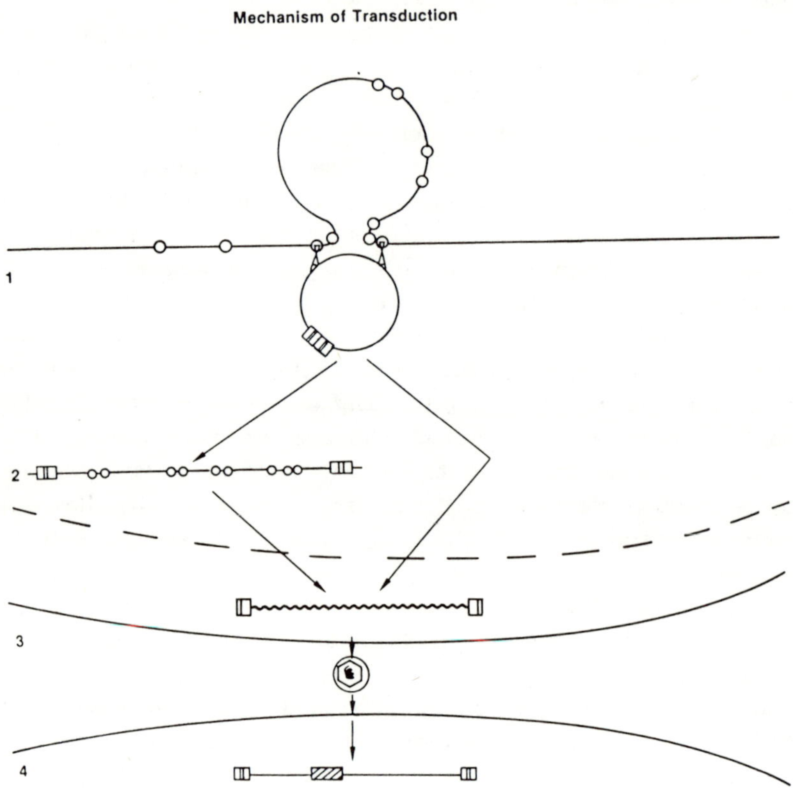

Figure 2. A possible mechanism of transduction. Homologous recombination, both 5' and 3', occurs between the unintegrated DNA intermediate of MoLV and the c-raf locus. The introns are stripped during transcription and the RNA is packaged by helper virus and shed. Reverse transcription establishes the 3611 MSV carrying the v-raf oncogene.

Primary hemopoietic cells from fetal liver or adult bone marrow and spleen are being immortalized in culture media supplemented with IL3. The immortalized cells remain continously dependent on IL3 (U.R. Rapp and J. Ihle, in preparation).

In vitro transformed fibroblastic and epithelial cells are induced for release of transforming growth factors TFGα and TGFβ and are blocked for the binding or epidermal growth factor (EGF). Transformed epithelial MMCE cells were analyzed for the production and deposition of pericellular glycoproteins by immunofluorescence and by radioactive metabolic and cell surface labeling techniques followed by analysis in polyacrylamide gels and fluorography (18). The pericellular fibronectin matrix was lost, but unlike in virus-transformed fibroblastic cells, the production of fibronectin was not affected. The major differences detected were decrease in collagen production and initiation of synthesis of two major glycoproteins with Mr 58,000 and 60,000. Cell surface carbohydrate labeling indicated that after 3611-MSV transformation the cells expressed Mr 100,000 and 68,000 polypeptides. It will now be interesting to determine the reationship of the 58,000- and 60,000-dalton peptides to either growth factors or growth factor-dependent transforming factors and whether the transformed epithelial cells release activity which preferentially transforms phenotypically epithelial cells.

In order to obtain a first indication as to the histologic type of natural tumors in which the raf oncogene might be involved we have determined the chromosomal location of raf genes in mouse and man. If tumor specific rearrangement activates oncogenes, it might be possible to use the chromosomal location of an oncogene to focus on a few types of tumors as the most probable candidates for involvement of the oncogenes.

We analyzed a set of hamster-mouse somatic cell hybrids by blot hybridization to find the chromosomal location of the mouse cellular homolog of c-raf (19). Hybrids were generated by fusing cells from three inbred mouse strains (BALB, A, and NGS.Akv-2) with cells of the Chinese hamster line E36. These hybrids contain all of the hamster chromosomes and different subsets of mouse chromosomes. Mouse chromosomes were identified in metaphase spreads by Giemsa-trypsin binding followed by staining with Hoechst 33258. High-molecular-weight DNA was prepared from hamster, mouse, and hybrid cells digested with BglI or PstI, electrophoresed, and examined in Southern blots with the v-raf probe. All 22 somatic cell hybrid lines tested after digestion with BglI contained a 4.45-kb hamster specific fragment, and seven of these hybrids also contained the 12-kb mouse specific band. Correlations with the mouse chromosome content of these 22 lines showed that the c-raf sequence is present in mouse chromosome 6. All seven hybrids with mouse c-raf sequences contained chromosome 6, and all of the remaining hybrids lacked both chromosome 6 and c-raf. All other mouse chromosomes showed discordant segregation with this sequence. This correlation was confirmed in experiments in which PstI instead of BglI was used for DNA restriction. Thus we have shown that the mouse c-raf gene is present on chromosome 6.

The two human genes, c-raf 1 and c-raf-2 were mapped in an analogous fashion with the help of thirthy-five somatic cell hybrids made with normal human lymphocytes and either mouse or Chinese hamster cell lines (20). The results obtained for the 22 Chinese hamster-human hybrids and 13 mouse-human hybrids indicate a clear correlation between the presence of c-raf-1 and chromosome 3 and the presence of c-raf-2 and choromosome 4. The presence of the pseudogene c-raf-2 on a different chromosome from the one containing c-raf-1, together with a lack of introns, is consistent with c-raf-2 being a processed pseudogene.

There are numerous reports of chromosome 3 abnormalities in human tumors that lack any clear specificity. There are, however, three types of tumors that involve specific rearrangements of chromosome 3, all on the short arm of the chromosome: familial renal cell carcinoma with translocations at 3p21 and 3p13-14, small-cell lung carcinomas with deletions of various sizes spanning the region 3p14-3pter, and mixed parotid gland tumors with translocations at 3p21 and 3p25 (cited in 20). All three tumors involve epithelial cells that might be expected to be transformed by raf. To determine the locus of the c-raf-1 gene more precisely and to evaluate whether it is near any of these tumor-specific rearrangements, we have mapped its position by chromosomal in situ hybridization. Analysis of 70 chromosomal spreads revealed that approximately 9 percent of all silver grains were located on or directly beside chromosome 3 at band p25 and that approximately 16 percent of all cells showed hybridization at 3p25. Statistical analysis of these data by the Poisson distribution with the number of grains per chromosome band adjusted for the relative size of the band in a 400-band idiogram revealed a highly significant (P | 10-33) distribution at 3p25. This location suggests that the c-raf-1 locus may be involved in the mixed parotid gland tumors with the t(3;8) (p25;q21) translocation. It is likely from its position that the c-raf-1 gene is not rearranged in either small-cell lung carcinoma or renal cell carcinoma. However, most 3p deletions in small-cell lung carcinoma could result in a hemizygous state for the c-raf-1 gene. Whether this alteration reveals the presence of a deleterious recessive gene, as has been proposed for retinoblastoma (21), remains to be determined. A recent examination of the exon-composition of c-raf mRNA from NIH 3T3 cells suggests that it is different from that in v-raf. Thus it appears that transformation of NIH fibroblast cells is the consequence of ecotopic expression of c-raf protein from alternately spliced c-raf mRNA. We are currently performing a similar analysis for mRNA from small cell lung carcinoma cells.

SYNERGYISM BETWEEN raf AND myc ONCOGENES

The avian carcinoma virus MH2 was recently shown to contain a second oncogene, v-mil, in addition to the v-myc gene which had previously been identified in this virus (22-25). Because of the possible association of v-raf with the induction of lung carcinoma (see above) we considered the possibility of homology between the v-raf and v-mil genes. The first indication of a possible sequence relationship between cloned v-mil and v-raf DNAs came from a comparison of their restriction site patterns. A direct demonstration of sequence homology was provided by digestion of cloned MH2 DNA with appropriate restriction enzymes, and hybridization of blotted DNA fragments to both v-mil and v-raf probes. Complete confirmation of the Southern blot data was obtained by heteroduplex between cloned integrated MH2 DNA and v-raf containing segment of 3611-MSV DNA subcloned in pBR322 which showed that v-raf and v-mil sequences annealed over a contiguous segment of 0.9 kb (26,27). Further confirmation of these hybridization data was obtained by comparison of the nucleotide sequences of v-raf and v-mil. The 80% homology between the nucleotide sequences and the 94% homology between the predicted amino acid sequences of the two viral genes clearly indicate that these are the avian and murine forms of the same gene (16). Comparison of the two sequences with that of human cellular homologue (12) indicates that v-raf has more 3' untranslated sequences while v-mil has additional sequences from two 5' exons of the cellular homologue. Although the mil/raf amino acid sequences reveal partial homology to that of the v-src product, no tyrosine-specific protein kinase activity is detected for the gag-mil and the gag-raf hybrid proteins which instead are associated with a ser/thr specific protein kinase (see above). The nucleotide sequence of v-mil is in agreement with that for v-mil (mht) reported by Kan et al., (28) and Galibert et al. (29). A summary of general properties of the raf oncogene is given in Table 1.

The mode of acquisition of two oncogenes, v-mil and v-myc, by the parent virus of MH2 is unclear. The oncogenes may have been combined first in cells by a chromosome rearrangement before retrovirus capture; they

Table 1. Properties of the raf oncogene

Transforming gene of 3611 MSV	Isolated from a mouse with lung and peritoneal tumors. Induces fibrosarcoma/histiocytoma in newborn mice.
Avian homolog of v-raf (v-mil) is part of MH2	An avian carcinoma virus which also contains v-myc.
Member of the src	Has associated ser/thr specific family protein kinase activity.
Two genes in man, an active gene and a pseudogene	The active gene maps on chromosome 3 at p25. Site is specifically altered in small cell lung carcinoma, ovarian carcinoma, and mixed salivary gland tumors.
Active gene has 15 exons transcribed into 2 alternately spliced mRNAs	11 exons homologous to v-mil and v-raf. At least 4 additional exons at 5' end spread over another 15 Kb A 3.1 kb message in human lymphocytes. A 3 kb message in NIH/3T3 cells does not contain the 3' terminal exon contained in the liver and placental RNAs and in v-raf.
One of the gene for is 65 K M.W.	Liver and placental mRNAs code a 648AA protein which contains no transmembrane region.
Cytoplasmic location	Located predominantly in cytoplasm. Minor fraction is membrane associated.

may have been transduced separately, giving rise to independent virus isolates which subsequently recombined; or they may have been acquired from cells in two steps by the same virus. In order to begin our investigation into the origin of MH2, we have sequenced its 3' terminal region and compared it to that of other avian retroviruses (30). This portion of the viral genome commonly has a structure that is unique for a given virus strain and is therefore useful for the determination of family relationships. From the nucleotide sequence of the 3' terminal region we conclude that MH2 contains a unique assembly of 3' terminal sequences which includes part of the helper virus derived SPC region of avian sarcoma virus Y73 and the complete F3 and F1 segments of Rous sarcoma virus (RSV) strain SR-A. We are currently involved in determining the sequence of the natural helper virus of MH2 to gain further insight into its role in the generation of this unique transducing avian retrovirus.

In contrast to three other viral isolates among avian acute transforming retroviruses which contain the v-myc oncogene, MH2 is distinguished by the predominant induction of liver and kidney carcinoma in fowl. Since only MH2 contains v-mil in addition to v-myc, the pathogenic specificities of MH2 may be due to the simultaneous expression of two oncogenes. Several types of data suggest possible interaction of the raf and myc genes in human tumors. Human mixed salivary gland tumors have a 3p25, 8q23 translocation (cited in 20) which may affect the activity of both the raf oncogene at 3p25 and the myc oncogene at 8q24. A subclass of the small cell lung carcinomas, the small cell/large cell (SC/LC) carcinomas which have a particularly poor prognosis, have amplififed myc gene DNA (31) and also express the c-raf-1 gene. Moreover, the avian homolog of v-raf, v-mil, is naturally linked to v-myc in the carcinoma virus MH2 where it presumably contributes to carcinoma induction since avian acute leukemia viruses which only contain v-myc have a much lower incidence of this tumor type. It therefore became important to test the effect of v-myc on the oncogeneity of 3611-MSV. We have approached this question by making constructs between DNA from 3611-MSV, MH2, and the v-myc transducing virus MC29. Two constructs have been compared, pHWJ-1, which contained a hybrid raf/mil oncogene but a defective myc gene and pHWJ-2, in which the defect in the v-myc gene was corrected by addition of the 3 half of MC29 v-myc. Foci that appeared after cotransfection of NIH/3T3 cells with construct DNA in the presence of helper virus DNA were isolated for growth of high titer virus stocks and the virus was titrated on NIH/3T3 cells. The transformed morphology of foci induced by pHWJ-2 was dramatically enhanced relative to those induced by pHWJ-1.

In order to determine the expression of the raf/mil and myc hybrid oncogenes in these cells, we have performed immunoprecipitation and indirect immunofluorescence experiments with antisera specific for p30, v-raf/mil and v-myc, respectively. Both viral oncogenes were expressed in NIH cells infected with pHWJ-2, whereas only v-raf/mil was expressed in cells infected with pHWJ-1. NIH/3T3 cells also expressed a low level of endogenous myc protein.

Having verified the proper expression of the v-raf/mil and v-myc oncogenes by both constructs we tested their ability to transform hemopoietic cells in vitro and induce tumors in newborn NSF/N mice. Consistent with their differential ability to transform fibroblasts in culture we observed a striking difference in the transformation of bone marrow cells. Virus derived from pHWJ-2 rapidly induce the emergence of transformed cells in these cultures in the absence of added CSF-1 or IL-3 in the culture medium, whereas pHWJ-1 virus and two other MuLV constructs containing the myc oncogene (H.W. Kansen et al., unpublished data) did not. Similarly, pHWJ-2 virus induced rapid tumor development (1-2 weeks latency) whereas pHWJ-1 and the v-myc transducing constructs did not induce tumors before a period of 7 weeks. The pathology of pHWJ-2-induced tumors differed from those induced by 3611-MSV in that malignant lymphomas developed in addition to the less frequent histiocytomas,

Table 2. Frequency of establishing long-term lines

		In vivo primary tumors		In vitro HPT cultures	
Virus	Oncogene	+IL3	-IL3	+IL3	-IL3
3611	raf	10/10	0/10	3/3	0/3
HaSV	ras	3/3	0/3	10/10	0/10
pHWJ-2	raf/mil+myc	10/10	10/10	2/2	8/8*

For tumor induction newborn NSF/N mice were inoculated with 3611/MSV Harvey SV and pHWJ-2 virus. Infection of hemopoietic tissue cells (HPT) in culture included fetal liver (3611 MSV, Harvey SV and pHWJ-2) and bone marrow (3611 MSV, pHWJ-2). Culture medium was supplemented with IL-3 at 20 U/ml. *Fraction of infected cultures showing homogeneous growth at 2-3 weeks post infection. These cells are not immortalized and differentiate at 4 weeks post infection.

fibrosarcoma, and erythroleukemias which also develop with 3611-MSV (6 and unpublished data). In parallel with the difference in transforming activity of pHWJ-1 and -2 for fibroblasts and hemopoietic cells in vitro, we found that permanent cell lines would be readily established from tumors induced by pHWJ-2 virus whereas 3611 virus-infected hemopoietic cells required IL-3 for maintenance of lines in culture (Table 2). The latter phenomenon, i.e., growth factor dependence of cells from virus-induced hematopoietic tumors, is not unique to 3611-MSV and was observed with Harvey sarcoma virus (Table 2) as well as Moloney sarcoma virus (Rein and Ihle, unpublished data). Typing tumor cell lines with a panel of differentiation specific markers has indicated that pHWJ-2 induced tumors consist predominantly of T and B lineage immunoblasts (U.R. Rapp, J. Cleveland, H.W. Jansen, K. Bister, K. Holmes, T. Gredericksen and H. Morse, in preparation). Cells from 3611-MSV and Ha-MSV-induced tumors as well as from in vitro infected liver cultures which have been established in the presence of IL-3 initially consist of a mixture of pre-B cells, pre-T cells, macrophages and mast cells which develop into homogenous IL-3-dependent permanent mast cell lines that continue to express virus specific oncogene products (U.R. Rapp and J.N. Ihle, in peparation). Bone marrow cells transformed in vitro with pHWJ-2 in the absence of a growth factor supplement may belong to the myeloid cell lineage (E. Blasi, L. Varesi, P. Borchert, H.W. Jansen, K. Bister and U.R. Rapp, in preparation). We conclude that combination of the v-raf with v-myc oncogene increases the transforming activity of either gene in NIH/3T3 and hemopoietic cells, respectively. In the presence of both genes, cells are transformed in vivo and in vitro to autonomous, factor-independent growth whereas the v-raf gene alone transforms hemopoietic cells in vivo to immortalized factor (IL-3) dependent lines.

The mechanism that underlies the cooperative interaction between the v-raf and v-myc oncogenes in fibroblasts and hemopoietic cells is not understood. It appears that either oncogene provides, directly or indirectly, a function that complements the other. The v-raf oncogene as well as the Ki-ras and several src family oncogenes including v-mos, v-abl, and v-fes are known to induce production of mitogenic signals such as TGFs upon transformation of fibroblast cells. v-myc, which does not morphologically transform mammalian fibroblast cell lines to a similar degree, is not known to cause secretion of such factors by these cells. Because of the induction of v-myc in fibroblastic and lymphoid cells (32) upon exposure to PDGF we have speculated that the complementation is between a progression signal coded for or induced by v-raf and a competence signal provided by v-myc (33). If induction of myc may be a common property of "competence" (for cell division) inducing growth factors which in turn may depend on myc for signal transduction from their cell surface receptors to the nucleus, then introduction of myc into cells which depend on such competence factors for growth should abrogate their factor dependence. Consistent with this hypothesis we have recently found that infection of IL-2 and IL-3 dependent lymphoblastoid cell lines with pHWJ-2 and other myc transducing MuLV did in fact abolish their specific growth factor requirements (U.R. Rapp, H.W. Jansen, K. Bister and J.N. Ihle, in preparation).

There are currently three oncogenes implicated in the development of small cell lung carcinoma. An activated Ki-ras gene was isolated by DNA transfection (34) and may be involved in a small fraction of these tumors. The myc protooncogene was found to be amplified in small cell/large cell carcinoma (31). And according to cytogenetic (20) observations, the c-raf-1 proto-oncogene may be involved in 90% of small cell lung carcinoma. It is tempting to speculate that two or more of these genes act jointly in this tumor type similar to the joint action of v-raf and v-myc in the virus constructs that we have presented. It therefore becomes important to study the transformation of primary lung cells in culture with these constructs in the hope of gaining insights into mechanisms involved in the transformation-associated hormone production that may be typical for these tumors.

ACKNOWLEDGMENTS

We would like to acknowledge the expert assistance of Carolyn Whistler and Linda Kesselring in the preparation of this manuscript.

REFERENCES

1. Rapp, U.R. & Todaro, G.J. (1978) Science 21, 821-824.
2. Rapp, U.R. & Todaro, G.J. (1980) Proc. Natl. Acad. Sci. USA 77:624-628.
3. Rapp, U.R., Reynolds, F.H., Jr., Stephenson, J.R. (1984) in gene Transfer and Cancer, eds. Pearson, M.L. & Sternberg, N.L. (Raven press, New York, pp. 169-177.
4. Rasheed, S., Gardner, M.D. & Huebner, R.J. (1978) Proc. Natl. Acad. Sci. USA 75:2972-2976.
5. Pavlish, O.A. & Mazurenko, N.P. (1984) Neoplasma 31:15-20.
6. Rapp, U.R., Reynolds, F.H., Jr. & Stephenson, J.R. (1983) J. Virol. 45:914-924.
7. Rapp, U.R., Goldsborough, M.D., Mark, G.E., Bonner, T.I., Groffen, J., Reynolds, F.H., Jr. & Stephenson, J.R. (1983) Proc. Natl. Acad. Sci. USA 80:4218-4222.
8. Mark, G.E. & Rapp, U.R. (1984) Science 224:285-288.
9. Schultz, A.M., Copeland, T.D., Oroszlan, S., Mark, G. & Rapp, U.R., Virology, submitted.
10. Wierenga, R.J. & Hol, W.G.J. (1983) Nature 302:842.
11. Moelling, K., Heimann, B., Beimling, P., Rapp, U.R. & Sander, T. Nature, submitted.
12. Bonner, T.I., Kerby, S., Sutrave, P., Gunnell, M., Mark, G. & Rapp, U.R. Nature, submitted.
13. Mueller, R. & Mueller, D. (1984) EMBO J. 3:1121-1127.
14. Van Beveren, C., Van Straaten, F., Curren, T., Muller, R. & Verma, I.M. (1983) Cell 32:1241-1255.
15. Klempnauer, K.H., Gonda, T.J. & Bishop, J.M. (1982) Cell 31:453-463.
16. Sutrave, P., Bonner, T.I., Rapp, U.R., Jansen, H.W., Patschinsky, T. & Bister, K. (1984) Nature 309:85-88.
17. Ihle, J.N. (1984) in Contemporary Topics in Molecular Immunology, in press.
18. Keski-Oja, J., Rapp, U.R. & Vaheri, A. (1982) J. Cell. Biochem. 20:139-148.
19. Kozak, C., Gunnell, M.A. & Rapp, U.R. (1984) J. Virol. 49:297-299.
20. Bonner, T.I. O'Brien, S.J., Nash, W.G., Rapp, U.R.,

Morton, C.C., & Leder, P. (1984) Science 223:71-74.
21.Benedict, W.F., Murphree, A.L., Benerjee, A., Spina, C.A., Sparkes, M.C. & Sparkes, R.S. (1983) Science 219:973.
22.Jansen, H.W., Patshinsky, T. & Bister, K. (1983) J. Virol. 48:61-73.
23.Jansen, H.W., Ruckert, B., Lurz, R. & Bister, K. (1983) EMBO J. 2:1969-1975.
24.Kan, N.C., Flordellis, C.S., Garon, G.F., Duesbeg, P.H. & Papas, T.S. (1983) Proc. Natl. Acad. Sci. USA 80:6566-6570.
25.Cole, J., Righi, M. de Taisne, C., Dissous, C., Gegonne, G. & Stehelin D. (1983) EMBO J. 2:2189-2194.
26.Jansen, H.W., Lurz, R., Bister, K., Bonner, T.I., Mark, G.E. & Rapp, U.R. (1984). Nature 307:281-284.
27.Bister, K. et al. (1984) UCLA Symp. Molec. Cell. Biol., in press.
28. Kan, N.C. et al. (1984) Science 223:813-816.
29.Galibert, F., Dupoint de Dinechin, S., Righi, M. & Stehelin D. (1984) EMBO J. 3:1333-1338.
30.Sutrave, P., Jansen, H.W., Bister, K. & Rapp, U.R. (1984) J. Virol. in press.
31 Little, C.D., Nau M.M., Carny, D.N., Gazdan, A.F. & Minna, J.D. (1984) Nature 306:194-196.
32.Kelly, K., Cochran, B.H., Stiles, C.D. & Leder, P. (1983) Cell 35:603-610.
33.Rapp, U.R., Bonner, T.I., Moelling, K., Jansen, H.W., Bister, K. & Ihle, J.N. in Recent Results in Cancer Research, eds. Havemann, K., Sorenson, G. & Gropp, C. in press.
34.Santos, E., Martin-Zanca, D., Reddy, E.P., Pierotti, M.A., Della Porta, G. & Barbacid, M. (1984) Science 223:661-664.

ROLE OF RETROVIRAL ONCOGENES IN THE ATTACHMENT OF CELLS TO NATURAL SUBSTRATA.

B. Azzarone[1], G. Carloni[2], M. Mareel[3], O.E. Varnier[4], and A. Macieira-Coelho[1].

1. Laboratoire de Pathologie Cellulaire, I.C.I.G., 94804 Villejuif Cedex; 2. Laboratoire de Genetique Cellulaire, E.R.278 du CNRS, IRSC, C.N.R.S., 94802 Villejuif, France ; on leave from Istituto Medicina Sperimentale, C.N.R., Roma, Italy; 3. Laboratory of Experimental Cancerology, Dept. Radiotherapy and Nuclear Medicine, Academic Hospital, Ghent, Belgium; 4. Institute of Microbiology, School of Medicine, V.le Benedetto XV°, 10 16132 Genova, Italy

In vivo cell fibrin interactions play an important role in tissue repair processes and in cancer spread. These properties can be analyzed in an in vitro assay which quantifies cell-induced fibrin clot retractile (FCR) activity and cellular spreading within the fibrin clot. In several cell systems from different species, loss of FCR and spreading ability within fibrin are correlated with the acquisition of a malignant potential. These changes in cell fibrin interactions seem to take place late during the multistep process which leads eventually to the acquisition of the tumorigenic potential. In certain models, they are related to changes in the invasive and proliferative capacity of the tumor cells and to the presence of retroviral oncogenes. The invasive potential can be measured in vitro through the comparison of putative malignant cells with normal tissues.

SIGNIFICANCE OF IN VIVO CELL FIBRIN INTERACTIONS

Fibrin seems to play an important role in normal tissue organization which is manifested during wound healing. One of the first events during wound healing is the creation of fibrin threads along which fibroblasts proliferate and which seem to constitute contact guidance for the movement of cells filling the wound. The fibrin clots so formed are rapidly invaded by fibroblasts that appear to migrate within them, contributing to the contraction of the wound (1,2). Recently, a similar in vivo interaction between epithelial cells and fibrin has been described, also suggesting a biological role during tissue repair and organization (3,4).

On the other hand, it has been proposed that altered interactions between tumor cells and fibrin could play some role in the mechanisms of cancer spreading (5,6). Dvorack et al. (5) have shown that tumor cells of the hepatocarcinoma 10 line, contrary to normal cells, secrete molecules capable of activating the host's clotting system, causing the formation of a fibrin gel around the tumor cells within a few hours after implantation. They suggested that such a gel would provide tumors with a selective advantage in their interactions with the host, creating a mechanical barrier that isolates tumors from either afferent or efferent limbs of the host's immunologic system. Evidence suggesting that fibrin may play such a role was presented by Schlager and Dray (6) who reported that locally-injected anti-fibrin fragment E antibodies induced the complete regression of the hepatocarcinoma 10 cell line. These results are related to previous observations dealing with the production of procoagulation activities in murine and human tumors (for review, see ref. 5) and the presence of fibrin deposits in the immediate vicinity of many spontaneously arising tumors of animals and man (5,7).

ANALYSIS OF IN VITRO CELL-FIBRIN INTERACTIONS

Pertinent to the biological events associated with the neoplastic process, are the in vitro observations that neoplastic cells and cells transformed by oncogenic viruses show a decreased fibrinogen-fibrin binding ability (8) and are unable to induce the retraction of a fibrin clot (9-13). On the contrary, normal cells from different species of fibroblastic as well as epithelial origin are able to induce the retraction of a fibrin clot (FCR) within a few hours. We also observed that changes in FCR activity were associated with the ability of the cells to spread within the fibrin gel: loss of FCR coincided with the inability of the cells to stretch out along the fibrin threads (11).

FCR assay allows in vitro simulation at least in part of the complex cell-fibrin interactions which take place in vivo and permits the evaluation of the effects of different oncogenic agents within 24 hours from the start of the test. We first analyzed the relationship between neoplastic transformation and loss of FCR in a well characterized model system. The ability of avian sarcoma viruses (ASV) to transform both avian and mammalian cells, the availability of viral mutants and the detailed knowledge of the viral genome made ASV ideal for the study of the events that accompany cell transformation. We could show (9) that chick embryo fibroblasts (CEF), transformed by different strains of ASV, almost completely lost FCR activity regardless of the cell cycle phase in which they were tested. The fact that CEF chronically infected by ASV mutants, lacking src genes, exhibited growth curves and FCR levels similar to those of control cultures shows that loss of FCR was associated with the presence of the transforming src gene. On the other hand, in CEF infected with temperature sensitive mutants, reversion to the non transformed phenotype without loss of the tumor-forming ability at the non permissive temperature, was not associated with the recovery of FCR activity. These data indicated that changes in the FCR ability were strictly related to the in vivo neoplastic potential and to the presence of the viral transforming gene. We also investigated the loss of FCR activity in avian cells transformed by avian retroviruses bearing the erb, mic and myb oncogenes and found that the acquisition of a transformed phenotype was always related to significant decreases in FCR activity (unpublished results).

Subsequently, since neoplastic transformation is a multistep process, we tried to find out at which stage changes in FCR activity could be detected. We used murine immortalized fibroblastic cultures which display many in vitro criteria of transformation but are unable to induce tumors when injected in vivo. We could show that in C3H 10T1/2 cultures the acquisition of the tumor forming ability, obtained after exposure to X-rays, was associated with the loss of FCR activity. Moreover, the induction of unstable or stable reversion of the non neoplastic phenotype was always related to the transient or definitive re-acquisition of FCR activity (10). These data show that changes in cell-fibrin interactions are associated with changes in the ability to form tumors in vitro and that loss of FCR and the inability of cells to spread within fibrin are rather tardy events in the multistep process which leads to the acquisition of the fully malignant potential. Finally, we could confirm in human epithelial cells which undergo "spontaneous transformation", the relationship between loss of FCR activity and the acquisition of in vivo neoplastic potential, and the tardiness of the event (12).

ROLE OF Ki-RAS VIRAL ONCOGENE IN THE CONTROL OF CELL FIBRIN INTERACTIONS AND INVASIVENESS

On the basis of these results, we decided to further investigate in human cells the possible relationship between tumor-forming ability, changes in cell fibrin interactions, and expression of the activated form of the ras family oncogene (13). This was done in an established, non tumorigenic, human osteosarcoma (HOS) cell line (Te85 clone F5), which does not express endogenous active "c-oncogenes" (14), in its MSV (Kirsten strain) transformed tumorigenic counterpart (KHOS/NP), whose transfected DNA produces transformed foci in the NIH 3T3 transfection assay (14), and in its morphological non tumorigenic revertant (HOS 240S) (15). In this cell system, we studied in parallel tumorigenicity, cell shape, proliferation and retractile activity in contact with fibrin and invasiveness in chick heart organ culture. This in vitro assay mimics tumorigenicity in vivo and allows to distinguish proliferative potentials in spheroids of tumor cells (16).

We first investigated the presence and the number of integrated copies of Ki-MSV proviral DNA in the different HOS cell lines. Southern blot hybridization, performed using as a molecular probe, the KBE/2 plasmid, which contains only the viral transforming sequences (17), gives only one band of high molecular weight with KHSO/NP cellular DNA while no band was detected with 240S cellular DNA. These results are compatible with the presence of a single viral integration site in the KHOS/NP cell, and the loss of the Ki-ras viral sequences in the revertant cell lines.

Table I shows that while HOS cell lines were all invasive in the organ culture assay, they clearly differed in their proliferative potential within the invaded tissue: scant proliferation (Te85 and HOS 240S) coincided with lack of tumor-forming ability (Figure 1.). Incapacity to spread in contact with fibrin and to induce FCR (KHOS/NP) was also found to be correlated with the acquisition of malignancy. Finally, the parental HOS cell line and its MSV-transformed counterpart were able to proliferate in contact with fibrin even in the absence of growth factors in the medium while this property was lost in the revertant cell lines.

Table 1. Biological and molecular characterization of human established tumor-derived cell lines.

CELL LINE	HOS Te85 clone F5	KHOS/NP	HOS 240S
Number of integrated Ki-MSV Proviral DNA per cell*	0	1	0
Invasiveness in in organ culture	+	+	+
Proliferation within chick heart	±	++	±
Spreading on a fibrin gel	+	-	±
% FCR	70	1	50
Tumorigenicity in vivo/time of tumor appearance°	-	+	-

* Southern blot hybridization was performed using as a probe, the pKBE/2 plasmid (a pBR 322 plasmid containing an EcoRI-BamHI insert of 3,100 Bp of cloned Ki-MSV provirus) (17). Cellular DNAs of high MW were cleaved with EcoRI or HindIII restriction endonucleases which cleave respectively once and twice in the viral genome.

° $5x10^6$ cells were subcutaneously injected in the dorsal region of NIH nude mice. The inoculated mice were observed for tumor appearance over a period of 60 days.

These data suggest that the HOS cell lines examined are at different stages of an in vitro process that eventually leads to malignancy, and that progression to a

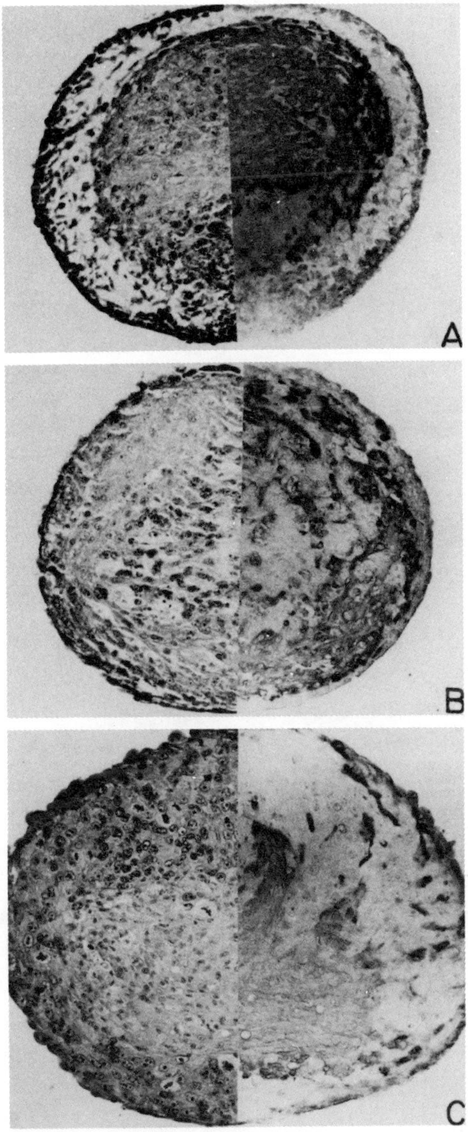
A
B
C

Figure 1. Light microphotographs of histological sections from spheroids of HOS cell lines confronted with a precultured fragment of cardiac muscle. A and B show the behaviour of HOS (Te85 clone F5) on the 3rd day (A), these cells slowly occupy the cardiac muscle, large part of which exists after 21 days incubation (B), mitotic figures are rare. The revertant HOS 240S behaves identically. C corresponds to 7 days incubation of KHOS/NP cells, these cells have almost completely replaced cardiac muscle, mitotic figures are frequent. Figures are composed of photographs from complementary areas on consecutive sections either (left) stained with hematoxilin and eosin (HOS cells have darker nuclei and larger nucleoli than cardiac cells) or right treated with antiserum against chick heart (HOS cells pale and cardiac cells dark). x200.

fully tumorigenic potential is obtained by the integration in the HOS DNA of a single Kirsten provirus. Acquisition of tumorigenicity is strictly dependent upon the presence of the V-Ki-ras oncogene, since its absence (Te85 cells) or its loss (HOS 240S line) is correlated with lack of tumor-forming ability. Finally, the V-Ki-ras oncogene seems to act primarily on the interactions with the organic substrata, with which HOS cells come in contact in vivo, improving the conditions of survival and proliferation. It is possible that these changes could create a protective fibrin barrier and a substratum for proliferation, to the HOS cells after in vivo injection.

On the basis of these results, we propose that the active form of the c-onc ras family could act in a similar way, inducing in the tumor cells similar last-step changes, which allow the expression of the tumor-forming ability.

POSSIBLE MOLECULAR TARGETS AND REGULATION OF FCR

For the moment, we cannot tell on which molecular target the v-Ki-ras oncogene acts in order to modify cell fibrin interactions. Fibrin clot retraction is a complex phenomenon which involves different cell structures: 1. membrane receptors for fibrinogen and fibrin different from fibronectin (8,18) are necessary for attachment to the substratum (8); 2. membrane calcium channels also play a role in the regulation of FCR (Azzarone et al., submitted for publication); 3. secretion of cellular factors such as trans-glutaminase are involved in the polymerization of fibrin (19) and 4. the turnover of cytoskeleton elements (18) also seems important since their inhibition causes a progressive decrease in FCR levels (unpublished results). Since these cellular structures can be disorganized by the action of oncogenic viruses (13,19,21), the loss of FCR activity in neoplastic cells may be caused both by single or combined damages induced on these structures.

PERSPECTIVES

The works described above have led to a better understanding of the cellular structure(s) involved in the regulation of the attachment of cells to their natural substrata. The availability of the cloned active forms of the viral and cellular oncogenes and of a human cell system (HOS cells) where the last step(s) towards the acquisition of malignancy can be induced will certainly be helpful in clarifying how these events can be stopped and (or) reversed.

ACKNOWLEDGMENTS

This work was supported by grants from ARC (N. 3050 and 3055), Euratom, CNRS (ATP N. 60.83.1208) and CNR (84.00838 and 84.01841).

REFERENCES

1. Banerjee, S.K., and Glynn, L.E. (1960): Ann. NY. Acad. Sci 86, 1064-1074.
2. Ross, R. (1968): Biol. Rev. 43, 51-96.
3. Clark, R.A., Della Pelle P., Lanigan, J.M., Dvorack, H.F., Colvin R.B. (1982): J. Invest. Dermatol. 79, 263-269.
4. Fujikawa, L.S., Foster, C.S., Marrist, J.J., Lanigan, J.M., Colvin, R.B. (1981): Lab. Invest. 45, 120-129.
5. Dvorack, H.F., Orenstein, N.S., Carvalho, A.C., Mallowel, C.W., Dvorack, A.M., Galli, S.J., Feder, J., Bitzer, A.M., Typisc, H. and Giovinco, P. (1979) J. Immunol. 122, 166-174.
6. Schlager, S.I. and Dray, S. (1975): Eur. J. Immunol. 115,976-981.
7. Dvorack, H.F., Dickersin, G., Dvorack, A.M., Manseav, E.J., Pyne, K. (1981): J.N.C.I 67, 335-345.
8. Colvin, R.B., Gardner, P.I., Roblin, R.O., Verderber, E.L., Lanigan, J.M., Mosesson, M.W. (1979): Lab. Invest. 41, 464-473.
9. Azzarone, B., Curatolo, L., Carloni, G., Donati, M.B., Morasca, L., Macieira-Coelho, A. (1981): J.Natl.Cancer Inst. 67:89-94.
10. Azzarone, B., Brouty-Boye, D., Macieira-Coelho, A. (1981): Int. J. Cancer 28, 799-803.
11. Curatolo L., Azzarone B., Failly-Crepin, C., Morasca, L., Macieira-Coelho, A. (1983): Int. J. Cancer 31, 249-255.
12. Azzarone, B., Macieira-Coelho, A., Curatolo, L., Brouty-Boye, D., Varnier, O.E., Donati, M.B. and Morasca, L. (1983): J.N.C.I. 71, 879-885.
13. Cooper, C.S., Blair, D.G., Oskersson, M.K., Tainsky, M.A., Eader, L.A. and Vande Woude, G.F. (1984): Cancer Res. 44, 1-10.
14. Pulciani, S., Santos, E., Lauver, A.V., Long, L.K.,

Robbins, K.C. and Barbacid, M. (1982): Proc. Nat. Acad. Sci. 79, 2845-2849.

15. Choh, Y, Cutchins, E.C., Rhim J.S., and Huebner R.J. (1976): Science 194, 951-953.
16. Mareel, M.M., Bruyneel, E.A., De Bruyne, G.K., Dragonetti, C.H., and Van Cauwenberge (1982): in Membranes and Tumor Growth, Elsevier Biomedical Press (Amsterdam) 223-232.
17. Ellis, R.W., DeFeo, D., Shih, I.Y., Gonda, M.A., Young, H.A., Tsuhida, N., Lowy, D.R., Scolnick, E.M. (1981): Nature 292, 505-511.
18. Daya-GrosJean, L., Azzarone, B., Maunoury, R., Zaech, P., Elia, G, Zaniratti, S. and Benedetto, A. (1984): Int. J. Cancer 33, 319-329.
19. Birckbichler, R., Orr, G.R., Conway, E., Patterson M.K., (1977): Cancer Res. 37, 1340-1344.
20. Azzarone, B.and Macieira Coelho, A. (1984): Exper. Cell Res.in press.
21. Balle, H, Singer S.J. (1981): Proc. Nat. Acad. Sci. 78:6986-6990.
22. Pollack, R., Osborn, M., Weber, K. (1975): Proc. Nat. Acad. Sci. 72, 994-998.

AMPLIFICATION OF CELLULAR ONCOGENES

IN COLON AND LUNG CANCER CELLS

K. Alitalo, J. Keski-Oja, K. Saksela and R. Winqvist.

Department of Virology, University of Helsinki, Haartmaninkatu 3, 00290 Helsinki 29, Finland.

Regulatory or structural alterations of cellullar oncogenes have been implicated in the causation of various forms of cancer. Oncogene alteration by point mutations can result in a protein product with strongly enhanced tumorigenic potential. Aberrant expression of cellular oncogenes may result from tumor-specific chromosomal translocations that dysregulate the normal function of a proto-oncogene. The amplification of cellular oncogenes can also enhance their expression by increasing the amount of DNA template available for the production of mRNA. It appears that the amplification of certain oncogenes is both a common correlate of the progression of some tumors and occurs as a rare sporadic event affecting various oncogenes in different types of cancer. Amplified copies of oncogenes may or may not be associated with chromosomal abnormalities that signify DNA amplification. Amplified oncogenes, whether sporadic or tumor type-specific, are expressed at elevated levels also in some cells where they are normally silent. Increased dosage of an amplified oncogene may contribute to the multistep progression of at least some forms of cancer. We summarize and discuss here several cases of oncogene amplification in cultured human colon and lung cancer cells.

CHROMOSOMAL ABNORMALITIES AND DNA AMPLIFICATION

Somatic amplification of specific genes has been implicated in an increasing variety of adaptive responses of cells to environmental stresses (21). Two cytogenetic abnormalities, double minute chromosomes (dmin:s) and homogeneously staining chromosomal regions (HSR:s) associated with DNA amplification were discovered in tumor cells and in cells selected for drug-resistance (10,15). In metaphase spreads, dmin:s appear as small, spherical, usually paired chromosome-like structures that lack a centromere (5). Homogenously staining chromosomal regions stain with intermediate intensity throughout their length rather than with the normal pattern of alternating dark and light bands in trypsin-Giemsa stained preparations (6). Both kinds of abnormalities are occasionally found in metaphases of freshly isolated cancer cells but not of normal cells (5,6).

DMIN:s and HSR:s are apparently rare in tumor cells in vivo, although exact data are difficult to obtain. These abnormalities are easily missed in routine cytogenetic analysis (5). DMIN:s and HSR:s have been found frequently in cultured malignant cells and with a notable frequency in neuroblastoma cell lines (6). Establishment of growth in culture apparently selects for tumor cells that contain either dmin:s or HSR:s. Moreover, in culture dmin:s are frequently lost concomitantly with the appearance of clonal populations of cells that have developed in HSR, suggesting that the two cytogenetic abnormalities are alternative forms of gene amplification, and that HSR:s may confer a selective advantage on cells over dmin:s (28). It has been assumed that HSR:s can break down to form dmin:s and that dmin:s can integrate into chromosomes to generate HSR:s (9). Amplified genes may also occupy abnormally binding regions, ABR:s (18).

Experimental work on drug-resistant cells has shown

that in the absence of a selection pressure (drug), dmin:s and the amplified genes that they contain are lost, whereas amplified DNA in the form of HSR:s is retained in the cells (22). This is explained by the fact that dmin:s are segregated unevenly in mitosis and frequently are lost from the nucleus due to their lack of centromeres (21,22). HSR chromosomes carry centromeres and are therefore divided equally at mitosis. If dmin:s and HSR:s contain amplified genes that encode growth-stimulating protein products, it would follow that the more stable chromosomal form, the HSR, confers a greater selective growth advantage for cells. Although dmin:s and HSR:s have been predominantly described in tumor cells selected for resistance to cytotoxic drugs, it is also clear that dmin:s and HSR:s can be present in cancer cells prior to the initiation of any form of therapy (5,6). It was in this setting that we and others first chose to explore the possible amplification of cellular oncogenes.

DMIN:S AND HSR:S CONTAIN AMPLIFIED ONCOGENES

Cases of oncogene amplifications that we have found in tumor cells are summarized in Table 1. Amplification has been found to affect at last four out of twenty known cellular oncogenes and the degree of gene amplification varies from ten to fifty-fold over the single haploid copies found in normal cells. The oncogene c-myc is amplified in a neuroendocrine cell line from a colon carcinoma, COLO 320 (Figure 1A). In these cells, the about 30-fold amplified c-myc copies were mapped either to HSR:s of a marker chromosome (2) or to dmin:s (16), depending on the particular subline studied. Since dmin:s were present already in the primary tumor cells from this colon carcinoma, it is very likely that also c-myc had been amplified during the growth of the tumor in vivo.

Extensive search for changes in other oncogenes and tumor cells has since revealed amplifications that do not show up as dmin:s or HSR:s. Thus, for example, the c-myb

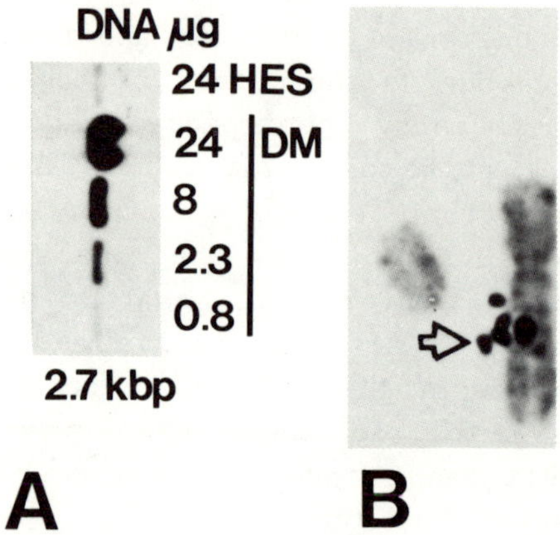

Figure 1A. Amplification and rearrangement of c-myc in COLO 320 cells. Different amounts of DNA from COLO 320 DM cells or primary cells from human embryonic skin, as indicated, were mixed with calf thymus DNA to give 24 ug of total DNA, digested with Sst I, electrophoresed, blotted and probed with a fragment of 3' human c-myc sequences. The intensities of the 2.7 kbp c-myc fragment in different samples were compared to assess its copy number, estimated to be about 30 in COLO 320 DM cells (DM). HES: human embryonic skin cells. 1B. Localization of amplified c-myc in COLO 205 cells by in situ hybridization. A characteristic, large marker chromosome (mar1) and the associated c-myb autoradiographic grains is shown. No HSR:s are found in the marker. Mar1 has probably evolved from chromosome number 6 (3, 29), the resident site of the c-myb oncogene in normal cells.

Table 1. Amplification of cellular oncogenes

Tumor cells	Oncogene	Fold	Chromosomal Location	Refs
Sporadic:				
COLO 320*	c-myc	30x	DM, HSR	(2)
COLO 201/205*	c-myb	10x	mar 1	(3,29)
Y1**	c-Ki-ras	50x	DM,HSR	(25)
Tumor specific:				
small-cell lung cancer	c-myc	up to 80x	n.d.	(17,20)
neuroblastomas	N-myc	up to 250x	DM, HSR	(23,24,26)

* Colon carcinoma; ** adrenocortical tumor. n.d., not determined; mar, marker chromosome.

oncogene is amplified in a characteristic marker chromosome of a colon carcinoma without evidence of HSR:s (3,29).

TRANSLOCATIONS AND DNA REARRANGEMENTS MAY ACCOMPANY ONCOGENE AMPLIFICATION

The evolution and progression of the karyotype of tumor cells is a complex process. Concomitant with amplification, DNA sequencs acquire an increased mobility in the genome with extrachromosomal intermediates visualized as dmin:s, transpositions and translocations to othe chromosomal segments, etc. (19). There may not be preferred chromosomal sites for the apparent reintegration of dmin:s as HSR:s (26). In at least one case oncogene amplification has, however, been observed in situ, in its resident chromosomal site (29). The finding of moderately amplified oncogenes also in chromosomal sites lacking HSR:s (see Fig; 1B) suggests that (onco)gene amplification may be more common than the structural alterations revealed by chromosome banding and microscopy (3,29).

In the colon carcinoma COLO 320, both damaged and normal forms of the c-myc gene are amplified (2). Although individual cell clones have not been examined yet, our unpublished experiments suggest that the same dmin-containing cells harbor and express both normal and rearranged forms of c-myc. However, the normal form of the amplified gene predominates in COLO 320 cells containing HSR:s; the rearranged version is present only in what appears to be a single copy (2). Although they have not been sequenced, other reported cases of amplified oncogenes are apparently structurally normal on the basis of mapping with restriction endonucleases (Table 1).Thus, mutation does not appear to be a necessary feature of oncogene amplification.

ENHANCED EXPRESSION OF AMPLIFIED ONCOGENES

In all cases where they have been studied, the amplified oncogenes have been found abundantly expressed at the RNA level, roughly in proportion to the amount of DNA amplification (2,3,25). Described cases of elevated RNA expression include examples of abnormal (2) and ectopic (3) transcription. In at least some cases this enhancement is not limited to synthesis of RNA: the Y1 cells that have amplified c-Ki-ras contain exeptionally large amounts of its protein product at the plasma membrane (25; Figure 2). High amounts of the c-myc encoded protein are also found in COLO 320 cells that have amplified the gene (12).

The myc oncogenes have recently been shown to encode nuclear proteins (1,11). Both the expression of the c-myc protein (14) and the subcellular localization of myc proteins are linked to the cell cycle (30). Elevated expression of specific c-myc functions may be necessary

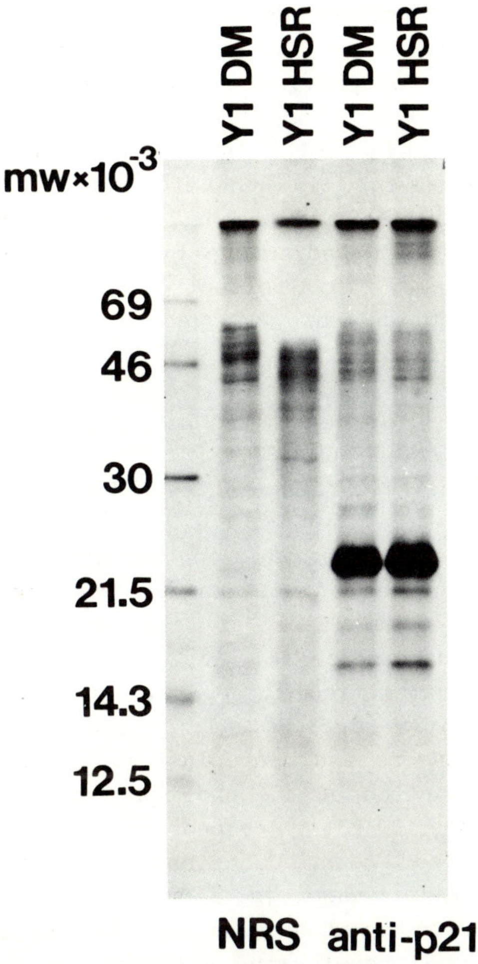

Figure 2. The Y1 DM and HRS cells which harbor a 50-fold amplified c-Ki-ras oncogene (25) and control cells were labeled with ^{35}S-methionine and p21 c-Ki-ras protein was immunoprecipitated (25), with normal rat serum (NRS) or rat monoclonal anti-p21 serum. The proteins were electrophoresed in a 15% polyacrylamide SDS gel. In addition to a major p21 band, a labeled band at about 16 KD was present in the immunoprecipitates. The amount of radioactivity in p21 in Y1 cells was about 50 fold that in normal rat kidney cells.

for cell cycle progression and the growth transformation aspect of the phenotype of cancer cells that may contribute to tumor progression (13). Elevated expression of c-myc has been shown to partially replace platelet-derived growth factor in induction of competence for DNA replication (4). In general, enhanced expression of an oncogene could be a necessary prerequisite for the acquisition of a growth advantage by cells having extra copies of the gene. This effect could also be the principal contribution of oncogene amplification to tumorigenesis.

TUMOR CELL AND STAGE SPECIFICITY OF ONCOGENE ACTIVATION AND AMPLIFICATION

Tumor cell specificity of oncogene amplification has been found in two types of malignancy. The c-myc oncogene is amplified in most cases of the variant form of small-cell lung cancer cells (17,20) and the putative N-myc oncogene is amplified in about a half of grade III and IV neuroblastomas (8,23,24,26). In addition to HSR:s, small-cell lung cancers and neuroblastomas frequently show a deletion of a portion of the short arm of chromosome 1 (7) and chromosome 3 (31), respectively. Two kinds of changes have also been described in neuroblastoma oncogenes. The first change is a mutation in the N-ras gene which was discovered because of its relatedness to other ras genes and transforming activity in transfection experiments (27). The second one is amplification of a distant homologue of the c-myc gene called N-myc (23,24,26). At present, these two events have not, however, been found in the same tumor cell line.

When does oncogene amplification occur during tumorigenesis? Amplification and enhanced expression of c-myc and N-myc apparently occur during the progression of human carcinoma of the lung and neuroblastoma cells to a more malignant phenotype (8,17,20). Gene amplification may not be an initiating event, although there may be no mandatory sequence of oncogene activations for the genesis of any particular tumor. Amplification of an oncogene could play its part in already initiated cells whenever it happened to occur.

ACKNOWLEDGMENTS

The studies of the authors have been supported by the Finnish Cancer Foundation and the Academy of Finland.

REFERENCES

1 Alitalo K., Ramsay G., Bishop J.M., Ohlsson-Pfeifer S., Colby W.W. & Levinson A.D. (1983) Nature 306, 274-277.
2. Alitalo, K., Schwab M., Lin C.C., Varmus H.E. & Bishop J.M. (1983) Proc. Natl. Acad. Sci. USA 80, 1707-1711.
3. Alitalo K., Winqvist R., Lin C.C., de la Chapelle, A., Schwab M. & Bishop J.M. (1984) Proc. Natl. Acad. Sci. USA 81, 4534-4538.
4. Armelin H.A., Armelin M.C.S., Kelly K., Stewart T., Leder P., Cochran B.H. & Stiles, C.D. (1984) Nature 310, 655-660.
5. Barker P.E. (1982) Cancer Genet. Cytogenet. 5, 81-94.
6. Biedler J.L., Meyers, M.B. & Stengler B.A. (1983) Adv. Cell. Neurobiol. 4, 268-301.
7. Brodeur, G.M., Green A.A., Hayes F.A., Williams K.J., Williams D.L.& Tsiatis A.A. (1981) Cancer Res. 41, 4678-4686.
8. Brodeur, G.M., Seeger R.C., Schawab M., Varmus H.E. & Bishop J.M. (1984), Science 224, 1121-1124.
9. Cowell J.K. (1982) Ann. Rev. Genet. 16, 21-52.
10. Cox, D., Yuncken C. & Spriggs A.I. (1965) Lancet I, 55-58.
11. Eisenman R.N., Tachibana C.Y., Abrams H.D., & Hann S.R. (1984) Submitted.
12. Hann .R., Abrams H.D., Rohrschneider L.R. & Eisenman R.N. (1983) Cell 34, 789-798.

13.Heldin C.H., & Westermark B. (1984) Cell 37, 9-20
14.Kelly K., Cochran B.H., Stiles C.D. & Leder P. (1983) Cell 35, 603-610.
15.Levan A., Levan G. & Mandahl N. (1981) In: Genes, Chromosomes, and Neoplasia (eds. F.E. Arrighi, P.N. Rao & E. Stubblefield) pp. 233-251 Raven press, New York.
16.Lin C.C., Alitalo K., Schwab M., George D., Varmus H.E. & Bishop J.M. (1984) Submitted.
17.Little C.D., Nau M.M., Carney D.N., Gazdar, A.F. & Minna J.D. (1983) Nature 306, 194-196.
18.Nowell, R.C., Finan J., Favera R.D., Gallo R.C., Ar-Rushdi A., Romanczuk G., Selden J.R., Emanuel B.S., Rovera G. & Croce C.M. (1983) Nature 306, 494-497.
19.Rowley J.D. (1983) Nature 301, 290-292.
20.Saksela K., Bergh J., Leehto V.P., Nilsson K. & Alitalo K. (1984) Submitted.
21.Schimke R.T. (1982) In: Gene Amplification. Cold Spring Harbor Press, CSH, New York.
22.Schimke R.T., Brown P.C., Kaufman R.J., McGrogan M. & Slate D.L. (1981) Cold Spring Harbor Symp. Quant. Biol. 55, 785-797.
23.Schwab, M., Alitalo K., Klempnauer K.H., Varmus H.E., Bishop J.M., Gilbert F., Brodeur, G., Goldstein M. & Trent J. (1983) Nature 305, 245-248.
24.Schwab M., Alitalo L., Varmus H.E. & Bishop J.M. (1984) In: The Cancer Cell, vol. 2, Cold Spring Harbor Press, in press.
25.Schwab M., Alitalo K., Varmus H.E., Bishop, J.M. & George D. (1983) Nature 303, 497-501.
26.Schwab M., Varmus H.E., Bishop J.M., Grezeschik K.H., Naylor S.L., Sakaguchi, A.Y., Brodeur, G. & Trent J. (1984) Nature 308, 288-291.
27.Shimizu K., Goldfarb M., Perucho M., & Wigler M. (1983) Proc. Natl. Acad. Sci. USA 80, 383-387.
28.Trent J.M., Thompson F.H., Rosenfeld S. & Ludwig C. (1984) Cancer Res., in press.
29.Winqvist R., Knuutila S., Leprince D., Stehelin D. & Alitalo K. (1984) Submitted.
30.Winqvist R., Saksela K. & Alitalo K. (1984) EMBO J. in

press.

31. Whang-Peng, J., Bunn P.A., Kao-Shan C.S., Lee E.C., Carney D.N., Gazdar A. & Minna J.D. (1982) Cancer Genet. Cytogenet. 6, 119-134.

THE NUCLEOTIDE SEQUENCE OF THE erbA GENE OF AVIAN ERYTHROBLASTOSIS VIRUS APPEARS UNRELATED TO OTHER KNOWN ONCOGENES

C. Henry, B. Debuire, M. Benaissa, G. Biserte, S. Saule[1], P. Martin[1], and D. Stehelin[1]

Inserm U. 124, Institut de Recherches sur le Cancer de Lille, Faculte' de Medecine, 59045 Lille Cedex, France, and [1]Inserm U. 186, Institut Pasteur, 15, rue Camille Guerin, 59019 Lille Cedex, France

Avian erythroblastosis virus carries two distinct oncogenes erbA and erbB. The erbB protein which is homologous to the C-terminal half of the epidermal growth factor receptor, is also related to the src family of oncogenic proteins and transforms erythroblasts whereas erbA potentiates the effects of erbB by blocking the differentiation of erythroblasts at an immature sequence. We sequenced this "potentiatior"; the deduced amino acid sequence of the erbA polypeptide appeared clearly different from the sequence of other known oncogene products and was related to carbonic anhydrases. These enzymes play an important role in the transport of carbon dioxide by erythrocytes, the precursors of which are main targets of avian erythroblastosis virus. Our results show that a src-related oncogene such as erbB, acting in synergy with an activated specific cell derived gene such as erbA, can profoundly affect early erythroid differentiation.

Considerable interest concerns the recent finding that two distinct oncogenes can act in synergy or complementation to transform normal cells (1,2); some retroviruses are interesting in that respect since they contain two specific cell-derived sequences in their genome (3,5) that probably led to their selection as highly transforming viruses. Avian erythroblastosis virus (AEV), a defective leukemia virus that transforms mainly erythroblasts (6,7), carries two host cell-derived oncogenes denoted erbA and erbB (8,9) expressed in transformed cells from two distinct messenger RNA's (mRNA's) (10,11). A 5.4 kilobase (kb) mRNA codes for a cytoplasmic $p75^{gag-erbA}$ fusion protein (12) while a subgenomic spliced 3.5 kb mRNA produces a membrane glycoprotein of 74,000 molecular weight (MW) (13). Recently, the v-erbB sequence (14) was identified as a portion of the epidermal growth factor (EGF) receptor (15). Both erbA and erbB are homologous to avian and mammalian chromosomal DNA sequences (c-erbA and c-erbB) (3,16) that may play a role in the differentiation of immature red blood cells (15). Wild type AEV-transformed erythroblasts are tightly blocked in their maturation (at the "colony forming unit" stage) (18); studies involving deletion mutants in erbA or erbB indicate that erbB is responsible for the transforming capacity of the virus whereas erbA potentiates this activity and appears to be responsible for the early blockage of cell differentiation within the erythroid lineage (19). We analyzed the nucleotide sequence of this "potentiator" (20). Our results provide a deduced amino acid sequence of the erbA stretch clearly distinct from other reported transforming proteins as attested to by computer analysis. Thus erbA appears to represent a genuinely distinct new member of the oncogene families.

A

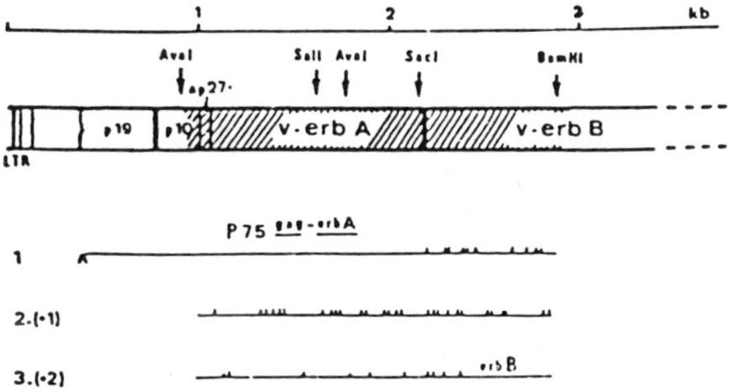

B

```
    GTG GTA GCC ATG CCT GTA GTG ATT AAG ACA GAG GGA CCC GCT TGG ACC
    Val Val Ala Met Pro Val Val Ile Lys Thr Glu Gly Pro Ala Trp Thr
    -20                                     -10
GAG<------------------ 1 ------------------>erbA
CCT CTG GAG CCA GAG GAC ACT CGG TGG CTG GAT GGC AAG CAC AAA AGA AAG AGC
Pro Leu Glu Pro Glu Asp Thr Arg Trp Leu Asp Gly Lys His Lys Arg Lys Ser
                1                                10

AGC CAA TGT TTG GTG AAG AGC AGC ATG TCA GGG TAC ATC CCT AGC TGC CTG GAC
Ser Gln Cys Leu Val Lys Ser Ser Met Ser Gly Tyr Ile Pro Ser Cys Leu Asp
                     20                                     30

AAA GAT GAA CAG TGC GTG GTG TGT GGG GAC AAA GCC ACC GGC TAC CAC TAC CGC
Lys Asp Glu Gln Cys Val Val Cys Gly Asp Lys Ala Thr Gly Tyr His Tyr Arg
                             40                                      50

TGC ATC ACC TGC GAG GGC TGC AAG AGC TTT TTC CGT CGG ACC ATC CAG AAG AAC
Cys Ile Thr Cys Glu Gly Cys Lys Ser Phe Phe Arg Arg Thr Ile Gln Lys Asn
                                     60

CTG CAC CCC ACC TAC TCC TGC ACG TAC GAT GGG TGC TGC GTC ATC GAC AAG ATC
Leu His Pro Thr Tyr Ser Cys Thr Tyr Asp Gly Cys Cys Val Ile Asp Lys Ile
     70                                      80

ACC CGC AAC CAG TGC CAG CTG TGC CGC TTC AAG AAG TGC ATC TCC GTG GGC ATG
Thr Arg Asn Gln Cys Gln Leu Cys Arg Phe Lys Lys Cys Ile Ser Val Gly Met
            90                                      100

GCC ATG GAC CTG GTG CTG GAC GAC TCG AAG CGC GTA GCC AAG CGG AAG CTG ATC
Ala Met Asp Leu Val Leu Asp Asp Ser Lys Arg Val Ala Lys Arg Lys Leu Ile
                    110                                     120

GAG GAG AAC CGG GAG CGG CGA CGC AAG GAG GAG ATG ATC AAA TCC CTG CAG CAC
Glu Glu Asn Arg Glu Arg Arg Arg Lys Glu Glu Met Ile Lys Ser Leu Gln His
                            130                                     140

CGG CCC AGC CCC AGC GCA GAG GAG TGG GAG CTG ATC CAC GTG GTG ACC GAG GCG
Arg Pro Ser Pro Ser Ala Glu Glu Trp Glu Leu Ile His Val Val Thr Glu Ala
                                    150

CAC CGC AGC ACC AAC GCG CAG GGC AGC CAC TGG AAG CAG AGG AGG AAA TTC CTG
His Arg Ser Thr Asn Ala Gln Gly Ser His Trp Lys Gln Arg Arg Lys Phe Leu
    160                                     170

CTC GAA GAT ATC GGT CAG TCG CCC ATG GCC TCC ATG CTT GAC GGG GAC AAA GTG
Leu Glu Asp Ile Gly Gln Ser Pro Met Ala Ser Met Leu Asp Gly Asp Lys Val
            180                                     190
                                    Domain 1<------------------------
GAC CTG GAG GCG TTC AGC GAG TTT ACA AAA ATC ATC ACG CCG GCC|ATC ACC CGC
Asp Leu Glu Ala Phe Ser Glu Phe Thr Lys Ile Ile Thr Pro Ala Ile Thr Arg
                    200                                     210
-->Domain 2
GTG GTC GAC TTT GCC AAA AAC CTG CCC ATG TTC TCG GAG CTG CCG TGC GAG GAT
Val Val Asp Phe Ala Lys Asn Leu Pro Met Phe Ser Glu Leu Pro Cys Glu Asp
                            220                                     230
```

```
CAG ATC ATC CTG CTG AAG GGC TGC TGC ATG GAG ATC ATG TCG CTG CGC GCC GCC
Gln Ile Ile Leu Leu Lys Gly Cys Cys Met Glu Ile Met Ser Leu Arg Ala Ala
                                    240

GTG CGC TAC GAC CCC GAG AGC GAA ACG CTG ACG CTG AGC GGG GAA ATG GCC GTC
Val Arg Tyr Asp Pro Glu Ser Glu Thr Leu Thr Leu Ser Gly Glu Met Ala Val
    250                                     260

AAA CGC GAG CAG TTG AAG AAC GGA GGG CTG GGG GTC GTG TCT GAT GCC ATC TTC
Lys Arg Glu Gln Leu Lys Asn Gly Gly Leu Gly Val Val Ser Asp Ala Ile Phe
            270                                     280

GAC CTC GGC AAG TCG CTG TCT GCC TTC AAC CTG GAC GAC ACC GAG GTG GCC CTG
Asp Leu Gly Lys Ser Leu Ser Ala Phe Asn Leu Asp Asp Thr Glu Val Ala Leu
                    290                                     300

CTG CAG GCC GTG CTG CTC ATG TCC TCA GAC CGG ACG GGG CTG ATC TGC GTG GAT
Leu Gln Ala Val Leu Leu Met Ser Ser Asp Arg Thr Gly Leu Ile Cys Val Asp
                            310                                     320

AAG ATA GAG AAG TGC CAG GAG TCG TAC CTG CTG GCG TTC GAG CAC TAC ATC AAC
Lys Ile Glu Lys Cys Gln Glu Ser Tyr Leu Leu Ala Phe Glu His Tyr Ile Asn
                                    330

TAC CGC AAA CAC AAC ATT CCC CAC TTC TGG TCC AAG CTG CTG ATG AAG GTG GCG
Tyr Arg Lys His Asn Ile Pro His Phe Trp Ser Lys Leu Leu Met Lys Val Ala
    340                                     350

GAC CTG CGC ATG ATC GGC GCC TAC CAC GCC AGC CGC TTC CTG CAC ATG AAG GTG
Asp Leu Arg Met Ile Gly Ala Tyr His Ala Ser Arg Phe Leu His Met Lys Val
            360                                     370

GAG TGC CCC ACG GAG CTC CCC CCA AGG AGG TGT AGA GCC CTA CAG ATT TTG GGA
Glu Cys Pro Thr Glu Leu Pro Pro Arg Arg Cys Arg Ala Leu Gln Ile Leu Gly
                    380                                     390
                    1194
AGT ATA TTG CCC TTT GTA TAG TCCATCCTACAAGAGCAAAAACTTGTAAGCATTTCAGGTAGCA
Ser Ile Leu Pro Phe Val AM
                    398

AAGTAATGAAACCACAAAATGCTGAAAATGCTCCACAGTTGAATGCACAGATATTTATGTTCTGTGTTTAT
                                                            Sa↓ ———→ erbB
TCCTGAAGTGTAAGGAATGTAAGGAAATCATAGATTAGTTGTTTCTTTCCTTTTTGCAG GGC CCA GAC
                                                            Gly Pro Asp
                                                              1

CAC TGC ATG AAG TGT GCT CAT TTT ATA GAT GGT CCC CAC TGT GTG AAG GGC CCT
His Cys Met Lys Cys Ala His Phe Ile Asp Gly Pro His Cys Val Lys Gly Pro
                         10                                      20

GCC CCG CTG GGG TCC TGG GTG AGA ATG ATA CCC TGG TCT GGA AGT ATG CAG ATG
Ala Pro Leu Gly Ser Trp Val Arg Met Ile Pro Trp Ser Gly Ser Met Gln Met
                                 30

CCA ATG CTG TTT GCC AGC TCT GCC ATC CAA ACT GTA CAC GAG GGT GCA AGG GAC
Pro Met Leu Phe Ala Ser Ser Ala Ile Gln Thr Val His Glu Gly Ala Arg Asp
 40                                      50

CAG GTC TTG AAG GAT GCC CAA ATG GCT CCA AAA CTC CAT CTA TCG CGG CTG GTG
Gln Val Leu Lys Asp Ala Gln Met Ala Pro Lys Leu His Leu Ser Arg Leu Val
         60                                      70

TTG TCC GGA GGA CTC CTG TGC CTG GTT GTG GTT GGT CTA GGC ATC GGT CTT TAC
Leu Ser Gly Gly Leu Leu Cys Leu Val Val Val Gly Leu Gly Ile Gly Leu Tyr
                 80                                      90

CTG CGG CGA CGC CAT ATC GTG CGG AAG CGC ACC CTG CGC AGG CTG CTG CAA GAG
Leu Arg Arg Arg His Ile Val Arg Lys Arg Thr Leu Arg Arg Leu Leu Gln Glu
                        100                                     110
                                                                    1754
AGG GAG CTT GTC GAA CCA CTG ACA CCC AGT GGG GAG GCA CCA AAC CAG GCC CAC
Arg Glu Leu Val Glu Pro Leu Thr Pro Ser Gly Glu Ala Pro Asn Gln Ala His
                                120
```

Figure 1. Copyright 19 xx - June 29, 1984- by the AAAS.
1A.- Reading frame in the genome of AEV. The DNA sequence was determined (hatched) by the Maxam and Gilbert procedure (22). The recombination of erbA with the viral genome occured at the sites shown as thick vertical bars in the diagram of AEV DNA. p27 denotes the remaining coding domain for the p27 protein of the gag gene, which was truncated during the recombination events leading to capture of the erb insert. The open reading frames in erbA are shown below the AEV DNA. A different open reading frame was detected for erbB. Vertical bars denote stop codons. LTR indicates a long terminal repeat.

1B. Nucleotide sequence of the erbA gene and of the 5' end of erbB. The sequence of 1814 nucleotides encompassing the erbA gene is shown. The deduced amino acid sequence of the erbA domain of $P75^{gag-erbA}$ is indicated from nucleotides 1 to 1194 and the deduced amino acid sequence of the 5' end of the erbB is indicated from the putative splice acceptor site (Sa, nucleotide 1370) to nucleotide 1754. Every tenth amino acid is numbered.

Figure 2. Copyright 19 xx - June 29, 1984- by the AAAS
Relatedness of erbA domain to the carbonic anhydrase family. Using the sequence of the putative erbA polypeptide, exhaustive homology searches were performed on the NEWAT (28) and NBRF (29) protein data banks with a computer sy[illegible] described by Claverie, J.M. (31). These searches revealed a homology encompassing 180 amino acid residues between erbA domain 2 and the carbonic anhydrase family. The significance of this homology was further assessed by an alignment program (32). The amino acid sequence of the predicted erbA polypeptide and of sheep (CRSH2) (35), rabbit (CRRB2) (34), bovine (CRBO2) (35), and human (CRHU2) (30) carbonic anhydrases were compared. The optimal alignment was found when a deletion weight of 1 for each gap plus 0.2 times the number of residues in each gap was used. In this case, the Needleman-Wunsch

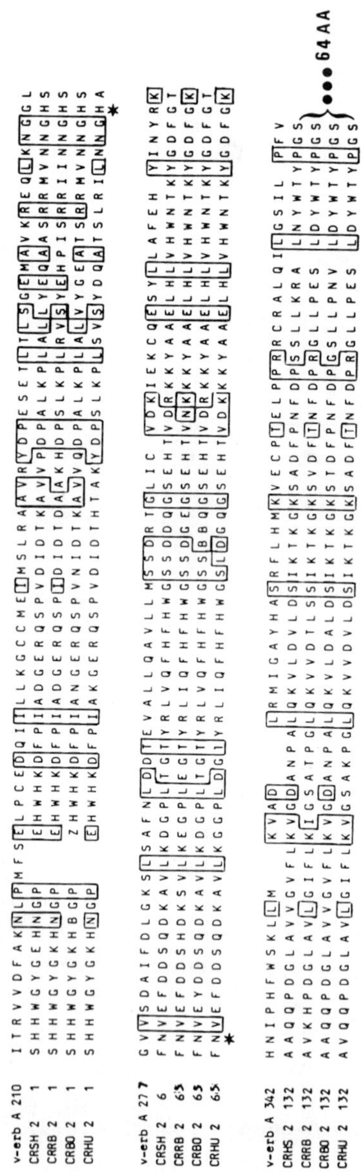
64 AA

Figure 2. (continued)
similarity value (36) was found 3.8 standard deviation units above the mean of 30 shuffled sequences. Scores that are three or more standard deviation units above the mean can reasonably be expected to represent authentic relationships (37). Common residues are boxed. Asterisks indicate amino acids known to be important in the active sites of carbonic anhydrases. The one-letter symbols for the amino acids are A, alanine; R, arginine; N, aspargine; D, aspartic acid; C, cysteine; Q, glutamine; E, glutamic acid; G, glycine; H, histidine; I, isoleucine; L, leucine; K, lysine; M, methionine; F, phenylalanine; P, proline; S, serine; T, threonine; W, tryptophan; Y, tyrosine; V, valine; B, asparagine or aspartic acid; and Z, glutamine or glutamic acid.

SEQUENCING OF THE erbA ONCOGENE

A molecular clone of avian erythroblastosis virus (pAEV 11) (21) bearing biological activity was used to sequence the erbA oncogene according to the Maxam and Gilbert procedure (22). The leftward boundary of erbA was assessed by comparison to the nucleotide sequence of the Prague-C strain (Pr-C) of Rous sarcoma virus (RSV) (23). The insertion of erbA is located within the coding domain for the virion protein $p27^{gag}$ (Figure 1A). The reading frame of erbA continues uninterrupted from the $p27^{gag}$ reading frame at position 1 (Figure 1B) until it is terminated by an amber codon at position 1195; a stretch of non coding sequences is following up to a putative splice acceptor (Sa in Figure 1B) site (24), TTTCCTTTTGCAG.G (T, thymidine; C, cytosine; G, guanine; A, adenine) for the erbB gene at nucleotide 1370. It is unlikely that the other two erbA reading frames are used because they are frequently closed by termination codons (vertical bars in Figure 1A). The consensus splice acceptor site at position 1370 could generate the subgenomic erbB mRNA in an open reading frame different from that of erbA and for which we present the deduced partial amino acid sequence (Figure 1B). Thus the erbB protein may start at the AUG (U, uracil) codon of gag used to produce $p75^{gag-erbA}$ (assuming that AEV and Pr-C use the same splice donor site in gag); alternatively the erbB product could initiate at the in-frame AUG codon at position 1386 in our sequence (Figure 1B). In the region we studied, the structure of erbB is virtually identical to the one recently described for another independent isolate of avian erythroblastosis virus (AEV-H) lacking the erbA oncogene (14). Importantly, erbB is closely related to the src gene of avian sarcoma virus (14) and to a portion of the EGF receptor (25).

THE PREDICTED erbA POLYPEPTIDE

The deduced amino acid sequence of erbA (398 amino acids) is indicated under the nucleotide sequence in Figure 1B. The calculated molecular weight of the erbA polypeptide is 45.4 kilodaltons (kl) yielding for $P75^{gag-erbA}$ (26) a deduced molecular size of 72 kD. There are no potential glycosylation sites Asn-x-(Thr or Ser) (27) in this polypeptide. Two domains can be defined within the erbA protein: the first domain (amino acids 1 to 209 in Figure 1B) exhibits elevated levels of cysteine and basic residues (10 percent and 21 percent, respectively, within amino acids 1 to 131) but shows no salient homology with other known proteins. A computer search for similarities between the erbA protein and the other proteins contained in the NEWAT (28) and NBRF (29) protein data bases revealed no obvious relationships with other oncogenes. However an intriguing relatedness was found between the carboxyl terminal half of erbA (domain 2 in figure 1B) and the carbonic anhydrase family (Figure 2). The homology begins with erbA amino acid residue 219 (amino acid residue 10 for the carbonic anhydrases) and extends across 180 residues up to the carboxyl terminus of the molecule (corresponding to residue 195 of the carbonic anydrases which continue for another 64 residues). When compared with the four mammalian carbonic anhydrases II available in the data banks we used, the overall homology was 27 percent but clustered in some portions of the molecule. For example, close to one of the known active sites of carbonic anhydrases (30) the homology increases to more than 51 percent (erbA residues 248 to 274) although the two residues reported to be important in the active site (His^{63} and Asn^{66}) (30) are not found in the erbA protein. This may imply a structural but not a functional relationship. Moreover, in human carbonic anhydrase I, which has a 61 percent homology with human carbonic anhydrase II, most of the homologies depicted in Figure 2 are conserved (not shown). Although, erbA domain 2 is related to carbonic anhydrases, we showed that it is not the enzyme itself. The human cellular erbA domain 2 was cloned, and a nucleotide sequence was determined (corresponding to nucleotides 675 to 936 in the erbA domain 2 of Figure 1B). Homology at the nucleotide level was 83 percent, and the deduced amino acid sequence in the corresponding open reading frame showed 96 percent homology (the two other reading frames were closed by stop codons). The homologies of the human erbA domain 2 with human carbonic anhydrase remained but were not augmented. Thus the erbA gene is related to but not identical to known carbonic anhydrases.

In conclusion, due to the synergistic action of two distinct oncogenes, erbA and erbB, AEV is an unusual retrovirus in that it can specifically block the maturation of erythroid cells at an immature stage of differentiation. It is of interest that the deduced erbA protein bears statistically significant relatedness, but not identity, with carbonic anhydrases because such enzymes play a fundamental role in the CO_2 transport by erythrocytes, the precursors of which are precisely the main targets of AEV. Our finding of this new type of oncogene also leads to the idea that, when acting in synergy with a specific activated cell-derived gene such as erbA, some src related oncogenes that were so far found - with the exception of AEV - as single transforming genes in retroviruses and transform mainly fibroblasts can profoundly affect early hematopoietic differentiation.

ACKNOWLEDGEMENTS

We thank Drs. B. Vennstrom and J.M. Bishop for providing the clone p-AEV 11; A. Begue and A. Schneeberger for helpful advice and discussion and A. Level for patient typing. This work was supported by the Institut National de la Sante et de la Recherche Medicale (U 124 CRL 822020; U 186 CRL 822033); Institut de Recherches sur le Cancer de Lille, Institut Pasteur de Lille and private foundations (Association pour la Recherche sur le Cancer; Fondation pour la Recherche Medicale).

REFERENCES

1. Land, H., Parada, L.F., & Weinberg, R.A. (1983) Nature (London) 304, 596-602.
2. Newbold, R.F. & Overell, R.W. (1983) Nature (London) 304, 649-651.
3. Vennstrom, B. & Bishop, J.M. (1982) Cell 28, 135-143.
4. Leprince, D., Gegonne, A., Coll, J., De Taisne, C., Schneeberger, A., Lagrou, C. & Stehelin, D. (1983) Nature (London) 306, 395-397.
5. Coll, J., Righi, M., De Taisne, C., Dissous, C., Gegonne, A. & Stehelin, D. (1983) EMBO J. 2, 2189-2194.
6. Graf, T., Royer-Pokora, B., Schubert, G.E., & Beug, H. (1976) Virology 71, 423-433.
7. Graf, T. & Beug, H. (1978) Biochim. Biophys Acta 516, 269-299.

8. Roussel, M., Saule, S., Lagrou, C., Rommens, C., Beug, H., Graf, T. & Stehelin, D. (1979) Nature (London) 281, 452-455.
9. Vennstrom, B., Fanshier, L., Moscovici, C. & Bishop, J.M. (1980) J. Virol. 36, 575-585.
10. Saule, S., Roussel, M., Lagrou, C. & Stehelin, D. (1981) J. Virol. 38, 409-419.
11. Sheiness, D., Vennstrom, B. & Bishop, J.M. (1981) Cell 23, 291-300.
12. Lai, M.M.C., Neil, J.C., & Vogt, P.K. (1980) Virology 100, 291-300.
13. Hayman, M.J., & Beug, H. (1984) Nature (London) 309, 460-462.
14. Yamamoto, T., Nishida, T., Miyajima, N., Kawai, S., Ooi, T., & Toyoshima, K. (1983) Cell 35, 71-78.
15. Downward, J., Yarden, Y., Mayes, E., Scrace, G., Totty, N., Stockwell, P., Ullrich, A., Schlessinger, J. & Waterfield, M.D. (1984) Nature (London) 307, 521-527.
16. Sergent, A., Saule, S., Leprince, D., Begue, A., Rommens, C., & Stehelin, D. (1982) EMBO J. 1, 237-242.
17. Coll, J., Saule S., Martin, P., Raes, M.B., Lagrou, C., Graf, T., Beug, H., Simon, I.E. & Stehelin, D. (1983) Exp. Cell Res. 149, 151-162.
18. Samarut, Y., & Gazzolo, L. (1982) Cell 28, 921-929.
19. Frykberg, L., Palmieri, S., Beug, H., Graf, T., Hayman, M.J. & Vennstrom, B. (1983) Cell 32, 227-238.
20. Debuire, B., Henry, C., Benaissa, M., Biserte, G., Claverie, J.M., Saule, S., Martin, P. & Stehelin, D. (1984) Science 224, 1456-1459.
21. Vennstrom, B., Fanshier, L., Moscovici, C. & Bishop, J.M. (1980) J. Virol. 36, 575-585.
22. Maxam, A.M. & Gilbert, W. (1980) Methods Enzymol. 65, 499-560.
23. Schwartz, D., Tizard, R. & Gilbert, W. (1983) Cell 32, 853-869.
24. Mount, S.M. (1982) Nucl. Acid. Res. 10, 459-472.
25. Ullrich, A., Coussens, L., Hayflick, J.S., Dull, T.J., Gray, A., Tam, A.W., Lee, J., Yarden, Y., Libermann,

T.A., Schlessinger, J., Downward, J., Mayes, E.L.V., Whittle, N., Waterfield, M.D. & Seeburg, P.H. (1984) Nature (London) 309, 418-425.

26. Hayman, M.J., Royer-Pokora, B. & Graf, T. (1979) Virology 92, 31-45.
27. Krebs, E.G. & Beavo, J.A. (1979) Annu. Rev. Biochem. 48, 923-959.
28. Doolittle, R.F. (1981) Science 214, 149-159.
29. Dayhoff, .M.O., Schwartz, R.M. & Orcutt, B.C. (1983) Protein Sequence Database Release 83: doc PRSD-0183C? National Biomedical Research Foundation, Washington D.C.
30. Liljas, A., Kannan, K.K., Bergsten, P.C., Waara, I., Firdborg, K., Strandberg, B., Carlbom, U., Jarup, L., Lovgren, S. & Petef, M. (1972) Nature New Biol. 235, 131-137.
31. Clavarie, J.M. (1984) Nucleic Acids Res? 12, 397-408.
32. Smith, T.F., Waterman, M.S., Fitch, W.M. (1981) J. Mol. Evol. 18, 385-391.
33. Tanis, R.J., Ferrell, R.E., & Tashian, R.E. (1974) Biochim. Biophys. Acta 371, 534-548.
34. Ferrell, R.E., Stroup, S.K., Tanis, R.J. & Tashian, R.E. (1978) Biochim. Biophys. Acta 533, 1-11.
35. Sciaky, M., Limozin, N., Filippi-Foveau, D., Gulian, J.M. & Laurent-Tabusse, G. (1976) Biochimie 58, 1071-1082.
36. Needleman, S.B., & Wunsch, C.D. (1970) J. Mol. Biol. 48, 443-450.
37. Barker, W.C., & Dayhoff, M.O. (1972) in Atlas of Protein Sequence and Structure (National Biomedical Research Foundation, Washington, D.C.) vol. 5, pp. 101-110.

CHARACTERIZATION OF A HUMAN OSTEOSARCOME ONCOGENE

H.G. Suarez, L. Grosjeachn, Y. Andeol and P.C. Nardeux

Institut de Recherches Scientifiques sur le Cancer B.P. N.°8, 94802, France

We present a characterization of an activated oncogene which we found to be present in DNA of the OHA human osteosarcoma cell line. This tumor oncogene is related to the ras-ki family of human oncogenes and seems to be amplified in the original tumor and some of the transfectants.

DNAs from different human tumors and tumor cell lines have been found to induce malignant transformation of the mouse contact-inhibited NIH 3T3 cells (1). The human DNA sequences responsible for transformation have been called "oncogenes" and it has been demonstrated that some of these genes are activated cellular homologs of retrovirus transforming genes. Each oncogene is closely related to a counterpart DNA sequence present in the normal cellular genome ("proto-oncogene"). For the ras family of oncogenes the mechanism of activation depends on alterations in the structure of the gene encoded protein (p21 protein). It has been shown that a single point mutation converted the ras proto-oncogenes into potent oncogenes. This substitution of one base for another results in the replacement of one aminoacid, normally present in the encoded p21 protein, by another. These changes do not always affect the level of expression of the genes (1).

Thus far, DNA sequences capable of inducing oncogenic transformation of NIH 3T3 mouse cells, have never been detected in human osteosarcoma tumors and/or cell lines (see Pulciani et al., 1982 and Land et al., 1983). Here we present results concerning a DNA sequence in a human osteosarcoma cell line (OHA), that is active in conferring a transformed phenotype to mouse 3T3 cells. The oncogene which seems to be responsible for it is related to the ras-ki (Kirstein) family of human oncogenes.

IDENTIFICATION OF THE OHA ACTIVATED ONCOGENE

The OHA human osteosarcoma cells had been derived from an explant of an osteorsacoma of a 16-yr-old boy. FNR-HOS (3) is a human osteorsarcome cell line obtained from Dr. B. Azzarone, Villejuif, France. HEL are normal human lung embryo cells (3). ESC are Swiss mouse 3T3 cells established in our laboratory by C. Lavialle. All the cells were routinely cultured in MEM medium in the presence of 10% adult calf serum, gassed with 5% CO^2. They are PPLO free.

High molecular weight (HMW) DNAs were extracted and purified from cells as described by Gross-Bellard et al. (1973) and were transfected on ESC cells as described by Perucho et al. (1981). The selective medium (MEM 5% adult calf serum) was changed twice weekly, the cells were cultured for at least 6 weeks and the colonies were isolated using glass cloning cylinders.

The OHA cell line HMW DNA induced transformation of mouse 3T3 cells with an efficiency of 0.01-0.1 transfectants/ug DNA. In contrast, DNAs of the FNR-HOS and HEL cells, lacked detectable transforming activity. DNAs from clones obtained in transfection assays were analyzed by Southern blotting for the presence of: 1) human repetitive Alu sequences and 2) an activated transforming gene. Procedures for: 1) digestion of cellular DNA (20 ug) with restriction endonucleases (100 U), electrophoresis in agarose gels (1%) and transfer to nitrocellulose filters;

2) ^{32}P-labelling of the probes by nick-translation and 3) detection of Alu sequences and ras-ki sequences, were performed as described by Maniatis et al. (1982). The Alu probe (containing mainly highly repetitive sequences) was prepared as described by Houck et al. (1979). The ras-ki probe was the PKBE 2 clone (8).

In 10/10 of the primary transfectants a large number of human Alu sequences were detected (Fig. 1 A). These DNAs were used in secondary transfection assays and all induced transformation of ESC cells with the same efficiency as the original osteosarcoma DNA. All secondary transfectants contained much lower levels of human Alu sequences than the primary ones (Fig. 1 B). As reported previously (2), several fragments 2.5- 7 Kb in size were more or less evident in the different clones.

It has been shown (2) that transfectants of different human tumor cell lines, bearing activated ras-ki genes, have acquired 3 and 6.6/6.8 kb Eco RI fragments hybridizing with a probe derived from the ras oncogene of Kirstein murine sarcoma virus. In our experiments, the OHA parental cell line contained an additional fragment of approximately 2.5 Kb. Only the 3 and 6.8 Kb ras-ki-containing EcO RI fragments were detected in ESC cells transformed by DNA of the OHA cell line. In one of the studied clones, the 3 Kb fragment was not detected. In the parental cell line and in some of the transfectants the transforming gene seems to be amplified.

EXPRESSION OF RAS GENE PRODUCTS IN OHA AND CONCLUSIONS

Thus the activated oncogene found in the OHA cell line appears to share homology with the ras-ki gene. This conclusion was corroborated by assaying for the p21 ras-encoded protein by immunoprecipitation. The immunoprecipitation technique was carried out as described by Der and Cooper (1983), using the broad spectrum rat monoclonal anti-21 antibody 259 (a gift from Dr. Marc Furth). The OHA cells and the transfectant clones were

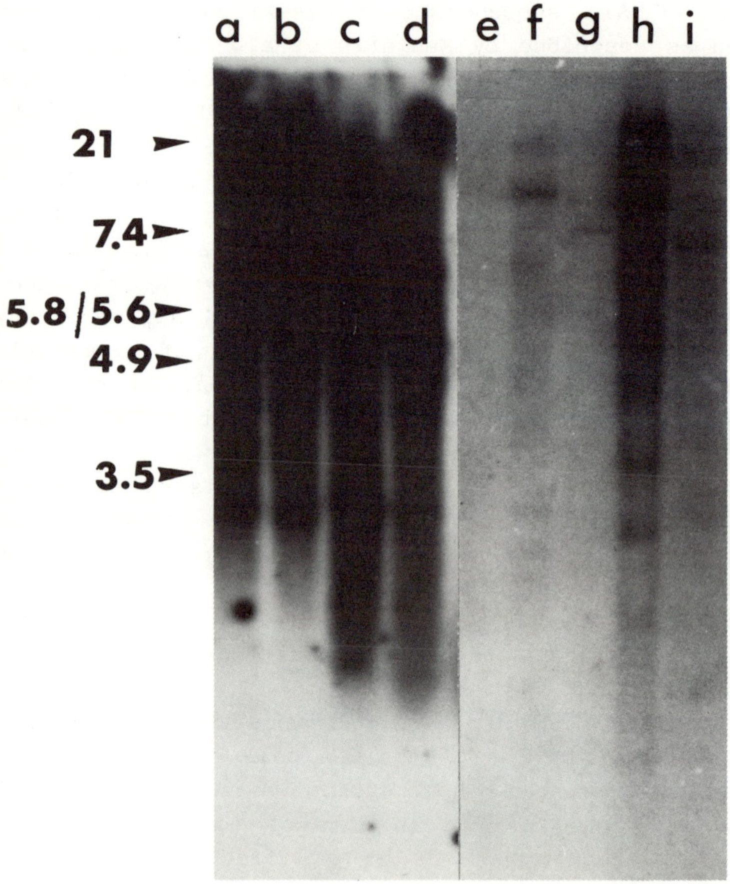

Figure 1a. DNA samples (20 ug each) of primary (lanes a, b, c, and d) and secondary transformants (lanes f, g, h, and i) were digested with Eco RI, electrophoresed in 1% agarose gels and hybridized with ^{32}P-labeled (2x10^{8} cpm/ug) Alu probe. Lane e: ESC DNA. The Alu probe contains mainly highly repetitive sequences. Transfer to nitrocellulose filters and hybridization with nick translated probes were performed as described (6). Molecular weights in Kbp of lamda Eco RI fragments are indicated.

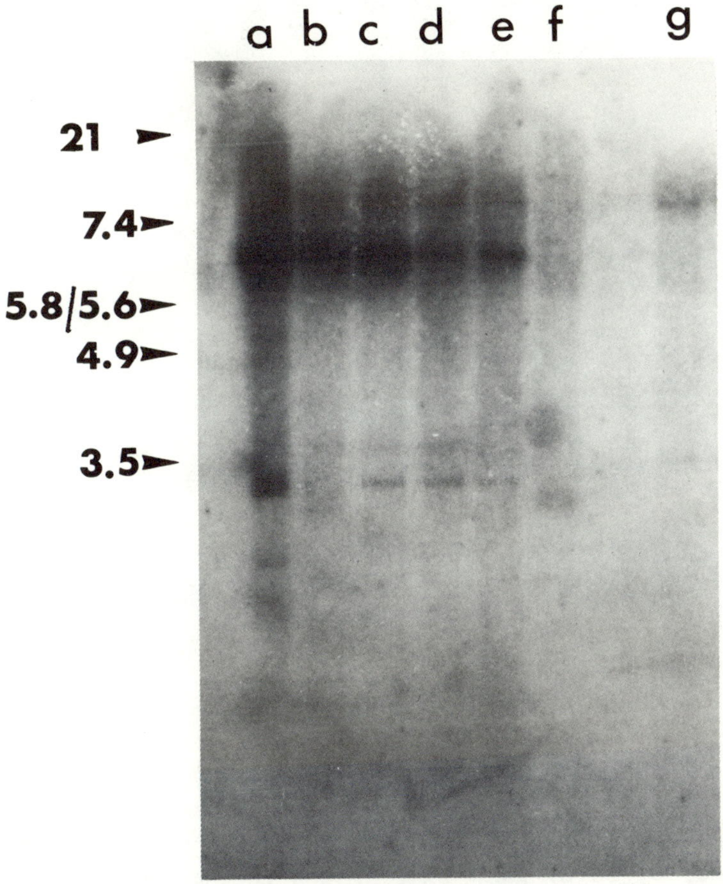

Figure 1b. DNA samples (20 ug each) of OHA (lane a), ESC secondary transformants (lanes b, c, d and e), HEL (lane f) and ESC (lane g) were digested with Eco RI, electrophoresed in 1% agarose gels and hybridized with the ^{32}P-labeled (4X10^{8} cpm/ug) PKBE 2 ras-ki probe. See figure 1a for other details.

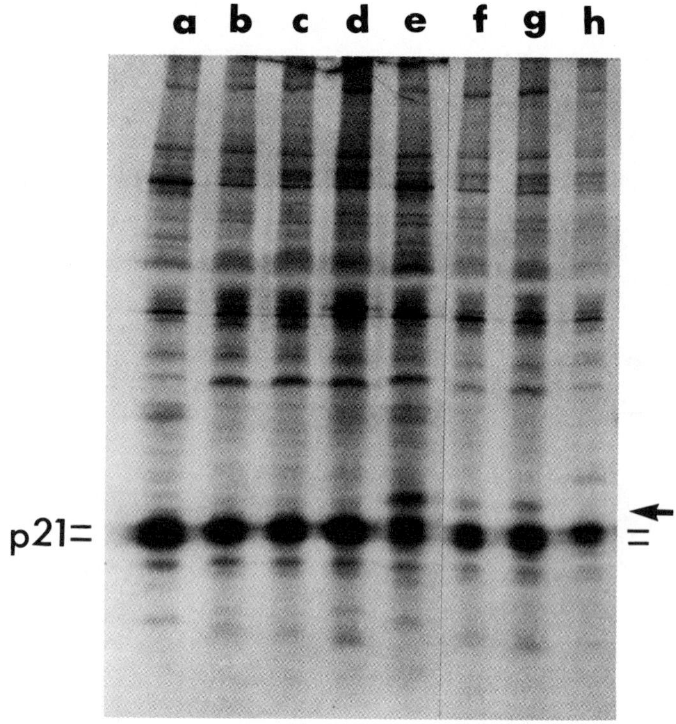

Figure 2. ^{35}S-methionine-labeled cell extracts were immunoprecipitated with 259 anti-p21 antibody and analyzed on 12% SDS-polyacrylamide gels. Lane a: SA 87 stomach adenocarcinoma cells; lanes b, c and d: ESC cells transformed by SA 87 DNA; lane e: OHA cells; lanes f and g: ESC cells transformed by OHA DNA; lane h: ESC cells. The SA 87 cells bear an activated ras-Ha gene (Suarez et al., unpublished results). Dashes: p21 doublet; arrow: altered p21 of OHA. The gels were calibrated according to the following molecular weight standards: myosin (200 K), phosphorylase B (93 K), bovine serum albumin (68 K), carbonic anhydrase (30 K), soybean trypsin inhibitor (21.5 K), alfa-lactalbumin (14 K).

found to produce protein in the size range expected for ras-encoded products (Fig. 2). This protein was an altered species of p21, recalling the abnormal forms found by Der and Cooper (1983) in three carcinomas carrying an activated ras-ki gene.

Our results indicate that in the OHA human osteosarcoma cell line, the transforming sequence(s) is related to the ras-ki oncogene. Tumor sources in which actived ras-ki gene has been identified include: lung, colon, bladder, biliary vesicle and pancreas carcinoma cell lines and a biopsy from an adenocarcinom of the large bowel (1, 2). Active genes of the ras family (Kirstein, Harvey and N-ras), have been more often identified by transfection of DNA derived from tumors of epithelial cell origin. However, there are some rare communications describing detection of these genes in sarcomas (1,2). Our present results together with data from Pulciani et al.(1982) concerning a solid rhabdomyosarcoma human tumor, show that ras-ki, though less frequently, can be activated in more than one tissue type. OHA is the first osteosarcoma in which an activated oncogene has been detected. Work is in progress to clone the OHA oncogene and to determine whether this gene is similar to the previously characterized active form of the ras-ki oncogene.

ACKNOWLEDGEMENTS

The expert technical assistance of J. Stevenet is gratefully acknowledged.

REFERENCES

1. Land, H., Parada, L.F., and Weinberg, R.A. (1983) Science, 222, 771-777.
2. Pulciani, S. et al. (1982) Nature, 300, 539-542.
3. Azzarone, B. et al. (1984). J. Cell. Biol.98, 1133-1137.

4. Gross-Bellard, M., Oudet, P. and Chambon, P. (1973) Europ. J. Bioch., 36, 32-38.
5. Perucho,M. et al. (1981) Cell, 27, 467-476.
6. Maniatis, T., Fritsch, E.F. and Sambrook, J. (1982) "Molecular cloning: A laboratory manual", Cold Spring Harbor Lab. Ed.
7. Houch, C.M., Reinehart, F.P. and Schmid, C.W. (1979) J. Mol. Biol. 132, 289-306.
8. Ellis, R.W. et al. (1981) Nature, 292, 506-511.
9. Der, C.J. and Coope, G.M. (1983) Cell 32, 201-208

COORDINATED REGULATION OF THE C-MYC GENE AND A TUMOR-RELATED MULTIGENIC SET IN HUMAN NEOPLASTIC CELLS TREATED WITH DIFFERENTIATION INDUCERS INCLUDING TUMOR PROMOTERS.

N. Hanania , D. Shaool, D. Zeliszewski, M.Castagna and J. Harel

GR 8 C.N.R.S., I.R.S.C. 94800 Villejuif, France

We previously showed (1,2) that one subfraction of the human genomic DNA, roughly corresponding to 2,000 non repeated sequences of 3 Kbs each, is activated in all the human neoplasias studied (leukemias, sarcomas or carcinomas), in tissue cultured cells as well as in primary tumours. By contrast, this subfraction, designated tumor activated DNA (TaDNA), was found very slightly, if at all, expressed in various normal cells, or tissues in the process of proliferation, including normal lymphocytes immortalized with Epstein Barr virus (EBV). We show here that the treatment of 2 Burkitt-lymphoma derived lines, Raji and Namalwa and of the myeloid leukemic derived HL-60 cell line, characterized by an abnormal activation of the c-myc gene, with several chemically unrelated differentiation inducers (TPA, teleocidin, mezerein, retinoic acid and DMSO) resulted in a drastic reduction in the levels of both c-myc and TaDNA - transcripts. On the contrary, the majority of TaDNA sequences are TPA-activated in normal EBV-immortalized lymphoid cells and cultured normal fibroblasts.

A growing body of evidence supports the concept that oncogenic transformation may depend on abnormal activation of cellular oncogenes (see general reviews 3,4), resulting from gene amplification, chromosomal rearrangements (5) or point mutations (6) and possibly involving cooperative oncogenes (7). This leaves open the question as to whether changes in the expression of many other genes occur in relation with, or as a result of carcinogenesis. The aim of the present study was to search for possible correlations between TaDNA activation and abnormal activation of oncogene(s). For this purpose we investigated the effects of various differentiation inducers in 3 lines of malignant hematopoietic cells characterized by translocation and/or an abnormal expression of c-myc.

The Raji and Namalwa cells (2 Burkitt lymphoma derived lines), the EBV-immortalized normal Priess cells and the HL-60 cells (a myeloid leukemia derived cell line) were grown in suspension in conditions already described (1,2). They were seeded at cell concentrations of $2.5\text{-}3.0 \times 10^5$ cells/ml, treated with different inducers 24 h after seeding and collected 24 h later for measuring the levels of TaDNA or myc-transcripts, or at different times for analysis of cell multiplication and differentiation. The HEL-cells (normal skin fibroblasts) were cultured in monolayers and treated before attaining confluence. We used various agents known as efficient differentiation inducers for HL-60 cells: DMSO, retionoic acid, mezerein, TPA (8, 9) and teleocidin (10). Phorbol esters induce macrophage characteristics whereas DMSO or retinoic acid favor the appearance of granulocytic or megakaryocytic cells (8,9). TPA is of particular interest because this potent tumor promoter for skin cancer can modulate cell phenotypes in opposite directions depending on the cell line studied (9). In particular, TPA can induce various different markers in Burkitt lymphoma lines or provoke in normal cells, pleiotropic changes which mimic those associated with oncogenic conversion. A chemical analog of

TPA, the 4 alfa-phorbol, 12, 13-didecanoate (4 alfa-PDD), almost devoid of activity (10), was used as control.

CELL DIFFERENTIATION

When treated with potent inducers like TPA in the range of 15-20 nM, 85-90% of the HL-60 cells became attached to the plastic support and the activities of 2 enzymatic markers (an esterase and an acid phosphatase) were increased 4-6 fold. The same treatment caused in Raji or Namalwa cells a significant decrease in the amounts of 2 antigenic markers (cALL and HLAdr) of the lymphoid precursor cells.

CELL MULTIPLICATION

Similar growth rates, at least for 48 h after seeding, were observed in all haemopoietic cell lines studied. Low concentrations (15-20 nM) of TPA, mezerein or teleocidin caused an almost complete arrest of multiplication of malignant cells but did not affect that of Priess cells. Greater concentrations of DMSO (1.3% = 60 nM) and retinoic acid (0.1 to 1 M) known to induce the differentiation of HL-60 cells resulted in a 50-55% reduction in the multiplication rates. In control assays, 4 alfa-PDD (10 to 100 nM) had no effect on cell differentiation and growth rates.

EFFECTS ON TaDNA TRANSCRIPTS

The percentages of TaDNA forming DNA-RNA hybrids at saturation levels, with an excess of total RNA from the various treated or not treated cells are summarized in the table 1.

It is clear that the various differentiation inducers caused in malignant cells a roughly dose-dependent

Table 1. TaDNA-RNA liquid hybridization data

Chemical Agent	Molar Concentration	% TaDNA bybridized to RNAs from malignant cells HL60	Raji	Namalwa	normal cells Priess	HEL
None		74+3	81+5	76+4	5+1.5	5+2
4alfaPDD	20 nM	70	76	73	-	-
TPA	3 nM	51	44.5	46	-	-
	16 nM	10.5	14	15.5	31	42.5
	50 nM	-	-	-	40.5	58
	160 nM	-	-	-	58	-
	1.6 uM	-	-	-	85	-
Teleoc.	4 nM	48	-	42.5	-	-
	20 nM	13	-	13	-	-
Mezerein	15 nM	68	-	-	-	-
	150 nM	11.5	-	-	28.5	-
	1.5 uM	9	-	-	45	-
Retinoic	400 nM	40	-	-	-	-
Acid	1 uM	12	-	-	22.5	-
	10 uM	-	-	-	35	-
DMSO	60 mM	16	-	-	-	-

Cellular RNAs and Raji cell DNA were prepared as described (1). A single-stranded DNA fraction, greatly enriched in transcribing sequences, was labelled with ^{125}I, and depleted of sequences shared with Priess cells by successive cycles of hybridization with RNA from Priess and Raji cells proliferating with similar growth rates (11). Centrifugation in cesium sulfate gradients allowed the separation of DNA-RNA hybrids from non hybridized DNA sequences (1,2). The percentages indicated are those obtained by the use of S1 nuclease at apparent saturation levels. In some crucial experiments, isopycnic centrifugation (in Cs sulfate gradient) confirmed that the S1 nuclease resistant molecules exclusively consisted of DNA-RNA duplexes (see 1,2). Teleoc. : teleocidin.

reduction in the population of TaDNA transcripts. We can notice that 10 fold higher concentration of mezerein than TPA is required to obtain the same level of inhibition of TaDNA activity, although these 2 agents are equipotent differentiation inducers. On the contrary, in normal cells, the TPA-treatment caused the occurence of RNA species hybridizable up to 85% of the Raji-cell TaDNA, in a dose-dependent manner, whereas only 4-5% for the latter could form hybrids with RNAs from untreated normal cells. At much higher concentrations, mezerein and retinoic acid produced enhancing effects.

EFFECTS ON C-MYC RNA

The treatment of HL-60 cells with optimal amounts of each differentiation inducer resulted in a drastic reduction (at least 10 fold) in the level of c-myc RNA (figure 1). This reduction in the level of c-myc RNA was also found in Namalwa cells treated with TPA whereas this level was not modified in Priess cells treated with higher amounts of TPA (not shown). We have checked with an actin-gene specific probe that none of the agents studied caused a significant reduction in the level of actin-specific RNAs (not shown).

We show here that the treatment of 3 distinct malignant cell lines, characterized by translocation and/or an abnormal activation of the c-myc gene, with several chemically-unrelated differetiation inducers, produces a drastic reduction in the levels of both c-myc RNA and TaDNA specific RNAs. This cannot be simply due to the cell growth inhibition caused by the differentiation inducers for several reasons, in particular because the majority of TaDNA sequences, which were silent in exponentially growing normal lymphoid cells and normal fibroblasts, become transcriptionally active within 24 h of treatment with TPA which did not change their proliferation rates. These opposite effects of TPA suggest that this agent (and probably other agents as well) may

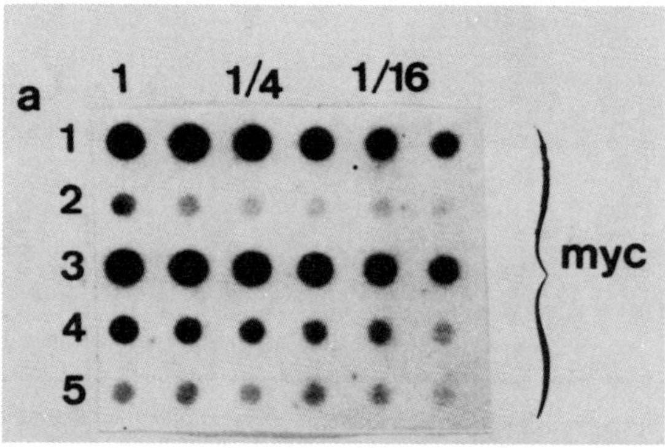

Figure 1. Dot blot hybridization showing the level of c-myc-RNA in HL-60 cells treated with various agents were performed following Thomas (12). The c-myc probe, consisting of a cloned 1.5 Kb Sac I restriction fragment containing most of the 2 exons (plasmid obtained from Dr. D. Stehelin) was nick-translated as described by Maniatis et al. (13) with ^{32}P-labelled dCTP (NEN) (3,000 Ci/mmol) to obtain specific activities in the range of 5-8x10^{8} cts/min/ug. From left to right the dots contained decreasing amounts (by 1/2) of total cellular RNAs : 2.5 ug, 1.25 ug, etc. Row No 1 : no treatment; No 2 : 15 nM mezerein; No 3 : 20 nM 4 alfa PDD; No 4 : 20 nM teleocidin; No 5 : 1 uM retinoic acid. 3A: the blots were prehybridized overnight at 42 C in 50% formamide (vol/vol), 0.75 M NaCl - 0.075 M Na citrate - 0.05 M Na phosphate buffer pH 6.5, containing 125 ug/ml of sonicated, denatured salmon sperm DNA and 0.02% each of bovine serum albumin, Ficoll and polyvinylpyrrolidone. They were thereafter hybridized for 24 h with the c-myc-specific probe (10^{6} cts/min/ml) in the same medium.

operate either as a tumor promoter or a differentiation inducer through a common control mechanism of the TaDNA-transcripts. Finally, our results suggest that TaDNA corresponds to a multigenic set which modulates the malignant phenotype, possibly in cooperation with c-myc or other oncogenes implicated in the initiation and genotypic maintenance of cancer.

REFERENCES

1. Hanania, N., Shaool, D., Poncy, C. and Harel, J. (1981) Proc. Natl. Acad. Sci. USA 78, 6504-6508.
2. Hanania, H., Shaool, D., Harel, J., Wiels, J., and Tursz T. (1983). EMBO J. 2, 1621-1624.
3. Cooper G.M. (1982) Science 218, 801-807.
4. Weinberg R.A. (1982) Adv. Cancer Res. 36, 149-163.
5. Klein G. (1983) Cell 32, 311-315.
6. Sukamar, S., Notario, V., Martin-Zanca D. and Barbacid M. (1983) Nature 306, 658-661.
7. Tabin, J.G. et al. (1982) Nature 300, 143-149.
8. Collins, S.T., Ruscetti, S.W., Gallagher R.E. and Gallo R.C. (1978) Proc. Natl. Acad. Sci. USA 75, 2458-2461.
9. Rovera, G., O'Brien, T.G., and Diamond, L. (1978) Science 204, 868-870.
10 Fisher, P.B., et al. (1982) Cancer Res. 42, 2829-2835.
11. Hanania, N., Shaool D., Poncy, C., Tapiero, H., and Harel, J. (1977) Cell Biol. Int. Rep. 1, 309-315.
12. Thomas, P. (1980) Proc. natl. Acad. USA 76, 5201-5205.
13. Maniatis, T., Kee, S.G., Efstradiatis, A., and Kafatos, F.C. (1975). Proc. Natl. Acad. Sci. USA 1154-1158.

TRANSCRIPTS OF c-fes ONCOGENE ARE PRESENT AT DETECTABLE LEVELS IN TOTAL CELLULAR RNA OF HUMAN MYELOID BUT NOT LYMPHOID NORMAL AND NEOPLASTIC CELLS.

S. Ferrari, L. Selleri, L. Moretti, D. Venturelli, A. Donelli, F. Narni, G. Ceccherelli, G. Torelli, U. Torelli

Center of Experimental Hematology, Second Medical Clinic, University of Modena, 41100 Modena, Italy

Total cellular RNA from a variety of normal and leukemic myeloid and lymphoid cell populations was analysed for the expression of a human cellular oncogene, c-fes, by Northern blot hybridization assays. The probe used was a molecularly cloned human DNA sequence homologous to the 5', terminal portion of the transforming gene of the feline sarcoma virus, Snyder-Theilen strain. All the myeloid cell populations studied express the c-fes gene as a single 3.5 Kb long mRNA species. The level of expression was found to increase during the myeloid differentiation process. No transcripts of the c-fes gene were detected in the different lymphoid populations studied. The occurence of an RNA complementary to the c-fes sequence appears limited to myeloid populations so a possible relation with myeloid differentiation can be suggested. Moreover it is possible to postulate the use of this sequence as a tool to distinguish normal or neoplastic lymphoid cells from any myeloid population. Neither evident genomic amplification nor genomic rearrangements were detected in the cell DNAs digested with restriction endonucleases using Southern blot hybridization experiments.

The oncogene v-fes of the acutely transforming feline sarcoma virus, Snyder-Theilen strain, causes fibrosarcomas in cats and transforms cultured fibroblasts of various mammalian species (1). This virus has homologous cellular sequences (c-fes) in all vertebrate species including humans. The genomic structure of the human c-fes genetic locus homologous to the onc sequence of Snyder-Theilen feline sarcoma virus has been described by G. Franchini et al. (2). The transformation-specific protein of v-fes is a fused gag-onc polypeptide which exhibits associated tyrosine protein kinase activity (3). Moreover the c-fes human oncogene has been sublocalized by M. Harper et al. (4), by the in situ hybridization technique, to the distal end of the long arm of chromosome 15 (15q 25-26).

Thus far, c-fes transcripts have not been detected in several types of human cells, although the protein has been found in some cells by M. Barbacid et al. (3). Only very recently data obtained by D.J. Slamon et al. (5) and by our laboratory (6) demonstrate the presence of c-fes related transcripts in human cells. In all cases in which an RNA hybridized to the labeled ^{32}P c-fes DNA probe was detectable, only a single band was observed. Our data indicate that the size of this molecular species, calculated assuming for the two ribosomal RNA subunits the value of 5.45 Kb and 2.2 Kb respectively for 28S and 18S RNA, was approximatey 3.5 Kb long.

Having found the specific messenger RNA for the c-fes oncogene in human cells, we decided to investigate the levels of its expression in various human normal and leukemic cell populations by Northern blot assay. Furthermore we were interested in studying the genomic structure of the c-fes genetic locus by Southern blot hybridization in order to explore a possible relation between the genomic organization,the level of the oncogene

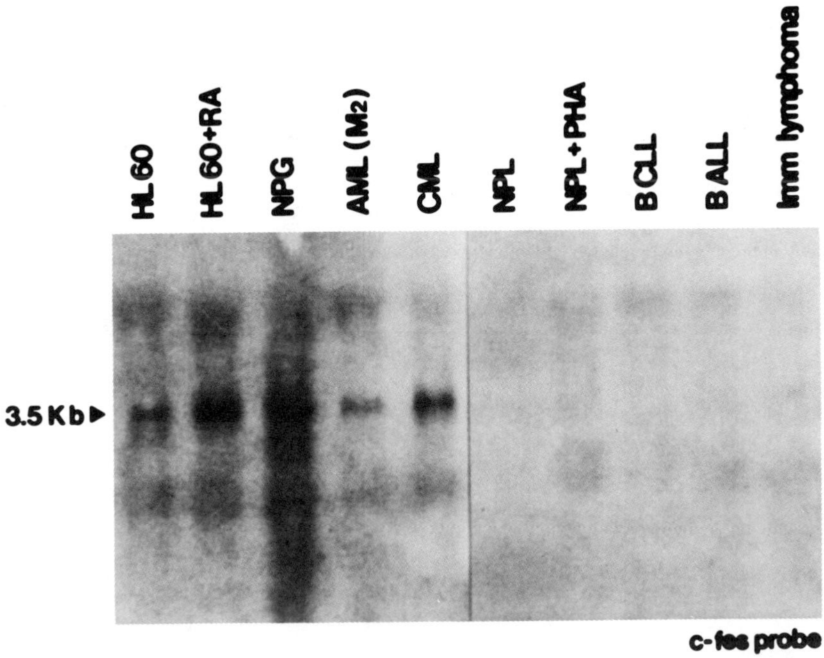

Figure 1. Total cellular RNA (10 ug/lane) was electrophoresed on 1.1% agarose-formaldehyde gel. The sample was prepared dissolving the RNA in 50% deionized formamide, 6% formaldeyde and 1xMOPS and incubating for 15' at 60 C. Transfer of the RNA to the hybridization membrane was done by using a Bio-Rad trans-blot cell. The cloned c-fes DNA was labeled to a specific activity of about 1.5 x 10^8 counts/min/ug using a commercial nick translation kit (NEN). The hybridization conditions were as described by S. Ferrari et al. (6). After the removal of excess probe by several washings, the membrane was autoradiographed at -70 C for 1-3 days in the presence of an intensifier screen (Quanta III). Autoradiograms were scanned using an image analyzer (Tesak VDC-501) to estimate the relative intensities of the bands.

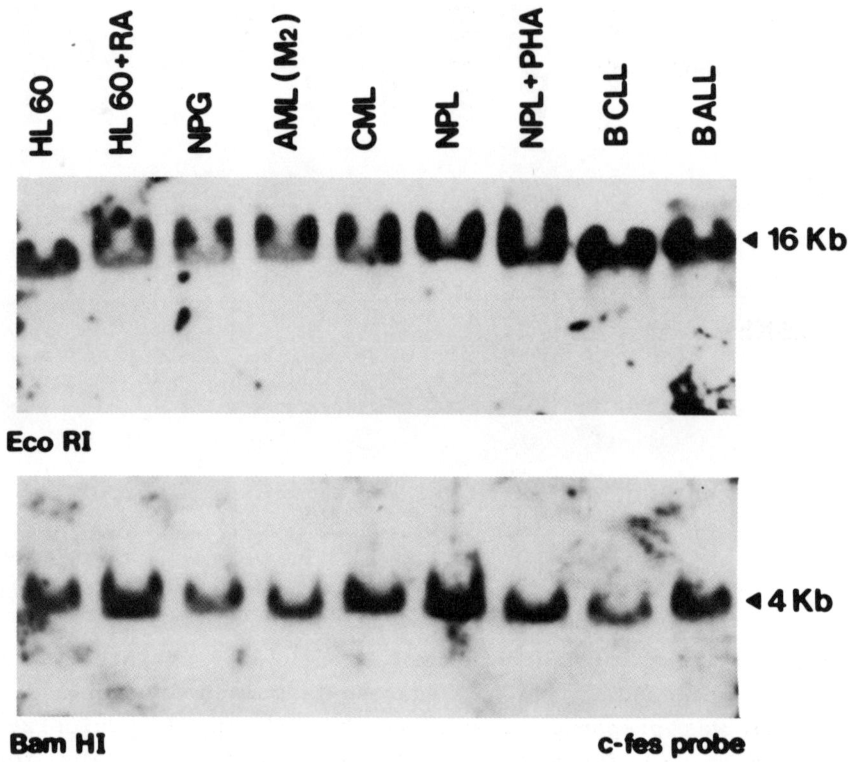

Figure 2. DNAs digested with different restriction endonucleases (20 ug/lane) were run in 0.8% agarose gel and transferred to a gene screen membrane (NEN) with a standard Southern blot procedure (9). Hybridization and washing conditions were as described (10). The hybridized blots were exposed at -70 C for 1-5 days as described in the legend to fig. 1.

product and the leukemic transformation.

The human c-fes clone (p26) was generously provided by Dr. G. Franchini from the Tumor Cell Biology Laboratory, NCI, Bethesda, Md. The clone represents a 4 Kb Bam HI restriction DNA fragment with 1.4 Kb homologous to the 5' terminal sequence of v-fes, inserted in the Bam HI site of the pBR322, transduced to E. coli MC 1061 (2). The plasmid DNA was purified and labeled to a specific activity of about $1.5x10^8$ counts/min/ug using the nick translation technique.

DNA and total cellular RNA were obtained from different normal and leukemia, myeloid and lymphoid, cell populations using a cell separator. In particular the myeloid cell populations were representd by circulating granulocytes from a normal donor, peripheral cells from 3 cases of CML, circulating blast cells from two patients with AML (one M2 and one M4). HL60 cells before and after induction of terminal differentiation by retinoic acid. Normal circulating lymphocytes were obtained from two normal donors. Normal peripheral lymphocytes from a third donor were stimulated for 72 hours with PHA. Leukemic lymphocytes were obtained from 2 patients with B CLL and 3 patients with ALL (two B and one T phenotype) and from a patient with immunoblastic lymphoma.

The DNAs obtained from the different cell populations were digested with Eco RI and Bam HI restriction endonucleases. Southern blot hybridization experiments showed that neither fragment length polymorphism (gene rearrangements) nor evident amplification events in the c-fes genomic locus were detectable in normal or leukemic DNAs. The methylation degree of the various lymphoid and myeloid DNAs is under investigation using Msp I and Hpa II restriction endonucleases.

With Northern blot hybridization experiments we were able to demonstrate that all the normal and leukemic myeloid cell populations studied expressed the c-fes gene. In some cell populations at an advanced stage of differentiation (normal peripheral granulocytes, circulating leukocytes from CML and HL60 cells induced to terminal differentiation by retinoic acid) the level of expression of c-fes messenger RNA was higher than in the immature myeloid cells. No transcripts of the c-fes gene were detected in the different, normal and leukemic, lymphoid populations studied. These data are fairly well in keeping with the data reported by G. Emilia et al (this book) using the in situ hybridization technique on normal and leukemic bone marrow cells as well as on circulating peripheral cells.

The reported pattern of expression of c-fes gene appears similar to that reported for c-abl and c-ras^{H}, since like these oncogenes c-fes expression is not reduced in late stages of myeloid differentiation. It has already been reported by several authors that c-myb and c-myc oncogenes, on the contrary, become less expressed during myeloid differentiation (7, 8).

Our data clearly show that the c-fes oncogene is expressed at detectable levels in myeloid but not in lymphoid cells. We believe that it could be used as a new molecular marker, in addition to the traditional morphological, cytochemical and immunological criteria, to distinguish myeloid from lymphoid cells. This distinction is probably based upon differences in the relative abundance of individual messenger RNAs which are at the very origin of the phenotype differences between different cell types.

REFERENCES

1. Snyder, S.P., Theilen, G.H. (1969) Nature 221, 1074-1075.
2. Franchini, G., Gelman, E.P., Dalla Favera, R., Gallo., R.C., Wong-Staal, F. (1982) Mol. Cell. Biol. 2, 1014-1019.
3. Barbacid, M., Beemon, K., Devare, S.G. (1980) Proc. Natl. Acad. Sci. USA 77, 5158-5162.
4. Harper, M.E., Franchini, G., Love, J., Simon, M.L., Gallo, R.C., Wong-Stahl, F. (1983) Nature 304,

169-171.

5. Slamong, D.J., deKernion, J.B., Verma, I.M., Cline, M.J. (1984) Science 224,256-262.
6. Ferrari, S., Torelli, U., Selleri, L., Donelli, A., Venturelli, D., Moretti, L., Torelli, G. (1984) British J. Haematology in press.
7. Westin, E.H., Wong-Staal, F., Gelmann, E.P., Dalla Favera, R., Papas, T.K., Lautenberger, J.A., Eva, A., Reddy, E.P., Tronick, S.R., Aaronson, S.A., Gallo, R.C. (1982) Proc. Natl. Acad. Sci. USA 79, 2490-2494.
8. Westin, E.H., Gallo, R.C., Arya, S.K., Eva, A., Souza, L.M., Baluda, M.A., Aaronson, S.A., Wong-Staal, F. (1982) Proc. Natl. Acad. Sci. USA 79, 2194-2198.
9. Southern, E.M. (1975) J. Mol. Bl. 98, 503-517.
10. Ferrari, S., Torelli, U., Selleri, L., Donelli, A., Venturelli, D., Narni, F., Torelli, G. (1984) submitted for publication.

HETEROGENEITY OF HUMAN NORMAL AND LEUKEMIC CELLS OF LYMPHOID AND MYELOID LINEAGE IN RESPECT TO THE EXPRESSION OF c-myc AND c-myb mRNA TRANSCRIPTS.

L. Selleri, S. Ferrari, D. Venturelli, A. Donelli, L. Moretti, G. Ceccherelli, G. Torelli, U. Torelli.

Center for Experimental Hematology, Second Medical Clinic, University of Modena, 41100 Modena, Italy.

The clones pMC41.5 and pMC41.3, representing respectively the 5' and the 3' terminal of c-myc and the clone F8, representing the 3' terminal of c-myb, were used to investigate the presence of myc and myb transcripts in Northern blot analysis of total cellular RNAs. The survey was carried out on the RNAs of different cell populations: leukemic cells of lymphoid and myeloid lineage, HL60 cells uninduced and induced to differentiation with retinoic acid (RA) and TPA, normal peripheral blood lymphocytes and PHA stimulated normal lymphocytes. c-myc expression, although at very different levels, occurs in many cell populations, being detectable only in 2 cases of ALL, in 2 cases of CLL and in 1 case of Hairy cell leukemia. On the other hand, c-myb RNA levels are either low or absent in most of the populations studied, except in 2 cases of ALL (one T and one B) and in 1 CML in blast crisis. The remarkable variations of c-myc and c-myb expression in different cases of the same pathology indicate that a possible correlaton between neoplasia and the expression of these oncogenes is at least not dose-dependent. In human normal lymphocytes, PHA stimulation strongly increases the expression of c-myb, whose mRNA, showing no detectable expression in resting lymphocytes, reaches a high concentration in the PHA stimulated cells.

A direct correlation between the level of expression of oncogenes and their transforming activity has been supported by several authors (reviewed in 1). However, most studies on c-onc expression have been made on cell lines in which the events occurring at the molecular level cannot be easily transferred to neoplastic cells in vivo. Furthermore a modulation of the expression of some c-onc has been found in normal cells (2) and this obviously hinders any correlation between the increase in oncogene expression and neoplastic transformation of the cell. In order to gain insight into the significance of c-onc expression in transformed cells in vivo, we carried out a survey in Northern blot analysis of many leukemic populations of both lymphoid and myeloid lineages and on human normal blood cells, with probes representing parts of the oncogenes c-myc and c-myb, which have been correlated by several authors to the hematopoietic malignancies (3,4,5). Lymphoid and myeloid leukemic cells were obtained from the patients by leukapheresis.

We studied 6 cases of CLL, 6 adult ALL, 5 AML, 1 CML blast crisis, 4 CML in the chronic phase, 1 case of idiopathic myelofibrosis and 1 case of dysemocytopoietic syndrome. The blast cells in all cases of acute leukemia were more than 90% of the population. Each phenotype was defined morphologically, cytochemically and immunologically. Human normal leukocytes, isolated onto Ficoll-Hypaque and then filtered through nylon columns (Leukopac), were finally more than 90% OKT1 and E rosette positive. Part of these normal T lymphocytes were stimulated with PHA for 72 hours.

RNAs were extracted from all these cell populations with a standard technique, run on denaturing agarose gel

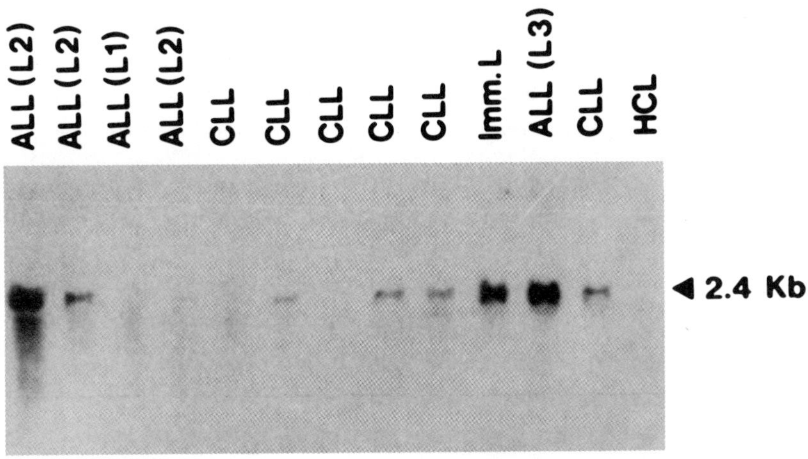

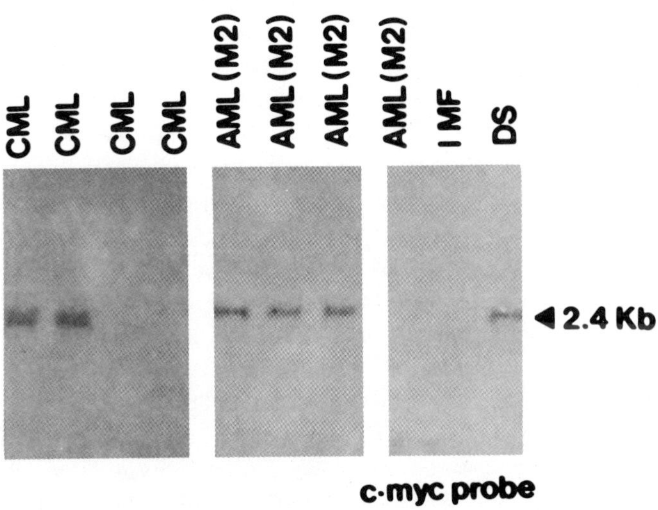

Figure 1. Northen blot analysis of 5' c-myc probe, nick translated with ^{32}P dCTP to a specific activity of 1.5x10^{8} cpm/ug and hybridized to total cellular RNAs, extracted from different human neoplastic cell populations (CML: chronic and AML: acute myeloid leukemia; DS: disemocytopoietic syndrome; IMF: idiopathic myelofibrosis; CLL: chronic and ALL: acute lymphatic leukemia; Imm.L.:

Figure 1 (continued).
leukemic phase of immunoblastic lymphoma; HCL: hairy cell leukemia). Electrophoresis of RNA was performed in 1.1% agarose gel in MOPS buffer, pH 7.0 and 6% formaldehyde. 10 ug of RNA, dissolved in 50% deionized formamide, 6% formaldehyde and 1 x MOPS, incubated for 15 min at 60 C, were run in each lane.

---

electrophoresis and transferred to Gene Screen sheets by electroblotting procedure.

The probes used in the hybridization assays were pMC41.5 and pMC41.3 corresponding respectively to the 5' and 3' terminal of the c-myc gene (6). The pMC41.5 recombinant plasmid has an inserted fragment of 2.0 kb, while the recombinant plasmid pMC41.3 has an inserted fragment of 1.6 kb. The F8 clone, corresponding to the 3' terminal of the c-myb gene, has an inserted fragment of 2.0 kb (7). (The clones were kindly provided by Dr. R.C. Gallo, Tumor Cell Biology Laboratory, NCI, Bethesda, Md., USA). The plasmid DNAs were purified, nick-translated with ^{32}P dCTP and hybridized to the blotted RNAs. After washings, the hybridized filters were exposed for 1-5 days at -80°C with an intensifier screen (Quanta III). Relative intensities of the hybridized bands were estimated with a computerized image analyzer (Tesak VDC501).

In all cases of positive hybridization, the mRNAs corresponding to c-myc and c-myb were respectively 3.8 kb for the c-myb probe and 2.4 kb for both the c-myc probes, the human ribosomal subunits having comigrated with the labelled 3' restriction fragments of DNA digested with EcoRI and HindIII, respectively 1900 NT for 18S and 4800 NT for 28S, in keeping with the data of Lewin (8).

Northern blot analysis of different acute and chronic lymphatic leukemias showed that c-myc was expressed at very different levels in many cell populations. However in 2 cases of ALL, 2 cases of CLL and 1 case of hairy cell

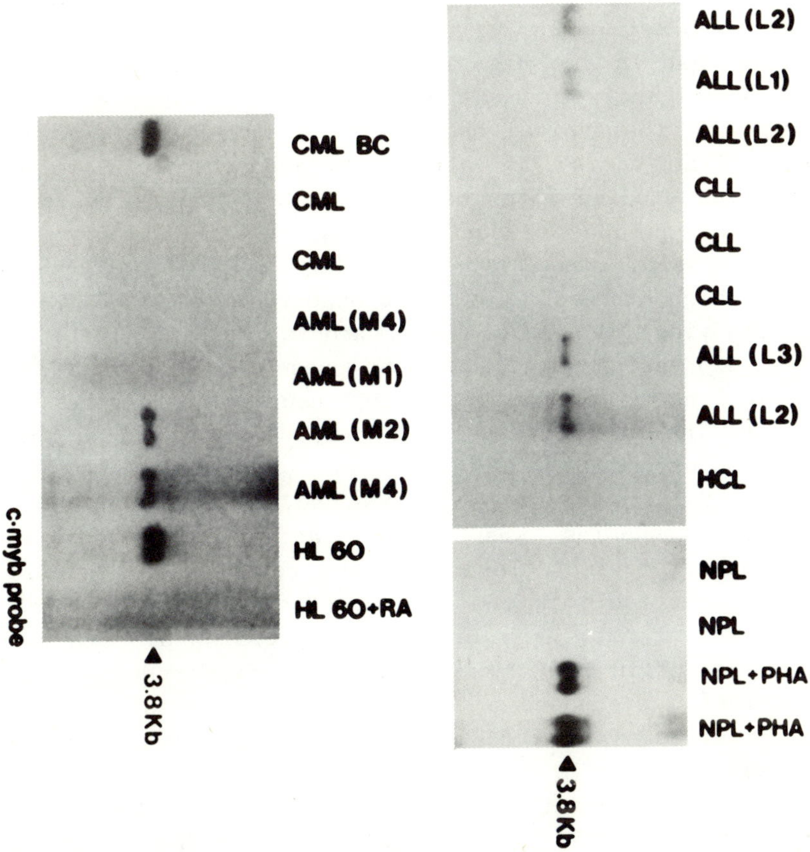

Figure 2. Northern blot analysis of 3' c-myb probe, nick translated with ^{32}P dCTP to a specific activity of 1.5x10^{8} cpm/ug and hybridized to total cellular RNAs. The RNAs were extracted from different human normal cells (normal peripheral blood resting -NPL- and PHA stimulated lymphocytes -NPL+PHA-), HL60 cells uninduced -HL60- and induced to differentiation with retinoic acid -HL60 + RA- and from neoplastic cell populations of lymphoid and myeloid lineage (abbreviations as in Fig. 1).

leukemia no detectable expression of this oncogene was found. On the contrary very high levels of expression were seen in blast cells of T and B phenotype. It is worth noting that in one case of B ALL (L_3 Burkitt-like type) the c-myc gene was very highly expressed, although in the absence of the typical chromosomal abnormalities described in similar cases. In all acute and chronic lymphatic leukemias studied with the c-myb probe, the expression of this oncogene was either very low or absent. Only in 2 cases of ALL, one T and one B (L_3 Burkitt-like), was a fairly high expression of c-myb observed.

Studying the acute and chronic myeloid leukemias, c-myc expression was found to be present in many different populations (7 out of 12) but usually at rather low levels. The highest levels of c-myc RNA were found in 2 CML populations.

As far as c-myb is concerned, its expression in myeloid leukemias was always absent or very low: completely undetectable in all the cases of CML studied, barely detectable in one case of CML blast crisis and in two cases of AML. High levels of expression of both c-onc were present in uninduced HL60 cells, while the expression drastically decreased after induction of these cells to differentiation with RA and TPA, in agreement with data already reported (3,4).

Eight different cell populations of human normal peripheral blood lymphocytes were studied for the expression of c-myc and c-myb. c-myc was detected in all the unstimulated lymphocytes examined; in contrast, no significant expression of c-myb was observed in the same unstimulated cells. Stimulation with PHA, while increasing mildly the expression of c-myc, activates very strongly the expression of c-myb, whose mRNA reaches a very high concentration in the stimulated cells. All data concerning this event have been reported elsewhere (9).

The activation of both c-myc and c-myb in normal lymphocytes by the action of PHA (2,9) hinders the direct correlation between the neoplastic state of the cell and the increase in oncogene expression. These oncogenes seem to be in some way related to the cell-cycle (10,11) and certainly further studies are needed to gain insight into the cell-cycle mechanisms at the molecular level and their possible alterations.

It seems rather interesting that cell populations strictly similar morphologically, cytochemically and immunologically show at the molecular level an impressive differential activity of a certain gene. This observation clearly underlines the notion that the conventional cytomorphologic and immunologic criteria define groups of malignancies in which a great heterogeneity in genomic expression is still present.

REFERENCES

1. Bishop, J.M. (1983) Ann. Rev. Biochem. 52, 301-354.
2. Kelly, K., Cochran, B.H., Stiles, C.D., Leder, P. (1983) Cell 35, 603-610.
3. Westin, E.H., Gallo, R.C., Arya, S.K., Eva, A., Souza, L.M., Baluda, M.A., Aaronson, S.A., Wong-Staal, F. (1982) Proc. Natl. Acad. Sci. USA 79, 2194-2198.
4. Westin, E.H., Wong-Staal, F., Gelman, E.P., Dalla Favera, R., Papas, T.S., Lautenberger, J.A., Eva, A., Reddy, E.P., Tronick, S.R., Aaronson, S.A., Gallo, R.C. (1982) Proc. Natl. Acad. Sci. USA 79, 2490-2494.
5. Rothberg, P.G., Erisman, M.D., Diehl, R.E., Rovigatti, U.G., Astrin, S.M. (1984) Mol. Cell. Biol. 4, 1096-1103.
6. Dalla Favera, R., Gelmann, E.P., Martinotti, S., Franchini, G., Pappas, T.S., Gallo, R.C., Wong-Staal, F. (1982) Proc. Acad. Natl. Sci. USA 79, 6497-6501.
7. Franchini, G., Woong-Staal, F., Baluda, M.A., Lengel, C., Tronick, S.R. (1983) Proc. Natl. Acad. Sci. USA 80, 7385-7389.
8. Lewin, B. (1980) in Gene Expression 2, ed. Lewin, B. (Wiley Interscience Pubblication, New York) pp 865-906.
9. Torelli, G., Ferrari, S., Donelli, A., Emilia, G.,

Selleri, L., Venturelli, D., Moretti, L., Torelli, U. (1984) submitted for pubblication.

10. Campisi, J. Gray, H.E., Pardee, A.B., Dean, M., Sonenshein, G.E. (1984) Cell 36, 241-247.
11. Gonda, T.J. & Metcalf D. (1984) Nature 310, 249-251.

DETECTION OF c-myc, c-myb AND c-fes ONCOGENE TRANSCRIPTS IN HUMAN MYELOID AND LYMPHOID NORMAL AND LEUKEMIC CELLS BY IN SITU HYBRIDIZATION.

G. Emilia, A. Donelli, S. Ferrari, L. Selleri, P. Zucchini, M. G. De Benedettis, G. Torelli, U. Torelli, A. Colò.

Center of Experimental Hematology, Second Medical Clinic, University of Modena, 41100 Modena, Italy.

The in situ hybridization technique was used to investigate the expression of the human cellular oncogenes, c-myc, c-myb and c-fes, simultaneously on different cell populations: normal resting and PHA stimulated T lymphocytes, leukemic resting and LPS stimulated B lymphocytes, AML, CML and IM cells. The probes used were the clones pCM 41.5 and pCM 41.3 corresponding to the 5' and 3' terminal of c-myc, the clone F8 corresponding to the 3' terminal of c-myb and the clone p 26 corresponding to the 5' terminal of c-fes, Snyder-Theilen strain. In all myeloid cell populations c-myc, c-myb and c-fes expression was detected, but while c-myc and c-myb were present at a higher level in immature cells and decreased during myeloid maturation, c-fes markedly increased in more mature elements. The expression of c-fes was not detected in normal and leukemic lymphoid cells, while c-myc and c-myb, detectable at a very low degree in resting lymphocytes, drastically increased in mitogen stimulated normal and leukemic cells.

These data suggest that the expression of c-myc and c-myb in hemopoietic cells may be linked to cell proliferation while c-fes expression seems to be related to myeloid maturation processes.

Much evidence has linked oncogene structure and expression with cancer (1). Recently it has been shown that some oncogenes are involved in normal cell functions as proliferation (2) and differentiation (3). In order to examine the level of expression of some c-oncs and its significance in normal and leukemic hematopoietic cells, we chose the in situ hybridization technique. This technique is a useful tool to simultaneously investigate the expression of RNA sequences in cell populations heterogeneous for lineage and maturation level. Furthermore it overcomes the problems related to the difficulty of performing a molecular hybridization by Northern blot technique from a mixture of different cell types. Therefore, even with a low number of cells, it is possible to correlate the abundance of a specific mRNA simultaneously with cells different in lineage and maturation level. By in situ hybridization analysis we carried out a survey on normal and leukemic hematopoietic cells with probes representing part of the oncogenes c-myc and c-myb which have been correlated to hematopoietic malignances (4,5,6) and c-fes whose related transcripts have been recently reported in human hemopoietic cells (7,8,3). We studied leukemic myeloid cells obtained from the peripheral blood of 1 patient with Acute Myelogenous Leukemia (AML) M_4 type (FAB classification), 1 patient with Chronic Myelogeneous Leukemia (CML), 1 patient with Idiopathic Myelofibrosis (IM); normal resting and PHA stimulated peripheral blood T lymphocytes obtained from 4 normal donors, leukemic resting and Lypopolysaccharide (LPS) stimulated B lymphocytes obtained from 2 B-Chronic Lymphocytic Leukemia (CLL) patients. The phenotype in each case was defined by morphological, cytochemical, cytogenetic and immunological criteria. HL60 cells, a human promyelocytic leukemia cell line, uninduced and induced with Retionic Acid (RA) and Phorbol Acetate (TPA) were also studied. The probes used in the hybridization assays were the pMC 41.5 and pMC 41.3 clones corresponding to the 5' and 3' terminal of the c-myc gene (9), the F8 clone corresponding to the 3' terminal of the c-myb gene (10) and the p26 clone corresponding to the 5' terminal of c-fes, Snyder-Theilen strain (11). (The clones were kindly provided by Dr. R.C. Gallo and Dr. G. Franchini, Tumor Cell Biology Laboratory, NCI, Bethesda, Md. USA). The cloned DNA was ^3H labeled to a specific activity of about $1\text{-}2 \times 10^7$ cpm/min/ug using a commercial nick translation kit (Amersham). In situ hybridization was performed on cells cytocentrifuged onto acid washed slides according to the technique of Brahic and Haase (12), with 7 ul buffer on $1\text{-}2 \times 10^5$ cells/slide and 2.5×10^5 cpm of ^3H nick translated probe. Hybridizations were carried out in a humidified thermostat at 43° C for 18 hours. At the end of incubation the slides, after extensive washing, were covered with Kodak NTB2 liquid emulsion. Autoradiographic exposure was done for 8 days; micrographs of cells counterstained with MGG were at a final magnification of 1000x. A total of approximately 1500 grains per slide were counted (three slides were used for each sample described).

All the myeloid cellular populations expressed the c-fes gene; this finding is in agreement with the data reported by Ferrari et al. (this volume) using Northern blot hybridization assays. Blast cells from AML (M_4) expressed a discrete level of c-fes in almost all the elements, while a low degree of uniform labelling was found for c-myc expression (Fig. 1, H,I). Marked changes in the level of c-fes expression were observed in leukemic cells from CML in the chronic phase (50% mature elements) and IM in which a substantial increase of labelling degree was present in more mature elements (Fig. 1, J,K,L). A similar pattern of c-fes expression was observed in uninduced (immature) and RA induced (mature) HL60 cells (Fig. 1, E,F). While uninduced HL60 cells showed a homogeneous low labeling degree, a two fold higher c-fes expression was found in RNA induced cells (more marked in bands and granulocytes). No significant variation was

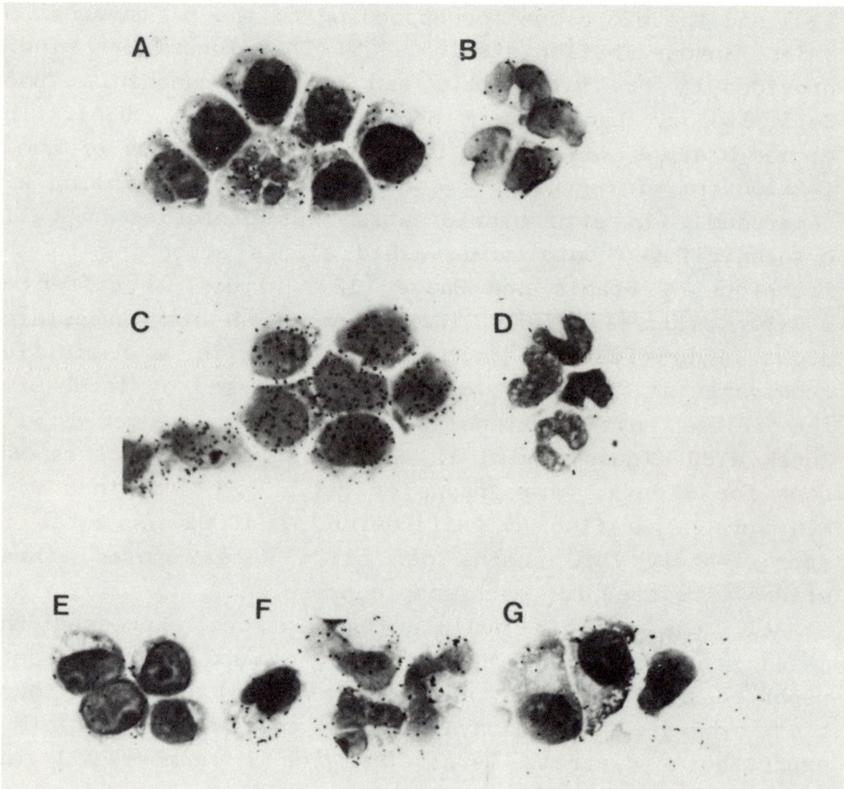

Figure 1. In situ hybridization of c-myb to uninduced (A) and RA induced (B) HL60 cells; c-myc to uninduced (C) and RA induced (D) HL60 cells; c-fs to uninduced (E), RA induced (F) and TPA induced (G) HL60 cells; c-fes (H) and c-myc (I) to AML (M_4) blast cells; c-fes to immature (J) and more mature cells (K, L) of a CML patient. Autoradiographic exposure: 8 days; magnification: x1000.

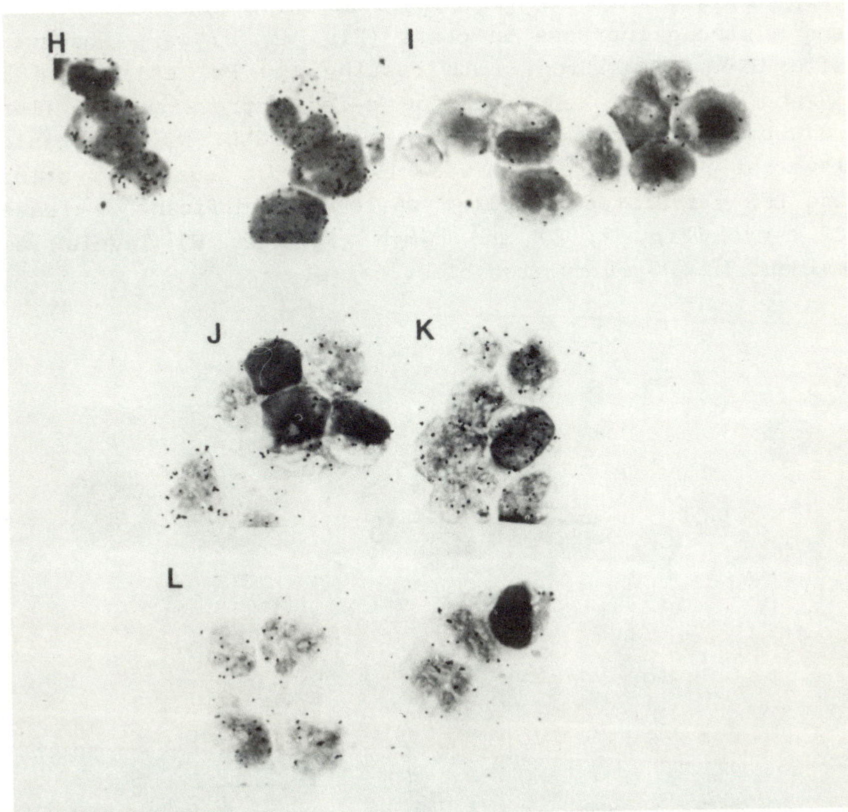

Figure 1. (continued)

observed in TPA induced HL60 cells (macrophages)(Fig.1, G). On the contrary uninduced HL60 cells showed a level of c-myc and c-myb expression dramatically higher than RA induced cells (Fig. 1, A,B,C,D) (a 14 fold and 6.4 fold decrease respectively in mature cells) in agreement with data already reported (5). A different pattern of c-myc and c-myb expression was observed before and after PHA lymphocyte stimulation: c-myc and c-myb expression was either extremely low or absent in resting lymphocytes (Fig. 2, A), while a mild increase in c-myc (Fig. 2, C) and a strong increase in c-myb (Fig. 2, B) were observed after PHA stimulation. Both resting and PHA stimulated T lymphocytes were negative for c-fes expression. Similar results were obtained in 2 cases of B-CLL. No detectable level of c-fes expression was observed in leukemic resting and LPS stimulated B cells, while a significant increase of c-myc (Fig. 2, E) and c-myb (Fig. 2, F) levels was evident in LPS stimulated blast cells.

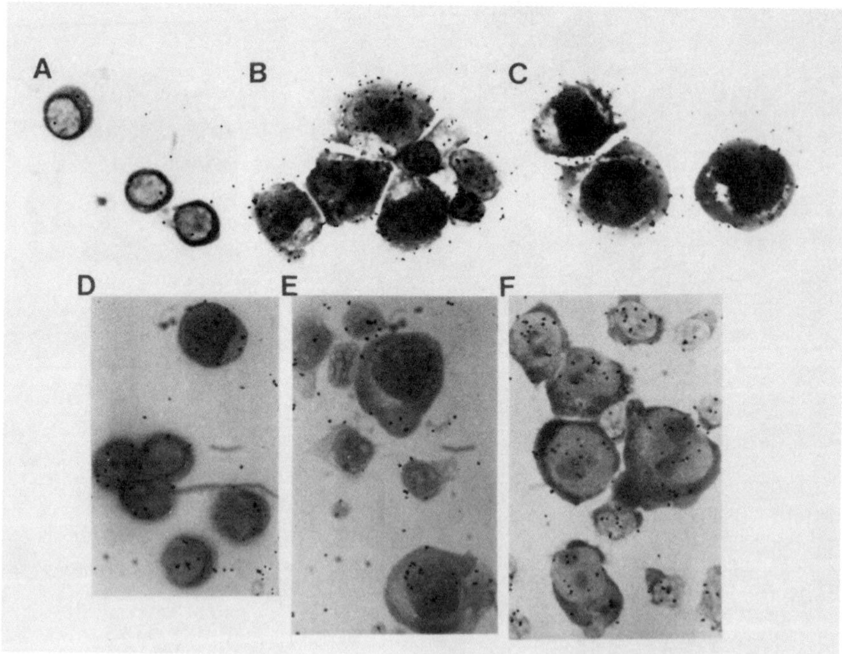

Figure 2. In situ hybridization of c-myb to normal resting (A) and PHA stimulated (B) peripheral blood T lymphocytes; c-myc to PHA stimulated normal peripheral blood T lymphocytes (C); c-myb to leukemic resting (D) and LPS stimulated (E) B-CLL lymphocytes; c-myc to LPS stimulated B-CLL lymphocytes.

The results obtained by the in situ hybridization technique for the expression of c-myc, c-myb and c-fes in resting and stimulated proliferating lymphocytes, are in keeping with the data obtained by Kelly et al. (2) and Ferrari et al. (3) in Northern blot experiments. Meanwhile the high expression of c-myc and c-myb in immature myeloid cells (HL60 cells) and its drastic decrease in mature cells (HL60 RA induced) may be correlated to the loss of proliferative activity of these cells. On the contrary, all the myeloid cells were found positive for c-fes expression and the labelling degree was seen to be increasing in maturing elements. To get insight into the expression of c-myc, c-myb and c-fes in normal hemopoietic cells we are now performing in situ hybridization on normal bone marrow cells (data not shown). The specificity of c-fes expression in myeloid cell populations and its lack of expression in lymphoid cell populations, easily detectable by the in situ hybridization technique, seem to be very useful tools in clnical diagnosis. Furthermore the possible correlation of c-myc and c-myb expression to the proliferation of the cell could be used in evaluating the growth fraction of a neoplastic hemopoietic population.

REFERENCES

1. Bishop, J.M. (1983) Ann. Rev. Biochem. 52, 301-354.
2. Kelly, K., Cochran, B.H., Stiles, C.D., Leder, P. (1983) Cell 35, 603-610.
3. Ferrari, S., Torelli, U., Selleri, L., Donelli, A., Venturelli, D., Moretti, L., Torelli, G. (1984) Br. J. Haemat. in press.
4. Westin, E.H., Gallo, R.C., Arya, S.K., Eva, A., Souza, L.M., Baluda, M.A., Aaronson, S.A., Wong-Staal, F. (1982) Proc. Natl. Acad. Sci. USA 79, 2194-2198.
5. Westin, E.H., Wong-Staal, F., Gelman, E.P., Dalla Favera, R., Pappas, .S., Lautenberger, J.A., Eva, A., Reddy, E.P., Tronick, S.R., Aaronson, S.A., Gallo,

R.C. (1982) Proc. Natl. Acad. Sci. USA 79, 2490-2494.

6. Rothberg, P.G., Erisman, M.D., Diehl, R.E., Rovigatti, U.G., Astrin, S.M. (19484) Mol. Cell. Biol. 4, 1096-1103.
7. Koeffler, H.P. (1983) Blood 62, 709-721.
8. Slamon, D.J., deKernion, J.B., Verma, I.M., Cline, M.J. (1984) Science 224, 256-262.
9. Dalla Favera, R., Gelman, E.P., Martinotti, S., Franchini, G. Papas, T.S., Gallo, R.C., Wong-Staal, F. (1982) Proc. Natl. Acad. Sci. USA 79, 6497-6501.
10. Franchini, G., Wong-Staal, F., Baluda, M.A., Lengel, C., Tronick, S.R. (1983) Proc. Natl. Acad. Sci. USA 80, 7385-7389.
11. Franchini, G., Gelman, E.P., Dalla Favera, R., Gallo, R.C., Wong-Staal, F. (1982) Mol. Cell. Biol. 2, 1014-1019.
12. Brahic, M., Haase, A.T. (1978) Proc. Natl. Acad. Sci. USA 75, 6125-6129.

SUBJECT INDEX